G000122524

THERAPY FOR HEPATOCELLULAR CARCINOMA

ETIOLOGY AND TREATMENT

CANCER ETIOLOGY, DIAGNOSIS AND TREATMENTS

Additional books in this series can be found on Nova's website under the Series tab.

Additional e-books in this series can be found on Nova's website under the e-book tab.

CANCER ETIOLOGY, DIAGNOSIS AND TREATMENTS

THERAPY FOR HEPATOCELLULAR CARCINOMA

ETIOLOGY AND TREATMENT

NOBUHIRO OHKOHCHI
EDITOR

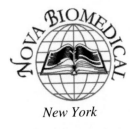

New York

Copyright © 2014 by Nova Science Publishers, Inc.

All rights reserved. No part of this book may be reproduced, stored in a retrieval system or transmitted in any form or by any means: electronic, electrostatic, magnetic, tape, mechanical photocopying, recording or otherwise without the written permission of the Publisher.

For permission to use material from this book please contact us:
Telephone 631-231-7269; Fax 631-231-8175
Web Site: http://www.novapublishers.com

NOTICE TO THE READER

The Publisher has taken reasonable care in the preparation of this book, but makes no expressed or implied warranty of any kind and assumes no responsibility for any errors or omissions. No liability is assumed for incidental or consequential damages in connection with or arising out of information contained in this book. The Publisher shall not be liable for any special, consequential, or exemplary damages resulting, in whole or in part, from the readers' use of, or reliance upon, this material. Any parts of this book based on government reports are so indicated and copyright is claimed for those parts to the extent applicable to compilations of such works.

Independent verification should be sought for any data, advice or recommendations contained in this book. In addition, no responsibility is assumed by the publisher for any injury and/or damage to persons or property arising from any methods, products, instructions, ideas or otherwise contained in this publication.

This publication is designed to provide accurate and authoritative information with regard to the subject matter covered herein. It is sold with the clear understanding that the Publisher is not engaged in rendering legal or any other professional services. If legal or any other expert assistance is required, the services of a competent person should be sought. FROM A DECLARATION OF PARTICIPANTS JOINTLY ADOPTED BY A COMMITTEE OF THE AMERICAN BAR ASSOCIATION AND A COMMITTEE OF PUBLISHERS.

Additional color graphics may be available in the e-book version of this book.

Library of Congress Cataloging-in-Publication Data

ISBN: 978-1-63117-929-7

LCCN: 2014938745

Published by Nova Science Publishers, Inc. † New York

Contents

Preface

Hepatocellular carcinoma (HCC) is the most common disease of the primary liver malignant tumor in the world. It is considered that the therapy for HCC is very troublesome because most of the HCC occur from the injured liver such as chronic hepatitis or cirrhosis. In Japan hepatitis C was prevalent after World War II and number of the patients with HCC remarkably increased compared with other countries. Under such circumstances of the limitation of cadaveric liver transplantation, various kinds of treatment have developed in Japan with clinical researches. A variety of important risk factors for the development of HCC have been investigated and high risk factors are as follows; hepatitis B carrier state, chronic hepatitis C virus infection, and nonalcoholic fatty liver disease, as well as various kind of cirrhosis. Numerous numbers of the patients with HCC have been found out because the diagnosing techniques using CT and MRI developed in the past two decades. A tumor smaller than 5mm diameter can be defined by an MRI. Up to the 20th century, the surgical resection and liver transplantation had been mainly carried out for the treatment of HCC. However, in the recent ten years, new therapies, i.e., radiofrequency ablation, transcatheter arterial chemo-embolization, and molecular-targeted drugs have developed and effectiveness of these therapies been recognized. Therefore, we have various powerful treatment options for HCC now. In this book we review the etiology and epidemiology of HCC and the diagnosis technique, and the indication and result of the treatments, i.e., radiofrequency ablation, molecular-targeted therapy, surgical resection, transplantation, trans-arterial chemo-embolization, and radiotherapy. In addition, proton beam therapy is introduced which is less invasive therapy for localized HCC. I hope that this book is helpful for the medical staff who treat the patients with HCC.

Nobuhiro Ohkohchi M.D., Ph.D.
Department of Surgery and Organ Transplantation
Faculty of Medicine
University of Tsukuba
1-1-1 Tennoudai, Tsukuba-city
Ibaraki-ken, Japan
Tel: +81-29-853-3221
nokochi3@md.tsukuba.ac.jp

In: Therapy for Hepatocellular Carcinoma
Editor: Nobuhiro Ohkohchi

ISBN: 978-1-63117-929-7
© 2014 Nova Science Publishers, Inc.

Chapter 1

Epidemiology and Etiology of Hepatocellular Carcinoma

Junichi Shoda, M.D., Ph.D., A.G.A.F.
Department of Gastroenterology, Faculty of Medicine, University of Tsukuba
Tsukuba, Ibaraki-ken, Japan

Abstract

The incidence of hepatocellular carcinoma (HCC) varies widely according to geographic location. The distribution of HCC also differs among racial and ethnic groups within the same country, and between regions within the same country. These extreme differences in distribution of HCC are probably due to regional variations in exposure to hepatitis viruses and environmental pathogens. Worldwide, men are more likely than women to develop HCC. The disparity is more pronounced in high-incidence regions, where men are affected much more frequently than women. A variety of important risk factors for the development of HCC have been identified. Among the most important are hepatitis B carrier state, chronic hepatitis C virus infection, hereditary hemochromatosis, and cirrhosis of almost any cause. Other factors such as environmental toxins and dietary factors, tobacco and alcohol abuse, and nonalcoholic fatty liver disease, etc. have been associated with an increased or decreased risk of HCC. Strict surveillance for HCC is indicated for subjects with disorders that put them at increased risk.

1. Introduction

Hepatocellular carcinoma (HCC), which accounts for 70% to 85% of all primary liver cancer cases, is a malignant tumor with poor clinical outcomes. This chapter describes the epidemiological characteristics of HCC and the etiology of HCC development.

2. Worldwide Epidemiology of HCC

Primary liver cancer is the sixth most common cancer in the world, with approximately 750,000 new cases diagnosed each year according to an estimation by the GLOBOSCAN 2008 database (http://www-dep.iarc.fr/) provided by the International Agency for Research on Cancer, an agency supported by the World Health Organization. The estimated incidence of new cases is approximately 520,000 per year in men and approximately 220,000 per year in women. It is the third most common cause of cancer mortality worldwide, with approximately 690,000 deaths per year. Because of its distinctive pathogenesis, HCC has been shown to have unique variations in geographic, age, and gender distributions.

Several reviews have summarized the global trends in the incidence of HCC. Chronic viral hepatitis, rather than dietary factors or alcohol consumption, has been shown to be the leading risk factor for HCC. Geographic variations in the incidence of HCC are thought to result from regional differences in the incidence and prevalence rates of hepatitis virus infection. More than 85% of all HCC cases occur in developing countries, particularly in sub-Saharan Africa and Southeast Asia [1]. In 2008, the age-standardized incidence rate of HCC per 100,000 individuals was more than 30 in Southeast Asia and 10 to 20 in Southern Europe, while it was less than 5 per 100,000 individuals in North America, South America, Northern Europe, and Oceania [2, 3]. In the United States, the incidence of HCC varies by ethnicity and reflects the incidence of HCC, particularly chronic infection of hepatitis B virus (HBV), in the patients' home countries.

HCC appears to be predominant in men globally, except in Iran. The overall male-to-female incidence ratio is 2.4:1 and tends to be higher in countries with higher incidences of HCC, with an exceptionally higher incidence rate among men in countries with a high prevalence. The average age at diagnosis of HCC is between 55 and 59 years in China and between 63 and 65 years in the United States and Europe. This difference in age at diagnosis is believed to be attributable to differences in etiologic virus types (i.e., HBV or hepatitis C virus [HCV]) and genotype, and the involvement of other etiologic factors.

3. Epidemiology of HCC in Japan

The epidemiological characteristics of HCC in Japan are reviewed below. Death rates due to HCC according to vital statistics reported annually [4] are shown in Figure 1.

Since the early 1950s, the number of deaths due to HCC in Japan was approximately 10 per 100,000 people, and this number gradually increased after the mid-1970s. Although the number of deaths seems to have slightly decreased from its peak in 2002 (27.5 per 100,000), it has remained largely unchanged in recent years. The number of deaths among men has been twice that among women; however, since 2002, this number has been showing a declining tendency, and the number of deaths in women has slightly decreased [5].

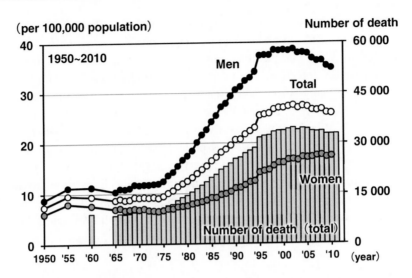

Figure 1. Chronological changes in the mortality numbers of hepatocellular carcinoma in Japan. The graphs were made according to the data of dynamic of population statistics from the Ministry of Health, Labor and Welfare in Japan. The figure was partly cited and modified from the reference 4.

Variations in death rates due to HCC according to etiology [5] determined according to reports by the Liver Cancer Study Group of Japan [6] and the number of deaths due to HCC reported according to vital statistics [4] are shown in Figure 2. The number of deaths related to chronic HBV infection has remained steady since the 1980s at approximately 3–4 per 100,000 people.

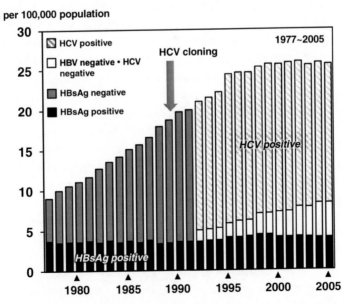

Figure 2. Chronological changes in the mortality numbers of hepatocellular carcinoma with respect to etiology. The graphs were made according to the data of dynamic of population statistics (from the Ministry of Health, Labor and Welfare in Japan) and those of the follow-up survey of hepatocellular carcinoma in Japan (from the Liver Cancer Study Group of Japan). The figure was partly cited and modified from the reference 5.

An increase in the HCC mortality rate observed from the 1970s to the 2000s was not due to infection by hepatitis viruses A and B but due to unidentified factors termed as non-A, non-B. A diagnostic test for HCV was developed in 1992; since then, most HCC deaths have been attributed to chronic HCV infection. The proportion of deaths caused by non-B, non-C HCC has been gradually increasing since 2000, presumably due to nonalcoholic fatty liver disease (NAFLD) [7, 8, 9]. Tokushige et al., conducted a nationwide survey of 14,530 HCC patients and showed that 14.1% of patients were positive for HBV, 66.3% were positive for HCV, and 3.7% were positive for both, while 7.2% of patients were diagnosed with alcoholic liver disease and 2.0% were diagnosed with NAFLD [10].

In summary, chronic HBV or HCV infection currently accounts for approximately 80% to 90% of HCC deaths in Japan. Meanwhile, the incidence of non-B, non-C HCC has been gradually increasing since 2000, accounting for 10% to 15% of all HCC cases. Non-alcoholic steatohepatitis (NASH) is assumed to be the underlying cause of this increase.

4. Risk Factors for HCC

Many risk factors for the development of HCC have been identified and include HBV infection, HCV infection, hereditary hemochromatosis, and cirrhosis due to various causes.

4.1. HBV Infection

Many studies have reported the role of chronic HBV infection in the development of HCC [11-16]. Approximately 5% of the world's population (350 to 400 million) is believed to be chronic carriers of HBV, of which 75% reside in Asia. While the infection rate in countries in Europe and America is as low as 0.3% to 1.5%, chronic HBV infection is a very prominent risk factor for HCC in sub-Saharan Africa and Asia, excluding Japan. Furthermore, approximately 50% to 80% of all HCC patients worldwide are assumed to be positive for HBV [17], whereas nearly all cases of HCC in children are thought to be due to HBV.

In addition, HBV carriers who have severe underlying liver diseases are more likely to develop HCC. Approximately 70% to 90% of HCC cases among chronic HBV carriers likely occur in the setting of cirrhosis [18]. Besides cirrhosis, other factors such as the virus titer and the presence of hepatitis B surface antigen (HBsAg) and hepatitis B e antigen (HBeAg) are implicated in the development of HCC in chronic HBV carriers.

HBV carriers with high serum HBV DNA levels have been reported to be at a higher risk for HCC development than those with low HBV DNA levels [19-23]. A community-based study in Taiwan evaluating the relationship between the serum HBV DNA level and the risk of HCC showed that the incidence rate of HCC was higher in cases with a high serum HBV DNA level at study entry. The authors reported that the cumulative incidence rate of HCC among cases with an HBV DNA level of $\geq$1,000,000 copies/mL was 14.9%, whereas it was only 1.3% among cases with an HBV DNA level of <300 copies/mL [19]. The serum HBV DNA level is an independent risk predictor of HCC even after adjustment for other HCC risk factors such as age, smoking, alcohol consumption, HBeAg status, the serum alanine transaminase level, and cirrhosis [24].

4.1.1. HBV Genotypes and the Risk of HCC

HBV has eight genotypes (A through H), and the prevalence of HBV genotypes vary by geographical area. Genotypes B and C are most commonly found in Asia. Genotype C, which affects nearly 85% of HBV carriers in Japan, is associated with more severe liver disease and a higher risk of HCC development than genotype B. In contrast, genotype B is strongly associated with HCC development at a younger age (≤50 years) and in children according to a study in Taiwan [25]. In North America and Western Europe, where genotypes A and D prevail, genotype D is associated with more severe liver disease and a higher incidence of HCC than genotype A.

4.1.2. Activity of Viral Replication and the Development of HCC

The presence of HBeAg in serum samples of HBV carriers indicates active viral replication and is associated with the development of HCC [26-31]. A large-scale 10-year prospective clinical study in Taiwan, which analyzed the association of HCC incidence with the HBsAg and HBeAg statuses determined at the time of enrolment, found that the incidence rate of HCC in subjects positive for both HBsAg and HBeAg was significantly higher than that in subjects positive for only HBsAg or negative for both [31]. Thus, HBeAg status is an independent risk predictor of HCC.

The risk of HCC in HBV inactive carriers who are positive for HBsAg but negative for HBeAg is significantly higher than that in non-carriers [32-36]. A population-based study conducted in Taiwan over a 13-year period also revealed that the annual incidence of HCC is markedly higher in HBV inactive carriers than in non-carriers [33].

Although HBV carriers who have seroconverted to HBsAg negative status due to host clearance of the virus generally have favorable prognosis, they remain at risk of developing HCC [37, 38]. A clinical study with a 20-year follow-up of patients with HBV infection with virus clearance and loss of HBsAg positivity showed that the incidence rate of HCC after clearance of HBsAg was higher than that in the general population, but lower than that in those who remained positive for HBsAg [39]. Another study suggested that patients with virus clearance at >50 years of age may remain at an increased risk of HCC development [40].

Several systematic reviews have reported that nucleoside/nucleotide analogues and interferon use in antiviral therapy against HBV can reduce the risk of HCC by 50%–60% in patients with HBV infection [41-44]. However, complete elimination of HCC risk by such antiviral therapy is difficult, and no reduction in HCC risk has been seen in patients who develop resistance to nucleoside/nucleotide analogues.

4.1.3. Molecular Mechanisms of HBV-Induced Hepatocarcinogenesis

Molecular mechanisms underlying the development of HCC have been extensively analyzed using human liver cancer tissues and various techniques such as HBV transgenic mouse and in vitro HBV overexpression systems in liver cell culture. Taken together, the data show that there are three major mechanisms of virus-induced hepatocarcinogenesis: the direct effect of the viral proteins, the indirect effect through chronic inflammation, and the integration of viral genetic material into the host DNA (Figure 3).

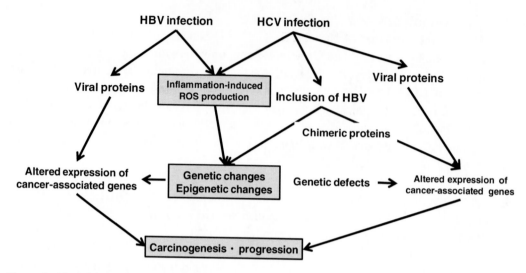

Figure 3. Altered expressions of cancer-associated genes induced by the infection of hepatitis viruses and hepatic carcinogenesis and cancer progression.

Transgenic mouse or *in vitro* overexpression systems to study the direct effect of viral proteins are useful since inflammatory reactions, the natural mechanisms of the body, are not involved. Transgenic mice harboring the viral regulatory gene *HBx* develop liver cancer [45]. The HBx protein is expressed in the nucleus and cytoplasm of hepatocytes and exerts its effect through i) transcriptional activation of proto-oncogenes such as the EGF receptor, c-myc, c-fos, and signaling molecules of the Ras pathway; ii) suppression of the cell cycle regulatory system; and iii) inhibition of DNA repair and apoptosis by tumor suppressor p53 via direct binding. Thus, the HBx protein is believed to promote hepatocarcinogenesis by enhancing cell proliferation and inhibiting apoptosis. Indeed, more than 95% of patients with HBV-positive cirrhosis and dysplasia, and more than 70% of patients with HBV-related HCC (HBV-HCC) are positive for HBx expression, suggesting that HBx plays a crucial role in hepatocarcinogenesis. Recently, HBx has been found to be associated with androgen receptors. The involvement of testosterone and androgen receptors in HCC has long been presumed since men have a much higher incidence of HBV-HCC than do women. Recently, HBx has been identified as a cause of the male predominance of HBV-HCC. In addition, transgenic mice harboring the viral *preS2* gene, which encodes one of the HBV surface proteins, develop liver cancer at a high frequency. The preS2 protein is thought to promote hepatocarcinogenesis through i) the induction of cell proliferation by activating mitogen-activated protein kinase, a signaling molecule that regulates cellular growth, and ii) the induction of the unfolded protein response (stress response) by accumulation in the endoplasmic reticulum of hepatocytes, which ultimately may lead to DNA damage.

The second mechanism of virus-induced hepatocarcinogenesis is via the indirect effect of the virus through chronic inflammation. Inflammation is thought to sustain aberrant expression of multiple genes that promote oncogenesis and progression during multistep hepatocarcinogenesis. Impaired expression of oncogenic genes generally results from genetic alternations that involve changes to the genomic sequence as well as epigenetic alterations that do not change the DNA sequence. Inflammation induces such genetic or epigenetic alterations through the overproduction of reactive oxygen species (ROS) by hepatocytes, which is recognized to play an important role in hepatocarcinogenesis [46].

The third mechanism of virus-induced hepatocarcinogenesis is the integration of viral genetic material into host DNA. HBV replicates by reverse transcription of an RNA intermediate called pregenomic RNA (pgRNA). During DNA synthesis from pgRNA, double-stranded linear HBV DNA can be integrated into host chromosomes. Integration of viral genes including *HBx* and truncated *PreS* genes can occur at early stages of chronic infection. In fact, such integration can be seen in approximately 90% of HBsAg-positive HCC cases. Moreover, many host genes mutated by the integration of viral DNA (insertional mutagenesis) have recently been identified [47], including genes encoding cell cycle proteins and signaling pathway molecules. Integration of viral DNA adjacent to the gene encoding telomerase reverse transcriptase (hTERT), a telomere-synthesizing enzyme that is associated with cellular immortalization, has also been frequently reported. Thus, integration of viral genes into the host genome can cause insertional mutagenesis resulting in deletion, translocation, and instability of the host genome, and occasionally, production of chimeric proteins created through the joining of viral and host genes. For example, deleterious mutations have been reported to occur in tumor suppressor genes such as *p53*, *Rb*, and *p16^{INK4A}*, leading to impairment in the tumor suppressing and cell cycle regulatory systems. In addition, HBV chimeric proteins and host components can activate oncogenes or inactivate tumor suppressor genes of the host. Development of HCC in non-symptomatic HBV carriers is driven by such integration of viral DNA, which is a distinct mechanism of HBV. In contrast, HCV does not integrate into host DNA since it replicates without reverse transcription.

4.1.4. Prevention of HCC

The multistep process of HBV-induced hepatocarcinogenesis involves aberrant expression of multiple genes implicated in oncogenesis. HBV promotes hepatocarcinogenesis directly through viral proteins or indirectly through chronic inflammation. Therefore, rigorous interventions in patients with HBV that suppress inflammation and eliminate or reduce the virus titer are crucial for the prevention of HCC.

4.2. HCV Infection

It is estimated that approximately 1% to 3% of the world's population has been infected with HCV. The incidence rate of HCC in HCV carriers is believed to be 15 to 20 times higher than that in non-carriers [48-50]. A prospective cohort study in 23,820 residents of Taiwan (30 to 65 years of age) positive for HCV showed a cumulative incidence rate of HCC of 24% in men and 17% in women [51]. That study also showed a cumulative incidence rate of HCC of 38% in male HBV carriers and of 27% in female HBV carriers. In the United States, HCV-related HCC (HCV-HCC) accounts for one-third of all HCC cases [52]. In addition, HCV-HCC generally develops against the background of advanced liver fibrosis or cirrhosis [53]. The annual incidence rate of HCV-related cirrhosis (HCV-cirrhosis) is estimated to be 7% to 8% in Japan and 1% to 4% worldwide. Studies have implicated heavy alcohol consumption, diabetes, and obesity as risk factors for HCC in HCV carriers [54-58].

HCV has six genotypes, of which genotypes 1a and 1b are the most common in America and Europe. Although an association between different genotypes of HCV and worldwide HCC incidence has not been fully clarified, a recent study reported that genotype 1b is associated with a two-fold higher risk of HCC compared to other genotypes [59]. Another study in Taiwan reported that viral load was associated with HCC risk [60]. However, this association has not been found in the United States and Europe; thus, definitive conclusions are pending.

HCV infection induces increased hepatocyte turnover and chronic inflammatory conditions in the liver. Chronic inflammatory status and the extent of necrosis in the liver are thought to be critical factors for the development of HCV-HCC, while involvement of specific oncogene activation is insignificant [61, 62]. Chronic inflammatory status is also an important predictor of clinical outcomes in HCC patients. Other predictors of clinical outcomes are the amounts of 8-hydroxydeoxyguanosine (8-OHdG) DNA adducts and 4-hydroxynonenal (4-HNE) protein adducts, which are biomarkers of oxidative stress and inflammation, in the liver. In fact, a previous study showed that elevated levels of 8-OHdG and 4-HNE are associated with poor clinical outcomes in patients with HCV-HCC [63]. Host immunity against HCV also plays important roles in cirrhosis and its progression to HCC [64].

Antiviral therapy with interferon or a combination of interferon and ribavirin can reduce the risk of HCC in HCV carriers [65-67]. According to a meta-analysis of observational studies, patients who have successfully achieved sustained virologic response (viral clearance) have a lower HCC risk than those who have failed to achieve such a response.

4.2.1. Molecular Mechanisms of HCV-Induced Hepatocarcinogenesis

HCV is the most common cause of HCC. HCV-associated hepatitis often becomes chronic, causing persistent inflammation, which induces progressive liver fibrosis leading to cirrhosis and ultimately to HCC. Although it has long been known that chronic inflammation plays a critical role in oncogenesis by inducing the expression of proinflammatory cytokines and ROS, the molecular mechanisms underlying hepatocarcinogenesis by HCV were not well understood until recently. Studies using transgenic mice that constitutively express the core protein, a structural protein of HCV, have revealed that these transgenic mice developed steatosis and cancer in the absence of inflammation, demonstrating that HCV itself has the ability to directly induce hepatocarcinogenesis [68, 69]. A further study revealed that the HCV core protein induces oxidative stress, which may contribute to hepatocarcinogenesis [70]. The underlying cause of oxidative stress is thought to be mitochondrial dysfunction. The HCV core protein localizes in the mitochondria and induces structural changes [69], resulting in the inhibition of electron transport complex I, which leads to oxidative stress [71]. The HCV core protein has also been shown to affect the expression of a mitochondrial protein chaperon, which may lead to impaired function of the mitochondrial respiratory chain with the overproduction of oxidative stress mediators [72]. Recently, the association between oxidative stress due to defects in iron metabolism and the development of HCC has drawn attention [73]. Many studies have demonstrated the molecular mechanisms underlying HCV-mediated defects in iron metabolism, showing that the virus can alter the expression of heme oxygenase-1, an important enzyme in iron metabolism, resulting in hepatic iron overload [74-77]. Indeed, it has been shown that iron overload is associated with a higher risk of HCC in HCV carriers [78, 79]. Several studies have also demonstrated the ability of the HCV core protein to interact with host proteins to activate and regulate the expression of host genes. Among these, proteasome activator PA28 (gamma), a regulator of proteasome activity that is implicated in proteolysis, has been shown to interact with the core protein [80] and to be associated with steatogenesis, insulin resistance, and hepatocarcinogenesis [81, 82].

4.2.2. Prevention of HCC

HCV and HBV share similarities and differences in the course of disease progression from infection to the development of HCC, but both etiologies comprise a multistep process that involves aberrant expression of multiple genes implicated in oncogenesis. HCV promotes hepatocarcinogenesis directly through viral proteins or indirectly through chronic inflammation. Thus, rigorous intervention that suppresses inflammation and eliminates or reduces virus titers is crucial for the prevention of HCC in patients with HCV.

4.3. Co-Infection of HBV with HCV or Hepatitis D Virus (HDV)

Although few studies have been reported on the effect of combined HBV and HCV infection on hepatocarcinogenesis [83-86], a meta-analysis of data obtained in eight countries, including the United States, Spain, Taiwan, and Japan, showed that the incidence of HCC is 23 times higher in HBV carriers, 17 times higher in HCV carriers, and 165 times higher in HBV/HCV carriers than in non-carriers [87]. Similarly, a study in China showed that the incidence of HCC was 14.1 times higher in HBV carriers, 4.6 times higher in HCV carriers, and 35.7 times higher in HBV/HCV carriers than in non-carriers. Thus, co-infection of HBV and HCV is considered to have an additive effect on the risk of HCC.

HDV co-infection with HBV is also associated with an increased risk of HCC [88]. According to a retrospective clinical study of 200 patients with HBV-related cirrhosis, 20% of patients that were HDV positive at diagnosis had an HCC risk and mortality rate that were double and triple, respectively, of those in HDV-negative patients [88]. The estimated 5-year risk for HCC after adjustment for clinical and serological differences at baseline was 13% in HBV/HDV carriers, 4% in HDV-only carriers, and 2% in HBV-only carriers. A population-based study in Sweden showed similar results where HDV co-infection with HBV increases the risk of HCC [89].

4.4. Hereditary Hemochromatosis

Hereditary hemochromatosis is an autosomal recessive genetic disorder that usually results from genetic defects in the *HFE* gene. The HFE protein encoded by this gene functions to regulate iron absorption in the intestine. Clinical symptoms of hereditary hemochromatosis are related to iron overload in organs, particularly in the liver, heart, spleen, and pituitary gland. Progressive iron deposition in the liver induces hepatomegaly, elevated liver enzyme levels, and eventually liver fibrosis and cirrhosis [90, 91].

HCC is the most serious complication of hereditary hemochromatosis [92-95]. The risk of HCC in patients with hereditary hemochromatosis is 20 to 200 times higher than that in the general population [96-99]. In fact, a population-based study showed a 20 times higher risk in patients with hereditary hemochromatosis than in the general population [100]. The HCC risk is also higher in male patients.

4.5. Obesity and Metabolic Syndrome

In developed countries, the obese population has been steadily increasing, and immediate intervention for obesity-related diseases is urgently needed. Many epidemiological and experimental studies have revealed obesity, diabetes, and non-alcoholic steatohepatitis (NASH) as risk factors for HCC [101-104]. In these contexts, the association between obesity and hepatocarcinogenesis has been extensively analyzed.

A recent clinical study in the United States comparing subjects with a body-mass index (BMI) of at least 35 and those of normal weight showed that the relative risk of death due to liver cancers including HCC was 4.52 in the male obese group and 1.68 in the female obese group [105]. In addition, diabetes has been shown to double the risk of HCC. Furthermore, the number of NASH-induced HCC (NASH-HCC) cases has been increasing against the background of the soaring number of metabolic syndrome cases [106]. According to a clinical study in the United States and Europe aimed at determining the etiology of HCC, NASH accounted for at least 13% of the 105 HCC cases analyzed [107]; thus, NASH has been recognized as an important underlying liver condition in the development of HCC. In Japan, NASH currently accounts for 2% of all HCC cases based on a nationwide survey [108]. However, it is expected to become the most common etiology of HCC overtaking HCV in 20 to 30 years.

A "two-hit" theory has been proposed for the developmental mechanism of NASH [109]. This theory describes two processes in disease pathogenesis: the "first hit" results in fatty liver through the effects of insulin resistance associated with diabetes or obesity and sensitizes the liver to a variety of factors that constitute the "second hit", which include oxidative stress and the accumulation of endotoxins, iron, and fatty acids [109, 110]. Approximately 5% to 25% of NASH cases usually progress to cirrhosis within 5 to 15 years, of which 11.3% progress to HCC [111]. The primary risk factors for NASH include age, male gender, cirrhosis, advanced liver fibrosis, diabetes, obesity, and iron deposition [106].

There have been many reports on the incidence of NASH in HCC patients. A clinical study in England aimed at investigating the underlying etiology of HCC showed that among 162 HCC patients recruited between 2007 and 2008, 23.3% were positive for HCV, 19% were positive for HBV, 12.7% had alcohol-induced liver disease, and 24% had NASH, indicating that HCC was most commonly associated with NASH [112]. In contrast, another study in Japan showed that among 1,168 HCC patients who underwent hepatectomy between 1990 and 2006, only 8 cases (1%) were associated with NASH [113]. Thus, the incidence of NASH in HCC patients varies largely by region.

Many studies have investigated the incidence of HCC in patients with NASH-related cirrhosis (NASH-cirrhosis). Ascha et al. compared the incidence of HCC in patients with NASH-cirrhosis (195 cases) and in those with HCV-cirrhosis (315 cases), and reported that patients with NASH-cirrhosis have a significantly lower annual incidence rate (2.6%) than do HCV-cirrhosis patients (4.0%) [114]. The proportion of NASH-cirrhosis cases progressing to HCC is approximately one-third to half that of HCV-cirrhosis cases. A prospective clinical study in Japan with age- and sex-matched NASH-cirrhosis and HCV-cirrhosis patients showed a 5-year incidence rate of HCC of 11.3% in the NASH group and 30.5% in the HCV group [115]. Although the incidence rate of HCC in Japanese NASH-cirrhosis patients is lower than that in HCV-cirrhosis patients, it is still significantly higher than that reported in the United States and Europe.

Obesity, diabetes, and the progression status of liver fibrosis are considered the primary risk factors for NASH-HCC. As described above, obese patients with a BMI of more than 35 have a higher relative risk of death due to liver cancers including HCC (4.52 in men and 1.68 in women) than do patients with normal BMI [105]. Diabetes also doubles the risk of HCC according to a meta-analysis in the United States and Europe [116]. Advanced liver fibrosis is another risk factor for NASH-HCC. A comparative, histological study in Japan showed that a higher proportion (80%) of patients with NASH-HCC had liver fibrosis of an advanced stage (F3-4) than those with NASH alone, supporting the notion that an advanced stage of liver fibrosis is a key risk factor for NASH-HCC [117]. Another histological study in Europe and the United States investigated the incidence of cirrhosis in NASH-HCC patients by analyzing non-cancerous lesions and reported that cirrhosis was detected in only 53% of NASH-HCC patients [112].

The clinical outcomes of NASH-HCC have been analyzed by many groups. Reddy et al. reported a comparative study conducted in Europe and the United States on 303 patients who underwent curative treatment for HCC such as liver transplantation, hepatectomy, and radio frequency ablation aimed to determine differences in long-term survival and recurrence outcomes between patients with NASH (17.2%) and those with HCV-cirrhosis (53.5%) [118]. According to that study, there were no differences in recurrence-free survival between the two groups, although NASH patients had longer overall survival. Another study by Hernandez-Alejandro et al. investigated the clinical outcome of patients who had HCC at the time of liver transplantation [119]. The authors reported that NASH-HCC patients, in comparison with HCV-HCC patients, showed significantly less vascular invasion and poorly differentiated HCC cells. The recurrence-free 5-year survival rate tended to be better in patients with these less aggressive tumor features of NASH-HCC than in HCV-HCC patients, although statistical significance was not achieved.

In Japan, Hashimoto el al. investigated the long-term survival and recurrence outcomes of 34 NASH-HCC patients and 56 age- and sex-matched HCV-HCC patients [120]. The study reported that the 5-year survival rate and the cumulative recurrence of HCC at 5 years in NASH-HCC patients were 55.2% and 69.8%, respectively, which were similar to those in HCV-HCC patients. The size of the primary tumor and the stage of liver fibrosis were identified as significant risk factors for HCC recurrence in NASH-HCC patients.

4.6. Gender

Men have a higher incidence of HCC than do women worldwide [121]. The influence of male gender is greater in areas of high HCC incidence, as shown by a higher male-to-female patient ratio in such regions (3.7:1). The ratio in areas of moderate incidence is 2.4:1, which is even lower in areas where HCC is rare. In 2008, the incidence rate of HCC per 100,000 people in North America was reported to be 6.8 in men and 2.2 in women [121].

The male predominance of HCC is reflected by the higher risk of hepatitis virus infection and higher consumption of alcohol in men. However, HCC incidence is higher even in men without such backgrounds, and this is thought to be attributable to the effect of male hormones such as androgens and testosterone [122, 123]. A clinical study in Taiwan and China showed significantly higher incidences of HCC in male HBV carriers with high serum testosterone levels [123]. High serum testosterone is also known to cause relatively rapid progression of liver fibrosis and severe inflammatory conditions. In contrast, there is insufficient data of a similar relationship in HCV carriers.

In women, the female hormone estrogen has been reported to reduce the risk of HCC through the inhibition of interleukin-6 [124, 125]. Increased incidence of HCC with increasing age in women is believed to be partly due to the reduction of estrogen levels after menopause [124, 125].

4.7. Alcohol Consumption

Heavy alcohol consumption alone is known to increase the risk of developing various cancer types [126-132], yet the threshold for the quantity and the duration of alcohol intake has not been determined. HCC can be induced by ethanol directly in non-cirrhotic livers or indirectly through prior induction of cirrhosis [133]. Furthermore, heavy drinking is associated with a higher risk of HCC in obese individuals with diabetes [134-138]. In hepatitis virus carriers, alcohol intake has a synergistic effect on the risk of HCC [139-141]. HCV carriers are considered to be more vulnerable to the effects of alcohol than are HBV carriers [142]. According to case-control studies in Italy on 464 HCC patients and 824 controls, alcohol intake increased the risk of HCC in a linear fashion when alcohol consumption was above 60 g per day, and the risk of HCC in hepatitis virus carriers was twice as high as in non-carriers [143].

4.8. Smoking

Data on the role of smoking as a risk factor for HCC are conflicting. Some studies support smoking as a risk factor for HCC [144-146], whereas others have not found an association [147-149]. Although the effect of smoking on the risk of HCC remains inconclusive, it has been clearly shown that smoking has an additive effect on the risk of hepatocarcinogenesis in HBV carriers and a synergistic effect in HCV carriers [150].

4.9. Dietary Factors

Betel nut chewing is a common cultural practice in some regions of Asia and is known to have carcinogenic effects in humans. Betel nut chewing has been shown to result in a higher risk of cirrhosis and HCC in case-control studies [151-153]. However, intake of white meat [154], fish/omega-3 fatty acid [155, 156], and vitamin E [157] has been shown to reduce the risk of HCC in population-based studies. Coffee has been shown to be another dietary factor that reduces the HCC risk in observational studies. A 43% reduction in the risk of HCC has been observed among coffee drinkers who consume more than two cups a day according to a meta-analysis [158, 159]. This favorable effect of coffee intake is thought to be attributable to the high amount of antioxidant substances in coffee that potently suppress oncogenesis and progression to cirrhosis by improving liver function.

4.10. Aflatoxins

The presence of aflatoxins against a background of HBV is a common cause of HCC in Asia and sub-Saharan Africa. Aflatoxins are mycotoxins that are commonly found contaminants of foods such as corn, soybeans, and peanuts. Frequent exposure to aflatoxins is correlated to the development of HCC. A clinical study in China showed that 65% of HCC patients were seropositive for aflatoxin B1-albumin adducts, whereas only 37% of age-matched controls were seropositive [160]. Another clinical study in China showed that exposure to aflatoxins and exposure to HBV individually were linked to a four- and seven-times higher risk of HCC, respectively, compared to non-exposed controls, whereas exposure to both factors increased the risk of HCC by 60 times [161-163], suggesting that aflatoxins augment the risk of HCC against the background of HBV infection. Furthermore, mutations in the tumor suppressor gene p53 have been found in patients who have been chronically exposed to aflatoxins [164, 165]. Similar results were found in HCC animal models of exposure to both aflatoxins and HBV [166].

5. Future Trends in the Epidemiology of HCC

In recent years, the incidence of HCC has been decreasing in countries where HCC is highly prevalent such as China and Japan, whereas it has been increasing in countries where HCC is relatively rare such as the United States and Canada [167]. The number of HCC cases worldwide will continue to increase in the near future, but this is expected to stabilize by 2015 to 2020 and gradually decrease thereafter. Although the proportion of HCC cases involving HBV or HCV infection shows a declining trend, the proportion of HCC cases caused by obesity or diabetes is predicted to increase. Therefore, it is important to immediately address these causative issues in order to reduce the incidence of HCC in the foreseeable future.

Conclusion

This chapter has reviewed recent acquisitions in the epidemiological characteristics of HCC and the etiology of HCC development.

References

[1]   International Agency for Research on Cancer (IARC), *Liver cancer incidence, mortality and prevalence worldwide in 2008*. Lyon: GLOBOCAN, 2008.

[2]   El-serag HB. Epidemiology of viral hepatitis and hepatocellular carcinoma. *Gastroenterology* 142:1264-73, 2012.

[3]   Wild CP. The role of cancer research in noncommunicable disease control. *J Natl Cancer Inst* 104:1051-8, 2012.

[4]   The Minister's Secretariat Statistics and Information Department of Ministry of Health, Labour and Welfare: *Dynamic of population statistics in Japan from 1975 to 2009.*

[5]   Tanaka J. Epidemiology and counterplan of hepatocellular carcinoma. Frontlines of Hepatic Cancer Survey. *Naika* 109:386-692, 2012.

[6]   Liver Cancer Study Group of Japan: *The 5th to 18th reports of follow-up survey of hepatocellular carcinoma in Japan.* 1982-2009.

[7]   Hashimoto E, Tokushige K. Hepatocellular carcinoma in non-alcoholic steatohepatitis: Growing evidence of an epidemic? *Hepatol Res* 42:1-14, 2012.

[8]   Okanoue T, Umemura A, Yasui K, et al. Nonalcoholic fatty liver disease and nonalcoholic steatohepatitis in Japan. *J Gastroenterol Hepatol.* 2011; 26 Suppl 1: 153-62. doi: 10.11 11/j.1440-1746.2010. 06547.x.

[9]   Yang JD, Roberts LR. Epidemiology and management of hepatocellular carcinoma. *Infect Dis Clin North Am* 24:899-919, 2010.

[10] Tokushige K, Hashimoto E, Hrie Y, et al. Hepatocellular carcinoma in Japanese patients with nonalcoholic fatty liver disease, alcoholic liver disease, and chronic liver disease of unknown etiology: report of the nationwide survey. *J Gastroenterol* 46:1230-7, 2011.

[11] Beasley RP, Hwang LY, Lin CC, Chien CS. Hepatocellular carcinoma-United States, 2001-2006. *MMWR Morb Mortal Wkly Rep* 59:17:517-520, 2010.

[12] Tsukuma H, Hiyama T, Tanaka S, et al. Risk factors for hepatocellular carcinoma among patients with chronic liver disease. *N Engl J Med* 328:675:1788-1801, 1993.

[13] Yu MW. Chen CJ. Hepatitis B and C viruses in the development of hepatocellular carcinoma. *Crit Rev Oncol Hematol* 17:71-91, 1994.

[14] Sherman M. Peltekian KM. Lee C. Screening for hepatocellular carcinomain chronic carriers of hepatitis B virus: incidence and prevalence of hepatocellular carcinoma in a North American urban population. *Hepatology* 22:432-438, 1995.

[15] Villeneuve JP, Desrochers M, Infante-Rivard C, et al. A long-term follow-up study of asymptomatic hepatitis B surface antigen-positive carriers in Montreal. *Gastroenterology* 106:1000-1005, 1994.

[16] Chen JD, Yang HI, lloeje UH, et al. Carriers of inactive hepatitis B virus are still at risk for hepatocellular carcinoma and liver-related death. *Gastroenterology* 138:1747-1754, 2010.

[17] Block TM, Mehta AS, Fimmel CJ, et al. Molecular viral oncology of hepatocellular carcinoma. *Oncogene* 22:5093-5107, 2003.

[18] Beasley RP. Hepatitis B virus. The major etiology of hepatocellular carcinoma. *Cancer* 61:1942-1956, 1988.

[19] Chen CJ, Yang HI, Su J, et al. Risk of hepatocellular carcinoma across a biological gradient of serum hepatitis B virus DNA level. *JAMA* 295:65-73, 2006.

[20] Chen CJ, Yang HI, lloeje U, et al. Models to predict hepatocellular carcinoma in patients with chronic hepatitis B injection: The REVEAL HBV study (abstract). *Hepatology* 42 Suppl 1:714A, 2005.

[21] Chen CF, Lee WC, Yang HI, et al. Changes in serum levels of HBV DNA and alanine aminotransferase determine risk for hepatocellular carcinoma. *Gastroenterology* 141:1240-1248, 2011.

[22] Yu MW, Yeh SH, Chen PJ, et al. Hepatitis B virus genotype and DNA level and hepatocellular carcinoma: a prospective study in men. *J Natl Cancer Inst* 97:265-272. 2005.

[23] Tseng TC, Liu CJ, Yang HC, et al. High levels of hepatitis B surface antigen increase risk of hepatocellular carcinoma in patients with low HBV load. *Gastroenterology* 142:1140-1149, 2012.

[24] Chen CJ, et al. Risk factors for hepatocellular carcinoma across a biological gradient of serum hepatitis B virus DNA level. *VAMA* 295:66-73, 2006.

[25] Kao JH, Chen PJ, Lai MY et al. Basal core promoter mutations of hepatitis B virus increase the risk of hepatocellular carcinoma in hepatitis B carriers. *Gastroenterology* 124:327-334, 2003.

[26] Lu SN, Lin TM, Chen CJ, et al. A case-control study of primary hepatocellular carcinoma in Taiwan. *Cancer* 62:2051-2055, 1988.

[27] Chen CJ, Liang KY, Chang AS, et al. Effects of hepatitis B virus, alcohol drinking, cigarette smoking and familial tendency on hepatocellular carcinoma. *Hepatology* 13:398-406, 1991.

[28] LinTM, Chen CJ, Lu SN, et al. Hepatitis B virus e antigen and primary hepatocellular carcinoma. *Anticancer Res* 11:2063-2065, 1991.

[29] Yu MW, You SL, Chang AS, et al. Association between hepatitis C virus antibodies and hepatocellular carcinoma in Taiwan. *Cancer Res* 51:5621-5625, 1991.

[30] Tsai JF, Jeng JE, Ho MS, et al. Additive effect modification of hepatitis B surface antigen and e antigen on the development of hepatocellular carcinoma. *Br J Cancer* 73:1498-1502, 1996.

[31] Yang HI, Lu SN, Liaw YF, et al. Hepatitis B e antigen and the risk of hepatocellular carcinoma. *N Engl J Med* 347:168-174, 2002.

[32] Villeneuve JP, Desrochers M, Infante-Rivard C, et al. A long-term follow-up study of asymptomatic hepatitis B surface antigen-positive carriers in Montreal. *Gastroenterology* 106:1000-1005, 1994.

[33] Chen JD, Yang HI, lloeje UH, et al. Carriers of inactive hepatitis B virus are still at risk for hepatocellular carcinoma and liver-related death. *Gastroenterology* 138:1747-1754, 2010.

[34] Tseng TC, Liu CJ, Yang HC, et al. High levels of hepatitis B surface antigen increase risk of hepatocellular carcinoma in patients with low HBV load. *Gastroenterology* 142:1140-1149, 2012.

[35] Yang HI, Lu SN, Liaw YF, et al. Hepatitis B e antigen and the risk of hepatocellular carcinoma. *N Engl J Med* 347:168-174, 2002.

[36] Dragosics B, Ferenci P, Hitchman E, Denk H. Long-term follow-up study of asymptomatic HBsAg-positive voluntary blood donors in Austria: a clinical and histologic evaluation of 242 cases. *Hepatology* 7:302-306, 1987.

[37] Chen CJ, Yang HI, lloeje UH, et al. Time-dependent relative risk of hepatocellular carcinoma for markers of chronic hepatitis B. *The REVEAL HBV study (abstract).* 2005; 42 Suppl 1: 722A.

[38] Tong MJ, Blatt LM, Kao JH, et al. Basal core promoter T1762/A1764 and precore A1896 gene mutations in hepatitis B surface antigen-positive hepatocellular carcinoma: a comparison with chronic carries. *Liver Int* 27:1356-1363, 2007.

[39] Simonetti J, Bulkow L, McMahon BJ, et al. Clearance of hepatitis B surface antigen and risk of hepatocellular carcinoma in a cohort chronically infected with hepatitis B virus. *Hepatology* 51:1531-1537, 2010.

[40] Yuen MF, Wong DK, Fung J, et al. HBsAg Seroclearance in chronic hepatitis B in Asian patients: replicative level and risk of hepatocellular carcinoma. *Gastroenterology* 135:1192-1199, 2008.

[41] Sung JJ, Tsoi KK, Wong VW, et al. Meta-analysis: Treatment of hepatitis B infection reduces risk of hepatocellular carcinoma. *Aliment Pharmacol Ther* 28:1067-1077, 2008.

[42] Papatheodoridis GV, Lampertico P, Manolakopoulos S, Lok A. Incidence of hepatocellular carcinoma in chronic hepatitis B patients receiving nucleos(t)ide therapy: a systematic review. *J Hepatol* 53:348-356, 2010.

[43] Shen YC, Hsu C, Cheng CC, et al. A critical evaluation of the preventive effect of antiviral therapy on the development of hepatocellular carcinoma in patients with chronic hepatitis C or B: a novel approach by using meta-regression. *Oncology* 82:275-289, 2012.

[44] Signal AK, Salameh H, Kuo YF, Fontana RJ. Meta-analysis: the impact of oral anti-viral agents on the incidence of hepatocellular carcinoma in chronic hepatitis B. *Aliment Pharmacol Ther* 38:98, 2013.

[45] Kim CM, et al. HBx gene of hepatitis B virus induces liver cancer in transgenic mice. *Nature* 351:317-320, 1991.

[46] Sasaki Y, et al. Does oxidative stress participate in the development of hepatocellular carcinoma? *J Gastroenterol* 41:1135-48, 2006.

[47] Minami M, et al. A novel PCR technique using Alu-specific primers to identify unknown flaking sequences from the human genome. *Genomics* 29:403-8, 1995.

[48] Bruix J, Barrera JM, Calvet X, et al. Prevalence of antibodies to hepatitis C virus in Spanish patients with hepatocellular carcinoma and cirrhosis. *Lancet* 2:1004-1006, 1989.

[49] Colombo M, Kuo G, Choo QL, et al. Prevalence of antibodies to hepatitis C virus in Italian patients with hepatocellular carcinoma. *Lancet* 2:1006-1008, 1989.

[50] Omland LH, Jepsen P, Krarup H, et al. Liver cancer and non-Hodgkin lymphoma in hepatitis C virus-infected patients: results from the DANVIR cohort study. *Int J Cancer* 130:2310-2317, 2012.

[51] Huang YT, Jen CL, Yang HI, et al. Lifetime risk and sex difference of hepatocellular carcinoma among patients with chronic hepatitis B and C. *J Clin Oncol* 29:3643-3650, 2011.

[52] Davila JA, Morgan RO, Shaib Y, et al. Hepatitis C infection and the increasing incidence of hepatocellular carcinoma: a population-based study. *Gastroenterology* 127:1372-1380, 2004.

[53] Lok AS, Seeff LB, Morgan TR, et al. Incidence of hepatocellular carcinoma and associated risk factors in hepatitis C-related advanced liver disease. *Gastroenterology* 136:138-148, 2009.

[54] Ikeda K, Marusawa H, Osaki Y, et al. Antibody to hepatitis B core antigen and risk for hepatitis C-related hepatocellular carcinoma: a prospective study. *Ann Intern Med* 146:649-656, 2007.

[55] Hassan MM, Hwang LY, Hatten CJ, et al. Risk factors for hepatocellular carcinoma: synergism of alcohol with viral hepatitis and diabetes mellitus. *Hepatology* 36:1206-1213, 2002.

[56] Ohki T, Tateishi R, Sato T, et al. Obesity is an independent risk factor for hepatocellular carcinoma development in chronic hepatitis C patients. *Clin Gastroenterol Hepatol* 6:459-464, 2008.

[57] Saunders D, Seidel D, Allison M, Lyratzopoulos G. Systematic review: the association between obesity and hepatocellular carcinoma – epidemiological evidence. *Aliment Pharmacol Ther* 31:1051-1063, 2010.

[58] Loomba R, Yang HI, Su J, et al. Synergism between obesity and alcohol in increasing the risk of hepatocellular carcinoma: a prospective cohort study. *Am J Epidemiol* 177:333-342, 2013.

[59] Raimondi S, Bruno S, Mondelli MU et al: Hepatitis C virus genotype 1b as a risk factor for hepatocellular carcinoma development: a meta-analysis. *J hepatol* 50:1142-1154, 2009.

[60] Hoshida Y, Villanueva A, Sangiovanni A, et al. Prognostic gene expression signature for patients with hepatitis C-related early-stage cirrhosis. *Gastroenterology* 144:1024-1030, 2013.

[61] Moriya K, Fujie H, Shintani Y, et al. The core protein of hepatitis C virus induces hepatocellular carcinoma in transgenic mice. *Nat Med* 4:1065-1067, 1998.

[62] Kamegaya Y, Hiasa Y, Zukerberg L, et al. Hepatitis C virus acts as a tumor accelerator by blocking apoptosis in a mouse model of hepatocarcinogenesis. *Hepatology* 41:660-667, 2005.

[63] Maki A, Kono H, Gupta M, et al. Predictive power of biomarkers of oxidative stress and inflammation in patients with hepatitis C virus-associated hepatocellular carcinoma. *Ann Surg Oncol* 14:1182-1190, 2007.

[64] Suruki RY, Mueller N, Hayashi K, et al. Host immune status and incidence of hepatocellular carcinoma among subjects infected with hepatitis C virus: a nested case-control study in Japan. *Cancer Epidemiol Biomarkers Prev* 15:2521-2525, 2006.

[65] Shen YC, Hsu C, Cheng CC, et al. A critical evaluation of preventive effect of antiviral therapy on the development of hepatocellular carcinoma in patients with chronic hepatitis C or B: a novel approach by using meta-regression. *Oncology* 82:275-289, 2012.

[66] Morgan RL, Baack B, Smith BD, et al. Eradication of hepatitis C virus infection and the development of hepatocellular carcinoma: a meta-analysis of observational studies. *Ann Intern Med* 158:329-337, 2013.

[67] Interferon-based therapy decreases risks of hepatocellular carcinoma and complications of cirrhosis in chronic hepatitis C patients. *PLoS One* 8: e70458, 2013.

[68] Moriya K, Yotsuyanagi H, Shintani Y, et al. Hepatitis C virus core protein induces hepatic steatosis in transgenic mice. *J Gen Virol.*78 (pt 7):1527-31, 1997.

[69] Moriya K, Fujie H, Shintani Y, et al. The core protein of hepatitis C induces hepatocellular carcinoma in transgenic mice. *Nat Med* 4:1065-7, 1998.

[70] Moriya K, Nakagawa K, Santa T, et al. Oxidative stress in the absence of inflammation in a mouse model for hepatitis C virus-associated hepatocarcinogenesis. *Cancer Res* 61:4365-70, 2001.

[71] Korenaga M, Wang T, Li Y, et al. Hepatitis C virus core protein inhibits mitochondrial electron transport and increases reactive oxygen species (ROS) production. *JBiol Chem* 280:37481-8, 2005.

[72] Tsutsumi T, Matsuda M, Aizaki H, et al. Proteomics analysis of mitochondrial proteins reveals overexpression of a mitochondrial protein chaperon, prohibitin, in cells expressing hepatitis C virus core protein. *Hepatology* 50:378-86, 2009.

[73] Furutani T, Hino K, Okuda M, et al. Hepatic iron overload induces hepatocellular carcinoma in transgenic mice expressing the hepatitis C virus polyprotein. *Gastroenterology* 130:2087-2098, 2006.

[74] Abdalla MY, Britigan BE, Wen F, et al. Down-regulation of heme oxygenase-1 by hepatitis C virus infection in vivo and by the in vitro expression of hepatitis C core protein. *J Infect Dis* 190:1109-18, 2004.

[75] Ghaziani T, Shan Y, Lambrecht RW, et al. HCV proteins increase expression of heme oxygenase-1 (HO-1) and decrease expression of Bach 1 in human hepatoma cells. *J Hepatol* 45:5-12, 2006.

[76] Wen F, Brown KE, Britigan BE, et al. Hepatitis C core protein inhibits induction of heme oxygenase-1 and sensitizes hepatocytes to cytotoxicity. *Cell Biol Toxicol* 24:175-88, 2008.

[77] Moriya K, Miyoshi H, Shinzawa S, et al. Hepatitis C virus core protein compromises iron-induced activation of antioxidants in mice and HepG2 cells. *J Med Virol* 82:776-792, 2009. 2010.

[78] Nahon P, Sutton A, Rufat P, et al. Liver iron, HFE gene mutations, and hepatocellular carcinoma occurrence in patients with cirrhosis. *Gastroenterology* 134:102-10, 2008.

[79] Soe K, Hishikawa Y, Fukuzawa Y, et al. Possible correlation between iron deposition and enhanced proliferating activity in hepatitis C virus-positive hepatocellular carcinoma in Myanmar (Burma). *J Gastroenterol* 42:225-35, 2007.

[80] Moriishi K, Okabayashi T, Nakai K, et al. Proteasome activator PA28gamma-dependent nuclear retention and degradation of hepatitis C virus core protein. *J Virol* 77:10237-49, 2003.

[81] Miyamoto H, Moriishi K, Moriya K, et al. Involvement of the PA28gamma-dependent pathway in insulin resistance induced by hepatitis C virus core protein. *J Virol* 81:1727-35, 2007.

[82] Moriishi K, Mochizuki R, Moriya K, et al. Critical role of PA28gamma in hepatitis C virus-associated steatogenesis and hepatocarcinogenesis. *Proc Natl Acad Sci USA* 104:1661-1666, 2007.

[83] Yu MW, You SL, Chang AS, et al. Association between hepatitis C virus antibodies and hepatocellular carcinoma in Taiwan. *Cancer Res* 51:5621-5625, 1991.

[84] Huang YT, Yang HI, Jen CL, et al. Suppression of hepatitis B virus replication by hepatitis C virus: combined effects on risk of hepatocellular carcinoma (abstract). *Hepatology* 42 (Suppl 1):230A, 2005.

[85] Benvegnu L, Fattovich G, Noventa F, et al. Concurrent hepatitis B and C virus infection and risk of hepatocellular carcinoma in cirrhosis. A prospective study. *Cancer* 74:2442-2448, 1994.

[86] Donato F, Boffeta P, Puoti M. A meta-analysis of epidemiological studies on the combined effect of hepatitis B and C virus infections in causing hepatocellular carcinoma. *Int Cancer* 75:347-354, 1998.

[87] Donato F, Boffeta P, Puoti M. A meta-analysis of epidemiological studies on the combined effect of hepatitis B and C virus infections in causing hepatocellular carcinoma. *Int Cancer* 75:347-354, 1998.

[88] Fattovich G, Giustina G, Christensen E, et al. Influence of hepatitis delta virus infection on morbidity and mortality in compensated cirrhosis type B. The European Concerted Action on Viral Hepatitis (Eurohep). *Gut* 46:420-426, 2000.

[89] Ji J, Sundquist K, Sundquist J. A population-based study of hepatitis D virus as potential risk factor for hepatocellular carcinoma. *J Natl Cancer Inst* 104:790-795, 2012.

[90] Adams PC, Deugnier Y, Moirand R, Brissot P. The relationship between iron overload, clinical symptoms, and age in 410 patients with genetic hemochromatosis. *Hepatology* 25:162-166, 1997.

[91] Fracanzani AL, Fargion S, Romano R, et al. Portal hypertension and iron depletion in patients with genetic hemochromatosis. *Hepatology* 22:1127-1131, 1995.

[92] Fargion S, Fracanzani AL, Piperno A, et al. Prognostic factors for hepatocellular carcinoma in genetic hemochromatosis. *Hepatology* 20:1426-1431, 1994.

[93] Deugnier YM, Guyader D, Crantock L, et al. Primary liver cancer in genetic hemochromatosis: a clinical, pathological, and pathogenetic study of 54 cases. *Gastroenterology* 104:228-234, 1993.

[94] Niederau C, Fischer R, Sonnenberg A, et al. Survival and causes of death in cirrhotic and in noncirrhotic patients with primary hemochromatosis. *N Engl J Med* 313:1256-1262, 1985.

[95] Niederau C, Fischer R, Purschel A, et al. Long-term survival in patients with hereditary hemochromatosis. *Gastroenterology* 110:1107-1119, 1996.

[96] Niederau C, Fischer R, Sonnenberg A, et al. Survival and causes of death in cirrhotic and in noncirrhotic patients with primary hemochromatosis. *N Engl J Med* 313:1256-1262, 1985.

[97] Yang Q, McDonnell SM, Khoury MJ, et al. Hemochromatosis-associated mortality in the United States from 1979 to 1992: an analysis of Multiple-Cause Mortality Data. *Ann Intern Med* 129:946-953, 1998.

[98] Bradbear RA, Bain C, Siskind V, et al. Cohort study of internal malignancy in genetic hemochromatosis and other chronic nonalcoholic liver diseases. *J Natl Cancer Inst* 75:81, 1985.

[99] Hsing AW, McLaughlin JK, Olsen JH, et al. Cancer risk following primary hemochromatosis: a population-based cohort study in Denmark. *Int J Cancer* 60:160-162, 1995.

[100] Elmberg M, Hultcrantz R, Ekbom A, et al. Cancer risk in patients with hereditary hemochromatosis and in their first-degree relatives. *Gastroenterology* 125:1733-1741, 2003.

[101] Calle EE, Rodriguez C, Walker-Thumond K, et al. Overweight, obesity and mortality from cancer in a prospectively studies cohort of US adults. *N Engl J Med* 348:1625-1638, 2003.

[102] El-serag HB, Tran T, Everhart JE. Diabetes increses the risk of chronic liver disease and hepatocellular carcinoma. *Gastroenterol* 126:460-468, 2004.

[103] Muto Y, Sato S, Watanabe A, et al. Overweight and obesity increase the risk for liver cancer in patients with liver cirrhosis and long-term oral supplementation with branched-chain amino acid granules inhibits liver carcinogenesis in heavier patients with liver cirrhosis. *Hepatol Res* 35:204-214, 2006.

[104] Pekow JR, Bhan AK, Zheng Hut, et al. Hepatic steatosis is associated with increased frequency of hepatocellular carcinoma in patients with hepatitis C-reltated cirrhosis. *Cancer* 109:2490-6, 2007.

[105] Calle EE, Rodriguez C, Walker-Thurmond K, et al. Overweight, Obesity, and Mortality from Cancer in a Prospectively Studied Cohort of U.S. Adults. *N Engl J Med* 348:1625-1638, 2003.

[106] Starley BQ, Calcagno CJ, Harrison SA. Nonalcoholic fatty liver disease and hepatocellular carcinoma: a weighty connection. *Hepatology* 51:1820-1832, 2010.

[107] Marrero JA, Fontana RJ, Su GL, et al. NAFLD may be a common underlying liver disease in patients with hepatocellular carcinoma in the United States. *Hepatology* 36:1349-1354, 2002.

[108] Tokushige K, Hashimoto E, Horie Y, et al. Hepatocellular carcinoma in Japanese patients with nonalcoholic fatty liver disease, alcoholic liver disease, and chronic liver disease of unknown etiology: report of the nationwide survey. *J Gastroenterol* 46:1230-1237, 2011.

[109] Day CP, James OF. Steatohepatitis: a tale of two "hits"? *Gastroenterology* 114:842-845, 1998.

[110] Rolo AP, Teodoro JS, Palmeira CM. Role of oxidative stress in the pathogenesis of nonalcoholic steatohepatitis. *Free Radic Biol Med* 52:59-69, 2012.

[111] Yatsuji S, Hashimoto E, Tobari M, et al. Clinical features and outcomes of cirrhosis due tu nonalcoholic steatohepatitis hepatitis C. *J Gastroenterol Hepatol* 24:248-254, 2009.

[112] Ertle J, Dechene A, Sowa JP et al.: Non-alcoholic fatty liver disease progresses to hepatocellular carcinoma in the absence of apparent cirrhosis. *Int J Cancer* 128:2436-2443, 2011.

[113] Kawada N, Imanaka K, Kawaguchi T, et al. Hepatocellular carcinoma arising from non-cirrhotic nonalcoholic steatohepatitis. *J Gastroenterol* 44:1190-1194, 2009.

[114] Ascha MS, Hanouneh IA, Lopez R, et al. The incidence and risk factors of hepatocellular carcinoma in patients with nonalcoholic steatohepatitis. *Hepatology* 51:1972-1978, 2010.

[115] Yatsuji S, Hashimoto E, Tobari M, et al. Clinical features and outcomes of cirrhosis due to non-alcoholic steatohepatitis compared with cirrhosis caused by chronic hepatitis C. *J Gastroenterol Hepatol* 24:248-254, 2009.

[116] Larsson SC, Orsini N, Wolk A. Diabetes mellitus and risk of colorectal cancer: a meta-analysis. *J Natl Cancer Inst* 97:1679-1687, 2005.

[117] Larsson SC, Mantzoros CS, Wolk A. Diabetes mellitus and risk of bladder cancer: a meta-analysis. *Diabetologia* 49:2819-2823, 2006.

[118] Reddy SK, Steel JL, Chen HW, et al. Outcomes of curative treatment for hepatocellular cancer in nonalcoholic steatohepatitis versus hepatitis C and alcoholic liver disease. *Hepatology* 55:1809-1819, 2012.

[119] Hernandez-Alejandro R, Croome KP, Drage M, et al. A comparison of survival pathologic features of non-alcoholic steatohepatitis and hepatitis C patients with hepatocellular carcinoma. *World J Gastroenterol* 18:4145-4149, 2012.

[120] Tokushige K, Hashimoto E, Yatsuji S, et al. Prospective study of hepatocellular carcinoma in nonalcoholic steatohepatitis in comparison hepatitis C. *J Gastroenterol* 45:960-967, 2010.

[121] Jemal A, Bray F, Center MM, et al. Global cancer statistics. *CA Cancer J Clin* 61:69-90, 2011.

[122] Okuda K. Epidemiology of primary liver cancer. In: *Primary Liver Cancer in Japan*, Tobe T (Ed), Springer-Verlag, Tokyo pp.3-15, 1992.

[123] Yuan JM, Ross PK, Stanczyk FZ, et al. A cohort study of serum testosterone and hepatocellular carcinoma in Shanghai, China. *Int J Cancer* 63:491-493, 1995.

[124] Naugler WE, Sakurai T, Kim S, et al. Gender disparity in liver cancer due to sex differences in MyD88-dependent IL-6 production. *Science* 317:121-124, 2007.

[125] Nakagawa H, Maeda S, Yoshida H, et al. Serum IL-6 levels and the risk for hepato-carcinomagenesis in chronic hepatitis C patients; an analysis based on gender differences. *Int J Cancer* 125:2264-2269, 2009.

[126] Trichopoulos D, Bamia C, Lagiou P, et al. Hepatocellular carcinoma risk factors and disease burden in a European cohort: a nested case-control study. *J Natl Cancer Inst* 103:1686-1695, 2011.

[127] Mayans MV, Calvet X, Bruix J, et al. Risk factors for hepatocellular carcinoma in Catalonia, Spain. *Int J Cancer* 46:378-381, 1990.

[128] Tanaka K, Hirohata T, Takeshita S, et al. Hepatitis B virus, cigarette smoking and alcohol consumption in the development of hepatocellular carcinoma: a case-control study in Fukuoka, Japan. *Int J Cancer* 51:509-514, 1992.

[129] Mohamed AE, Kew MC, Groeneveld HT. Alcohol consumption as a risk factor for hepatocellular carcinoma in urban southern African blacks. *Int J Cancer* 51:537-541, 1992.

[130] Donato F, Tagger A, Gelatti U, et al. Alcohol and hepatocellular carcinoma: the effect of lifetime intake and hepatitis virus infections in men and women. *Am J Epidemiol* 155:323-331, 2002.

[131] Lieber CS. Alcohol and the liver: 1994 update. *Gastroenterology* 106:1085-1105, 1994.

[132] Chiesa R, Donato F, Tagger A, et al. Etiology of hepatocellular carcinoma in Italian patients with and without cirrhosis. *Cancer Epidemiol Biomarkers Prev* 9:2130-2135, 2000.

[133] Tsukuma H, Hiyama T, Tanaka S, et al. Risk factors for hepatocellular carcinoma among patients with chronic liver disease. *N Engl J Med* 328:1797-1801, 1993.

[134] Ikeda K, Marusawa H, Osaki Y, et al. Antibody to hepatitis B core antigen and risk for hepatitis C-related hepatocellular carcinoma: a prospective study. *Ann Intern Med* 146:649-656, 2007.

[135] Hassan MM, Hwang LY, Hatten CJ, et al. Risk factors for hepatocellular carcinoma: synergism of alcohol with viral hepatitis and diabetes mellitus. *Hepatology* 36:1206-1213, 2002.

[136] Ohki T, Tateishi R, Sato T, et al. Obesity is an independent risk factor for hepatocellular carcinoma development in chronic hepatitis C patients. *Clin Gastroenterol Hepatol* 6:459-464, 2008.

[137] Saunders D, Seidel D, Allison M, Lyratzopoulos G. Systematic review: the association between obesity and hepatocellular carcinoma - epidemiological evidence. *Aliment Pharmacol Ther* 31:1051, 2010.

[138] Loomba R, Yang HI, Su J, et al. Synergism between obesity and alcohol in increasing the risk of hepatocellular carcinoma: a prospective cohort study. *Am J Epidemiol* 177:333-342, 2013.

[139] Donato F, Tagger A, Gelatti U, et al. Alcohol and hepatocellular carcinoma: the effect of lifetime intake and hepatitis virus infections in men and women. *Am J Epidemiol* 155:323-331, 2002.

[140] Brechot C, Nalpas B, Feitelson MA. Interactions between alcohol and hepatitis viruses in the liver. *Clin Lab Med* 16:273-287, 1996.

[141] Schiff ER. Hepatitis C and alcohol. *Hepatology* 26:39S-42S, 1997.

[142] Donato F, Boffeta P, Puoti M. A meta-analysis of epidemiological studies on the combined effect of hepatitis B and C virus infections in causing hepatocellular carcinoma. *Int J Cancer* 75:347-354, 1998.

[143] Donato F, Boffeta P, Puoti M. A meta-analysis of epidemiological studies on the combined effect of hepatitis B and C virus infections in causing hepatocellular carcinoma. *Int J Cancer* 75:347-354, 1998.

[144] Yu MC, Tong MJ, Govindarajan S, Henderson BE. Nonviral risk factors for hepatocellular carcinoma in a low-risk population, the non-Asians of Los Angeles County, California. *J Natl Cancer Inst* 83:1820-1826, 1991.

[145] Kuper H, Tzonou A, Kaklamani E, et al. Tabacco smoking, alcohol consumption and their interaction in the causation of hepatocellular carcinoma. *Int J Cancer* 85:498-502. 2000.

[146] Trichopoulos D, Bamia C, Lagiou P, et al. Hepatocellular carcinoma risk factors and disease burden in a European cohort: a nested case-control study. *J Natl Cancer Inst* 103:1686-1695, 2011.

[147] Mayans MV, Calvet X, Bruix J, et al. Risk factors for hepatocellular carcinoma in Catalonia, Spain. *Int J Cancer* 46:378-381, 1990.

[148] Tanaka K, Hirohata T, Takeshita S, et al. Hepatitis B virus, cigarette smoking and alcohol consumption in the development of hepatocellular carcinoma: a case-control study in Fukuoka, Japan. *Int J Cancer* 51:509-514, 1992.

[149] Mohamed AE, Kew MC, Groeneveld HT. Alcohol consumption as a risk factor for hepatocellular carcinoma in urban southern African blacks. *Int J Cancer* 51:537-541, 1992.

[150] Chuang SC, Lee YC, Hashibe M et al. Interaction between cigarette smoking and hepatitis B and C virus infection on the risk of liver cancer: a meta analysis. *Cancer Epidemiol biomarkers Prev* 19:1261-1268, 2010.

[151] Tsai JF, Chuang LY, Jeng JE, et al. Betel quid chewing as a risk factor for hepatocellular carcinoma : a case-control study. *Br J Cancer* 84:709-713, 2001.

[152] Tsai JF, Jeng JE, Chuang LY, et al. Habitual betel quid chewing as a risk factor for cirrhosis: a case-control study. *Medicine (Baltimore)* 82:365-372, 2003.

[153] Tsai JF, Jeng JE, Chuang LY, et al. Habitual betel quid chewing as a risk factor for hepatocellular carcinoma complicating cirrhosis. *Medicine (Baltimore)* 83:176-187, 2004.

[154] Feedman ND, Cross AJ, McGlynn KA, et al. Association of meat and fat intake with liver disease and hepatocellular carcinoma in the NIH-AARP cohort. *J Natl Cancer Inst* 102:1354-1365, 2010.

[155] Sawada N, Inoue M, Iwasaki M, et al. Consumption of n-3 fatty acids and fish reduces risk of hepatocellular carcinoma. *Gastroenterology* 142:1468-1475, 2012.

[156] Fedirko V, Trichopolou A, Bamia C, et al. Consumption of fish and meats and risk of hepatocellular carcinoma: the European Prospective Investigation into Cancer and Nutrition (EPIC). *Ann Oncol* 24:2166, 2013.

[157] Zhang W, Shu XO, Li H, et al. Vitamin intake and liver cancer risk: a report from two cohort studies in China. *J Natl Cancer Inst* 104:1173, 2012.

[158] Larsson SC, Wolk A. Coffee consumption and risk of liver cancer: a meta-analysis. *Gastroenterology* 132:1740-1745, 2007.

[159] Bravi F, Bosetti C, Tavani A, et al. Coffee drinking and hepatocellular carcinoma risk: a meta-analysis. *Hepatology* 46:430-435, 2007.

[160] Chen CJ, Wang LY, Lu SN, et al. Elevated aflatoxin exposure and increased risk of hepatocellular carcinoma. *Hepatology* 24:38-42, 1996.

[161] Qian GS, Ross RK, Yu MC et al. A follow-up study of urinary markers of aflatoxin exposure and liver cancer risk in Shanghai, People's Republic of China. *Cancer Epidemiol biomarkers Prev* 3:3-10, 1994.

[162] Qian GS, Ross RK, Yu MC, et al. A follow-up study of urinary markers of aflatoxin exposure and liver cancer risk in Shanghai, People's Republic of China. *Cancer Epidemiol Biomarkers* Prev 3:3-10, 1994.

[163] Bosch FX, Ribes J, Borras J. Epidemiology of primary liver cancer. *Semin Liver Dis* 19:271-285, 1999.

[164] Bressac B, Kew M, Wands J, Ozturk M. Selective G to T mutations of p53 gene in hepatocellular carcinoma from southern Africa. *Nature* 350:429-431, 1991.

[165] Unsal H, Yakicier C, Marcais C, et al. Genetic heterogeneity of hepatocellular carcinoma. *Proc Natl Acad Sci U S A* 91:822-826, 1994.

[166] Yan RQ, Su JJ, Huang DR, et al. Human hepatitis B virus and hepatocellular carcinoma. II. Experimental induction of hepatocellular carcinoma in tree shrews exposed to hepatitis B virus and aflatoxin B1. *J Cancer Res Clin Oncol* 122:289-295, 1996.

[167] Kanwal F, Hoang T, Kramer JR, et al. Increasing prevalence of HCC and cirrhosis in patients with chronic hepatitis C virus infection. *Gastroenterology* 140:1182-1188, 2011.

In: Therapy for Hepatocellular Carcinoma
Editor: Nobuhiro Ohkohchi

ISBN: 978-1-63117-929-7
© 2014 Nova Science Publishers, Inc.

Chapter 2

Diagnosis of Hepatocellular Carcinoma Using CT and MRI

Katsuhiro Nasu[*], M.D.[1], Manabu Minami, M.D.[1],
Kensaku Mori, M.D.[1], Masato Sugano, M.D.[2],
Yukio Morishita, M.D.[3] and Yoshifumi Kuroki, M.D.[4]

[1]University of Tsukuba, Faculty of Medicine,
Department of Radiology
[2]University of Tsukuba, Faculty of Medicine,
Department of Pathology
[3]Tokyo medical university Ibaraki medical center,
Division of Diagnostic pathology
[4]Tochigi Cancer Center, Department of Radiology

Abstract

Detection of hepatocellular carcinoma (HCC) in the early clinical stage is inclusively important to improve the prognosis of this malignancy. CT and MRI have greatly contributed to this purpose in the past 20 years. The diagnosing techniques using CT and MRI have enabled not only precise detection of HCC, but also visualization of the multistep carcinogenesis or adenoma-carcinoma sequence in the liver. The recent progress of MR imaging using liver-specific contrast agents represented by Gd-EOB-DTPA has succeeded in producing various novel findings regarding HCC. In brief, the technical developments of CT and MRI are still continuing, and their limits are unimaginable in the current era. In this chapter, we will discuss the current destinations of CT and MRI in diagnosing HCCs.

[*] Corresponding author. Tsukuba University, Faculty of clinical medicine, Department of radiology, 1-1-1 Tendoudai, Tsukuba, Ibaraki Japan 305-8577. Tel/Fax: +81-29-853-3205; E-mail address: kanasu-u3@md.tsukuba.ac.jp.

1. Introduction

Early detection of hepatocellular carcinoma (HCC) is highly important to perform proper treatment. The prognosis of HCC strongly depends on whether the patient can undergo curative local treatments [1]. During the past 30 years, the five-year survival rate for HCC has improved from 10% to over 40% [2]. This phenomenal success was brought about not only by the progress in treatments, but also by radiological developments that enabled detection of smaller HCCs whose clinical stage was suitable for local curative treatment. From these standpoints, CT and MRI have greatly contributed to the improvement in the prognosis of HCC, and the roles of these modalities are expected to increase in future. In this chapter, we will explain the current situation regarding CT and MRI, and the remaining problems in diagnosis of HCCs.

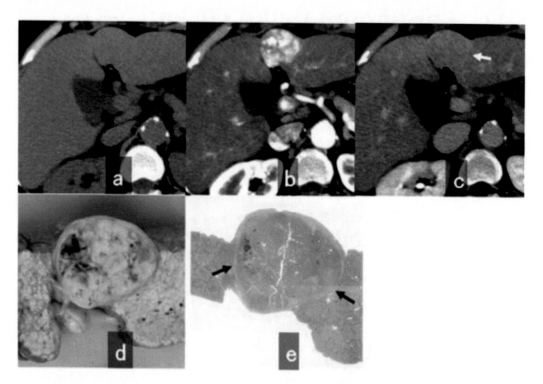

Figure 1. Dynamic CT scan of a typical classic HCC (margin distinct, simple nodular type) in a 69-year female is shown. The tumor in the lateral segment is isodense to the surrounding hepatic parenchyma on precontrast image (Figure 1a), enhances strongly on arterial-dominant phase image (Figure 1b) and becomes relatively hypodense to the surrounding hepatic parenchyma on equilibrium phase image (Figure 1c). Please notice that the fibrotic capsule is visualized as an enhancing thin linear structure around the tumor on equilibrium phase image (arrow). The fibrotic capsule is also clearly observed in pathological specimens (Figure 1d: the maximum section of undyed specimen, Figure 1e: macroscopic view of HE stain). The tumor is well-demarcated from the surrounding hepatic parenchyma by the fibrotic capsule which shows more prominent eosin stainability (black arrows).

2. Multistep Hepatocarcinogenesis and Hemodynamics

Small hepatic nodules are frequently found in cirrhotic levels (3). Nowadays, pathologists classify them into four groups: large regenerative nodule (LRN), low-grade dysplastic nodule (LGDN), high-grade dysplastic nodule (HGDN), and HCC [4, 5]. While LRNs are thought to be benign, DNs are considered as preneoplastic lesions, and HGDNs are the precursors of HCC. Pathologists also proposed the term "small HCC" for tumors measuring less than 2 cm. More recent studies reported that small HCCs should be divided into two subgroups: small HCCs with distinct margins, and small HCCs with indistinct margins. The former roughly correspond to small hypervascular simple nodular HCCs (Figure 1). The latter are ill-defined hypovascular nodules, consisting of well-differentiated malignant cells which correspond to the small nodular type with indistinct margin or so-called early HCCs (Figure 2). These hypovascular HCCs do not show invasion into the portal vein nor minute intrahepatic metastases [6].

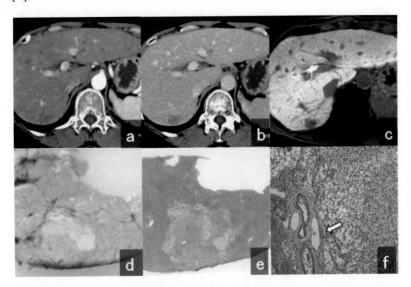

Figure 2. An early HCC (margin indistinct) with moderately differentiated HCC components in the center of the tumor in a 52-year-old female with autoimmune hepatitis. The tumor in the posterior segment does not show overt enhancement on arterial-dominant phase image (Figure 2a) and is observed as a relatively hypointense nodule on equilibrium phase image (Figure 2b) of dynamic CT scan. On hepatobiliary phase image of EOB-MRI (Figure 2c), the tumor is observed as a well-demarcated nodule but its margin is shaggy. These findings are typical for early HCC. On the maximum section of the undyed specimen (Figure 2d) and the macroscopic view of HE stain (Figure 2e), the margin of the tumor is irregular and the less demarcated that the tumor shown in Figure 1. On the low magnification macroscopic view of HE stain (Figure 2f) reveals that the tumor consists of well-differentiated HCC cells and these cancer cells invades into the Glisson`s sheath which are not usually seen in classic HCCs (arrow).

Current radiological examinations have succeeded in showing the multi-step carcinogenesis of HCC (hepatocarcinogenesis) occurring in DNs. This was because hepatocarcinogenesis is strongly related with hemodynamics, which was clearly depicted on imaging examinations using contrast medium [7-9]. The current consensus regarding hepatocarcinogenesis is the following: in the first place, DNs with slight cellular atypia emerge among LRNs. They have higher cellularity than the normal hepatic parenchyma, and the portal areas inside are compressed by the surrounding hepatic cells [10]. Consequently, the blood supply into DNs via normal portal veins and hepatic arteries decreases, and the hepatic cells in DNs become hypoxic [11]. Because of this hypoxia, some pre-neoplastic hepatic cells in DNs transform into well-differentiated cancer cells. However, these well-differentiated cancer cells are still hypovascular and do not have the potential of vascular invasion or intrahepatic metastasis. The nodules in this step are considered to be early HCCs. In the next step, these cancer cells induce some kinds of vascular endothelial growth factors (VEGF), and finally acquire an arterial blood supply [12]. The cancer cells having an arterial blood supply accelerate their speed of growth and finally replace the whole of the nodule from which the cancer originally emerged. The nodule replaced by hypervascular cancer cells is the equivalent of the so-called classic HCC. Not only classic HCCs but also hypervascular foci in DNs or early HCC are considered to have the potential of vascular invasion or intrahepatic metastasis.

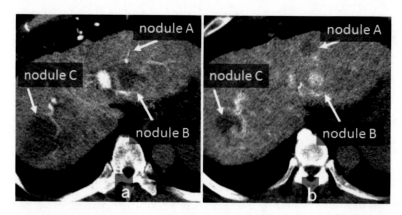

Figure 3. CTAP (Figure 3a) and CTHA (Figure 3b) of a 60-year-old male having multiple hepatic nodules. These images reveal the following issues; (i) the nodule-A has the same portal blood supply and decreased arterial blood supply as comparison with the surrounding hepatic parenchyma, (ii) the nodule-B has decreased the portal blood supply and increased arterial blood supply and (iii) the both blood supplies decreased in the majority of the nodule-C but the in rest of this nodule, the arterial blood supply has become increasing. These findings suggest that these three hepatic nodules are in the different steps of hepatocarcinogenesis.

This multi-step hepatocarcinogenesis accompanies dynamic changes in the portal and arterial blood supply in DNs. LGDNs have almost the same portal blood supply as the surrounding hepatic parenchyma. As the characteristics of DNs approach those of HCCs, both the portal and the arterial blood supplies decrease (these blood supply decreases may not be observed simultaneously) [7], and cancerous foci in the DNs lack portal blood supply and show overt arterial blood supply [8] (Figure 3). Finally, the whole of the nodule lacks portal blood flow and is completely supplied by arterial blood flow [9] (Figure 4). These processes can be clearly depicted by CT during arterial portography (CTAP) and CT during hepatic arteriography (CTHA) [7-9, 13]. The series of research studies revealing this multi-step hepatocarcinogenesis using CTAP and CTHA were not only epoch-making results in radiology but also monumental works of oncology, and proved the multi-step carcinogenesis of an internal organ in vivo.

However, about half of HCCs appear in the normal hepatic parenchyma without the above-described multi-step hepatocarcinogenesis [14]. They are considered to be de-novo HCCs. Their hepatocarcinogenesis processes cannot be visualized even by using CTAP and CTHA. At this time, it is still uncertain whether they really derive from usual hepatic cells, or whether they pass through multi-step hepatocarcinogenesis too rapidly to be detected by radiological methods. Additionally, the most important clinical issue in HCC management is not to find early HCCs without arterial neovascularization, but to detect classic HCCs or DNs/early HCCs with cancerous foci with arterial neovascularization. The recent development of non-invasive routine CT/MRI have high enough detectability for classic HCCs and DNs/early HCC with cancerous foci with arterial neovascularization. From these viewpoints, CTAP and CTHA, which are invasive imaging methods, have already become dispensable modalities in practical HCC management (See Column 1).

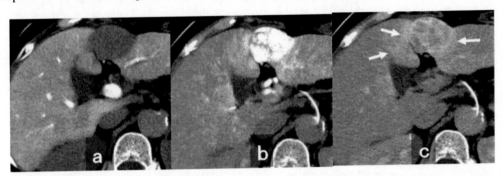

Figure 4. CTAP (Figure 4a), early phase (Figure 4b) and delayed phase (Figure 4c) of CTHA of the same patient presented in Figure 1 are shown. The tumor lacks the portal blood supply and is completely fed by arterial blood. These findings suggest that this tumor has reached the final step of hepatocarcinogenesis. The hepatic parenchyma around the tumor enhances like "corona" in the solar eclipse on delayed phase of CTHA. This finding is so-called corona enhancement. Please notice that the corona enhancement is observed in wider area than the fibrotic capsule depicted on Figure 1c-e.

Column 1. CTAP and CTHA

These imaging procedures are usually performed by using an IVR-CT system, combining both an angiography apparatus and CT. Of course, without an IVR-CT system, CTAP and CTHA can be performed, if patients with indwelling catheters in the superior mesenteric artery or common hepatic artery are moved from the angiography suite to the CT suite. However, such troublesome methods having an infection risk are not usually performed in an institute without an IVR-CT system.

CTAP is a CT scan obtained under arterial portography, which is a delayed image in superior mesenteric angiography. In CTAP, we can obtain pure information about portal flow in the liver which can never be acquired using usual dynamic CT. CTHA is a CT scan obtained under common hepatic angiography, and a useful modality to assess the hemodynamics of hepatic nodules or to detect small classic HCCs.

On the other hand, these modalities have many shortcomings; they are invasive, and pseudo-positive findings are frequent. When the high diagnostic ability of current routine non-invasive CT/MRI is taken into consideration, it is natural that the usage of CTAP/CHA is now decreasing.

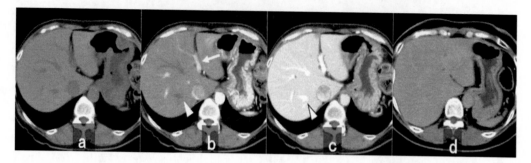

Figure 5. Typical four-phase dynamic CT scan (a: precontrast, b: arterial-dominant, c: portal-dominant, d: equilibrium) of a 60-year-old non-cirrhotic patient is shown. Please pay attention that on arterial-dominant phase image, the intravenously administered contrast material slightly opacities the portal vein (white arrow) but does not enhance the hepatic vein (arrowhead). These are the indispensable conditions of the proper arterial dominant phase. On portal-dominant phase image, the hepatic vein is opacified (black arrow) and the hepatic parenchyma shows the most strong contrast uptake. The enhancement effect of the hepatic parenchyma and vessels rapidly decrease on equilibrium phase image.

Column 2. Progress in CT Technology

About 30 years ago, it took more than five seconds to obtain one slice of CT scan. The single-slice helical CT adopting slip ring developed in the 1990s needed one second per slice. 10 years later after the advent of single-slice helical CT, MDCT was developed. In MDCT, a two-dimensional array of detector elements replaces the linear array of detector elements. This new type detector enables CT scanners to acquire multiple slices during one rotation of the X-ray tube. A high-end MDCT scanner can obtain 320 slices of 0.5mm-thickness within 0.275 second! Now, whole-liver scanning using MDCT only needs 3 seconds!

Column 3. Sophistication of Contrast Administration

Acceleration of CT scanning time brought major changes to the methods of administering contrast materials. Now, the following four devices are routinely used to optimize contrast administration at CT scanning of the liver: (i) dose optimization depending on body weight or body mass index of each patient; (ii) variable injection rate of contrast material to make the iodine dose per unit time, constant; (iii) saline flush after injection of contrast material; and (iv) optimization of scan start time by monitoring the CT value of the aorta using a low-dose CT scan during contrast injection.

---

3. Dynamic CT Scan and Classic HCCs

The modality that has most contributed to the improvement in the detection rate of classic HCCs is dynamic CT scan comprising several repeat scans performed before and after bolus intravenous administration of iodine contrast medium [15-17]. It usually consists of four phases: the precontrast, arterial-dominant, portal-dominant and equilibrium phases (Figure 5). Dynamic CT scan performed with multi-detector row CT (MDCT) having 16 rows or more and optimized injection protocols of contrast medium shows a 95% positive predictive value for classic HCCs [18]. This excellent record is almost the same with gadolinium-ethoxybenzyl-diethylenetriaminepentaacetic acid (Gd-EOB-DTPA) enhanced MR imaging (EOB-MRI) when the subjects of the examination are limited to classic HCCs [19]. Dynamic CT scan is inferior to EOB-MRI in the qualitative diagnosis of hepatic nodules or sensitivity to early HCCs [20-21]. However, there is no doubt that dynamic CT scan is the most powerful tool for diagnosis, staging, and decision-making in treatments for classic HCCs.

4. Transition in the Role of Dynamic MR Imaging in Diagnosing Classic HCCs

The main constituent of MR diagnosis for HCC is, similarly to CT, dynamic study using intraveneous bolus injection of gadolinium chelates. Liver-specific contrast agents typified by Gd-EOB-DTPA and several newly developed sequences such as diffusion weighted imaging (DWI) are changing the situation now. Hence, we will review the history of MR diagnosis for HCC.

Until the development of Gd-EOB-DTPA, dynamic MRI, like dynamic CT scan, had consisted of four-time repeated T1-weighted images before and after intraveneous bolus administration of gadolinium chelates such as Gd-DTPA, which is not an organ-specific contrast material and whose pharmacokinetics in the human body are almost the same as those of iodine contrast material [22] (Figure 6).

Before the development of MDCT, dynamic MRI was superior to dynamic CT scan in the detection rate of small classic HCCs [23, 24]. This may seem unlikely, because in these days the acquisition time of each phase of dynamic MRI was about 25 seconds and that of dynamic CT scan was about 20 seconds. However, the contrast determination time of MRI is about one third of the acquisition time [25] and the enhancement effect in all slices is uniform because the contrast enhancement effect of each phase of dynamic MRI is the average during the contrast determination time. When these characteristics of MRI are taken into consideration, we can understand that the arterial-dominant phase of dynamic MR imaging had a clear advantage over that of dynamic CT scan before MDCT was developed. There was a 20-second gap between the first and last slices of each phase of dynamic CT scan. The contrast enhancement effect of the arterial-dominant phase rapidly changed during this 20-second gap. Therefore, only a few slices of the arterial-dominant phase of dynamic CT scan had an optimal contrast enhancement effect suitable to detect classic HCCs. Additionally, gadolinium chelates have superior enhancement effect to iodine contrast material when their concentration is low [26]. These were the reasons why dynamic MR imaging had superior detectability for small classic HCCs than dynamic CT scan.

The development of MDCT reversed the situation. MDCT with a 16-row detector needs only seven seconds to obtain whole liver images and, thus, became equal to dynamic MRI in the contrast determination time. We guessed that the detectability for classic HCC in dynamic CT scan using MDCT with a 16-row detector would catch up with that in dynamic MRI [18], and the MDCT with a 64-row detector overtook MRI. At the beginning of this century, some radiologists seriously thought that dynamic MRI had become an old-fashioned, unnecessary modality for diagnosing HCCs (See Column 2 and 3).

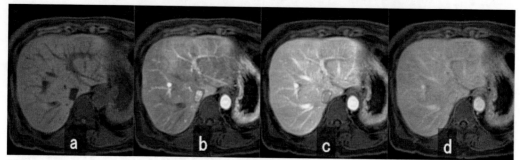

Figure 6. Typical four-phase dynamic MRI (a: precontrast, b: arterial-dominant, c: portal-dominant, d: equilibrium) of the same patient shown in Figure 5 are demonstrated. This dynamic MR is performed by using Gd-DTPA. The transition of the contrast enhancement of the portal veins, hepatic veins and hepatic parenchyma are almost the same with those in Figure 5. Please pay attention that the intravascular enhancement effect is far stronger on equilibrium phase image of dynamic MRI as comparison with that the same image of dynamic CT scan shown on Figure 5d. This phenomenon is due to the stronger enhancement effect of gadolinium chelate when its concentration is low as comparison with that of iodine contrast material used in CT scan.

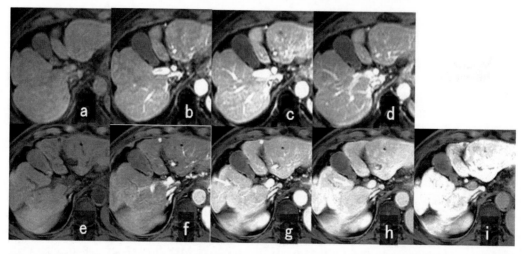

Figure 7. Comparison of a conventional four-phase dynamic MRI using Gd-DTPA (a: precontrast, b: arterial-dominant, c: portal-dominant, d: equilibrium) and typical EOB-MRI (e: precontrast, f: arterial-dominant, g: portal-dominant, h: delayed, i: hepatobiliary) of a same cirrhotic female patient (The conventional four-phase dynamic MRI was obtained at the age of 70 years old and EOB-MRI was performed at the age of 72). On conventional four-phase dynamic MRI, the hepatic parenchymal enhancement is strongest on portal-dominant phase image and shows rapid washout on equilibrium phase image on conventional dynamic MRI. On the other hand, the hepatic contrast uptake becomes higher on hepatobiliary phase image than on portal-dominant phase image of EOB-MRI. Please pay attention that the intravascular enhancement is much weaker on delayed phase image and hepatobiliary phase image of EOB-MRI than equilibrium phase image of conventional dynamic MRI findings. This finding means that there is no "equilibrium" phase in EOB-MRI.

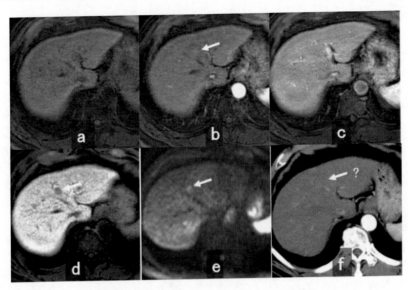

Figure 8. EOB-MRI (a: precontrast, b: arterial-dominant, c: portal-dominant, d: hepatobiliary, e: DWI) and arterial-dominant phase of dynamic CT scan (f) of a 64-year-old male suspected HCC are shown. A small well-demarcated nodule (arrows) is shown in segment 4 hypointensely on hepatobiliary phase image and hyperintensely on diffusion weighted image. With knowing these findings, it is not difficult to find a faint enhancement in the same location on arterial-dominant phase image; however, it may be impossible to point out this small nodule only on dynamic CT scan. In this manner, EOB-MRI has more sensitive method to screen HCC than dynamic CT. These are the reason why MRI still shows higher sensitivity to classic HCC than dynamic CT scan even in the MDCT era.

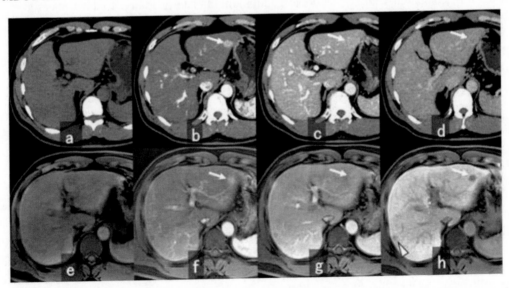

Figure 9. Dynamic CT scan (a: precontrast, b: arterial-dominant, c: portal-dominant, d: equilibrium) and EOB-MRI (e: precontrast, f: arterial-dominant, g: portal-dominant, h: hepatobiliary) of 62-year-old male suspected HCC. Both dynamic CT scan and EOB-MRI succeed to depict a classic HCC in the lateral segment (arrows). The hypointense nodule depicted on hepatobiliary phase image of EOB-MRI (arrowhead) is hardly pointed out on other images. This lesion is suspected as an early HCC (pathologically not proven). Such avascular hepatic nodules suspected early HCC have become frequently found after introduction of EOB-MRI in clinical setting.

Gd-EOB-DTPA reversed the situation once again. This novel contrast material for MRI has some special characteristics. With this contrast material, we can obtain arterial-dominant and portal-dominant phases that have almost the same quality as those of dynamic MRI obtained by using conventional gadolinium chelates [27]. Additionally, this contrast material is accumulated into the normal hepatic parenchyma by active transport. On the hepatobiliary phase of EOB-MRI, which is obtained 15 minutes or later after administration of Gd-EOB-DTPA, the majority of hepatic nodular lesions including HCCs are depicted as well-demarcated hypointense lesions among well-enhanced normal hepatic parenchyma [28] (Figure 7). With use of the hepatobiliary phase of EOB-MRI, more difficult HCCs whose arterial enhancements are subtle and hardly noticeable in dynamic CT scan or conventional dynamic MRI, can now be easily pointed out in clinical image interpretation (Figure 8).

Some recent reports mentioned that the many hepatic nodules in cirrhotic livers that were observed as well-demarcated hypointense nodules on hepatobiliary phase images and hardly noticeable on other images, including arterial-dominant phase, were early HCCs [20, 21, 29] (Figure 2, 9). Accordingly, the hepatobiliary phase of EOB-MRI is considered to succeed in depicting the first step of hepatocarcinogenesis without the use of CTAP/CTHA [29]. In the newest guidelines for liver cancer in Japan, the recommendation for EOB-MRI is grade B [30]. This is because the number of clinical experiences of EOB-MRI is still smaller than that of ultrasound or dynamic CT/MRI. However, for all abdominal radiologists, it is already the consensus that EOB-MRI plays a central role in the detection of HCC, while dynamic CT scan provides anatomical information and information on vascular invasion or distant metastasis that are indispensable to decide the treatment strategy.

However, we should recognize that Gd-EOB-DTPA is a really complicated contrast material as compared with conventional gadolinium chelate or iodine contrast material, and there are many unresolved problems in EOB-MRI (See Column 4, 5).

Except for EOB-MRI, T1-weighted in/opposed-phase images, T2-weighted images (T2WI), and DWI are routinely used in liver imaging, and each sequence has different important roles. Each of these is discussed below.

5. Other MR Sequences Used for Diagnosing HCCs

5.1. T1-Weighted In/Opposed-Phase Imaging

This sequence is a T1-weighted gradient recalled echo sequence with two different echo times (2.3 msec/4.6 msec at 1.5T, and 1.2 msec/2.3 msec at 3T). Two images with different TEs are simultaneously obtained in each slice level. Consider a steatotic tissue, which contains both fat and water. In longer-TE images, the magnetic vectors of fat and water face the same direction, and the signal intensity of this tissue is the sum of the signal intensities of fat and water. On the other hand, in shorter-TE images, the magnetic vectors of fat and water face opposite directions, and the signal intensity of this tissue is the balance between the signal intensities of fat and water [31]. We can easily understand that this tissue contains both fat and water when the signal intensity changes between these images are observed. This may be the most sensitive, non-invasive method to determine whether a tissue is steatotic. It is well- known that both HCC and the surrounding hepatic parenchyma frequently become steatotic [32, 33]. Accordingly, the clinical usefulness of this sequence is considerable (Figure 10).

This sequence can depict not only fat deposition but also iron deposition in a tissue. In a tissue with iron deposition, its signal intensity decreases in longer-TE images as compared with shorter-TE images [34] (Figure 11). Some recent reports mentioned that a quantitative analysis of fat and iron deposition in the liver can be performed with use of a similar sequence with T1-weighted in/opposed-phase imaging having six different TEs [35].

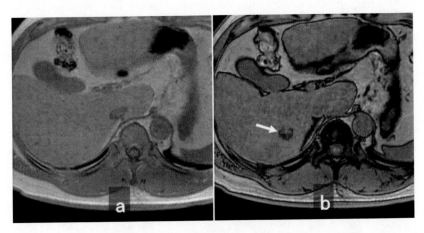

Figure 10. T1-weighted in/opposed-phase imaging (a: in-phase image, b: opposed-phase image) of a 59-year-old male diagnosed non-alcoholic steatohepatitis (NASH) is shown. On in-phase image, it is impossible to point out any abnormality in the liver except for the deformity due to NASH; however, on opposed-phase image, a small nodule advents in the posterior segment (arrow) as a hypointense area. These findings are consistent with a steatotic hepatic nodule suspected a HCC. Please pay attention that the surrounding hepatic parenchyma also shows signal drop on opposed-phase image because of fatty deposition.

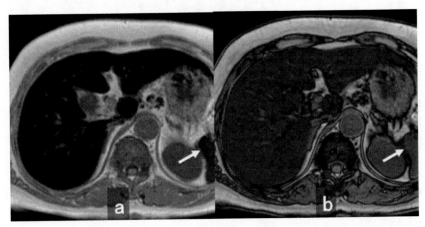

Figure 11. T1-weighted in/opposed-phase imaging (a: in-phase image, b: opposed-phase image) in a 76-year-old female diagnosed as secondary hemochromatosis due to over-dosage of ferric medicine. The hepatic parenchyma is shown more darkly on in-phase image than on opposed-phase image. These findings suggest strong iron deposition in the hepatic parenchyma. Generally speaking, in-phase images usually have longer echo time than opposed-phase images; therefore, the tissue with iron deposition more sensitively decreases its signal intensity on in-phase images than on opposed-phase images. Please pay attention that the iron deposition is also observed on the spleen (arrows).

5.2. T2-Weighted Imaging (T2WI)

The most important role of T2WI in diagnosing HCC is to differentiate hepatic cysts from other solid hepatic nodules including HCCs [36]. Small hepatic cysts measuring less than 5mm in diameter are often difficult to differentiate from solid nodules in dynamic CT/MRI. With the use of T2WI, we can easily differentiate such small hepatic cysts from other hepatic nodules.

T2WI, especially fat-presaturated T2WI, is also useful in detecting ascites, which is indispensable information to determine a Child-Pugh classification.

The signal intensities of HCCs on T2-weighted images are varied. However some reports mentioned that the signal intensities of HCCs on T2-weighted images tended to be higher as the pathological differentiation of each tumor became worse [37] (Figure 12).

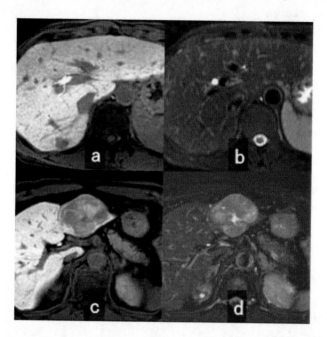

Figure 12. T2-weighted imaging findings of early HCC and moderately differentiated HCC are shown. An early HCC in a 69-year-old female (same case with Figure 2) is clearly depicted in the posterior segment on hepatobiliary phase image of EOB-MRI (Figure 12.a); however, it can hardly be pointed out on T2-weighted image because it is almost isointense to the surrounding hepatic parenchyma (Figure 12b). On the other hand, a moderately differentiated HCC in a 65-year-old male is relatively hypointense on hepatobiliary phase image (Figure 12c) and hyperintense on T2-weighted image (Figure 12d) to the surrounding hepatic parenchyma in the lateral segment.

5.3. Diffusion Weighted Imaging (DWI)

DWI can hyperintensely depict hypercellular tissues such as cancers [38]; therefore, it has high sensitivity to various malignant tumors including classic HCCs. It has the highest detectability for classic HCCs among the non-contrast imaging methods; however, its sensitivity for classic HCCs is inferior to that of dynamic CT/MRI [39].

DWI is considered to reflect the pathological grade more precisely than T2WI [39, 40]. In particular, it can depict poorly differentiated HCCs very brightly and may show higher detectability for poorly differentiated HCCs and portal venous tumor thrombi or their distant metastases than dynamic CT/MRI (Figure 13). On the other hand, DNs or early HCCs are usually observed as iso- to hypointense to the surrounding hepatic parenchyma (Figure 14).

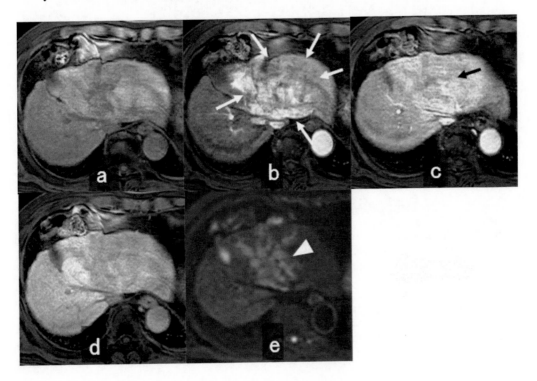

Figure 13. A 72-year-old male having diffuse tumor thrombi of poorly-differentiated HCC in the left hepatic lobe is shown. EOB-MRI (Figure 13a: precontrast, Fig.13b: arterial-dominant, Figure 13c: portal-dominant, Figure 14d: hepatobiliary) reveals that the whole of the left hepatic lobe shows strong arterial enhancement. This phenomenon is frequently seen in the hepatic parenchyma with tumor thrombi (white arrow), because the hepatic artery dilates and feeds more arterial blood to the hepatic parenchyma to compensate the decreased portal blood supply. Accordingly, HCCs can be hardly differentiated from surrounding hepatic parenchyma on arterial dominant phase in such patient. Additionally, the portal dominant phase is not effective to evaluate tumor thrombi because the intravascular enhancement effect rapidly decreases in EOB-MRI (black arrow). On the other hand, DWI can stably depict tumor thrombi (Figure 13e) (arrowhead).

However, the high signal intensities of DWI are basically non-specific. Not only tumors but also various abnormal conditions such as fresh infarctions abscesses and active inflammation may show positive findings in this sequence [41, 42]. Some normal tissues such as lymphatic tissues, adrenal glands, testes, or neural tissues are observed hyperintensely on diffusion weighted images.

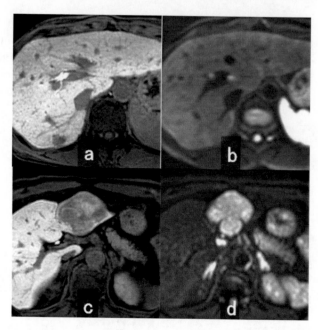

Figure 14. Comparison of DWI findings of early HCC and moderately differentiated HCC is shown. An early HCC in a 69-year-old female (same case with Figure 2, 12) is clearly depicted in the posterior segment on hepatobiliary phase image of EOB-MRI (Figure 14a); however, it can hardly be pointed out on diffusion weighted image because it is almost isointense to the surrounding hepatic parenchyma (Figure 14b). On the other hand, a moderately differentiated HCC in a 65-year-old male (same case with Figure 12) is relatively hypointense on hepatobiliary phase image (Figure 14c) and clearly hyperintense on diffusion weighted image (Figure 14d) to the surrounding hepatic parenchyma in the lateral segment. Please pay attention that the contrast between the tumor and surrounding hepatic parenchyma is more prominent on diffusion weighted image as comparison with that of T2-weighted image shown on Figure 12d.

6. Summary of Imaging Findings of Classic HCC

The imaging findings of classic HCCs in dynamic CT/MRI are already well known. The blood supply in normal hepatic parenchyma consists of 30% of arterial blood flow, and the remaining 70% of portal blood flow. On the other hand, classic HCCs are purely fed by the arterial blood flow and lack the portal blood flow. Reflecting these characteristics, classic HCCs are observed as relatively higher density/intensity lesions on arterial-dominant phase images and become relatively lower density/intensity lesions on portal-dominant or equilibrium phases than the surrounding hepatic parenchyma [12, 15]. Nowadays, hepatic nodules showing typical imaging findings of classic HCCs can be diagnosed as HCCs even though the tumor markers are low, and in such radiologically typical classic HCCs, percutaneous needle biopsy can be omitted before treatments (Figure 15). Of course, we should suspect classic HCCs when we find hypervascular hepatic tumors in cirrhotic livers. However, the above enhancement pattern in dynamic CT/MRI is not specific only to HCCs but is also observed in other hypervascular hepatic nodules such as hypervascular metastases, focal nodular hyperplasias, and perivascular endothelial cell tumors.

In the next part of this section, we describe other imaging characteristics of classic HCCs.

6.1. Fibrous Capsules and Septa

Fibrous capsules are the structures commonly found in the majority of classic HCCs measuring more than 2 cm in diameter, and can be usually observed in the imaging methods [16]. On the other hand, in HCCs measuring less than 1 cm in diameter, fibrous capsules are rarely seen either in the imaging methods or in the pathological examinations. Some past reports mentioned that capsular invasion was one of the risk factors of intrahepatic metastasis [43]. Accordingly, precise evaluation of the fibrous capsule is important to devise the proper treatment strategy for HCC.

Fibrous capsules are usually observed as well-enhanced ring-like structures surrounding classic HCCs on the equilibrium phase of dynamic CT scan or conventional dynamic MRI [16]. On precontrast T1WI, the fibrous capsules are seen as hypointense bands. On T2WI, the signal intensities of the fibrous capsules are varied [44]. In EOB-MRI, fibrous capsules are less frequently seen than in dynamic CT scan or conventional dynamic MRI, because the equilibrium phase does not exist in EOB-MRI [45] (Figure 1, 15).

Fibrous septa are also fibrous tissues penetrating inside of the tumors [46]. Each classic HCC often has different histopathological features in the bilateral sides of the septa. This is why classic HCCs often show the mosaic pattern described in the next section.

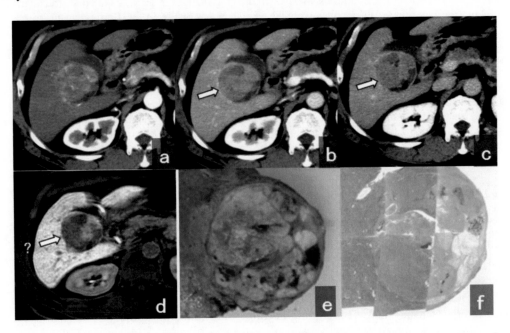

Figure 15. Dynamic CT scan (Figure 15a: arterial-dominant, Figure 15b: portal-dominant, Figure 15c: equilibrium) and hepatobiliary phase image of EOB-MRI (Figure 15d) of a typical HCC in a 64-year-old male (same patient with shown as Figure 7) are shown. The tumor in segment 5 shows strong inhomogeneous enhancement on arterial-dominant phase images of CT scan rapidly becomes relatively hypodense to the hepatic parenchyma on portal-dominant phase images of dynamic CT scan. The internal structure of the tumor shows typical mosaic appearance. The fibrous capsule is clearly depicted on portal dominant and equilibrium phase images of dynamic CT scan (arrows). Such typical tumor can be diagnosed as a HCC without needle biopsy. Please pay attention that the fibrous capsule can be hardly pointed out on hepatobiliary phase image. On the maximum section of the undyed specimen (Figure 15e) and the macroscopic view of HE stain (Figure 15f), the fibrous capsule and the mosaic internal structures are clearly seen.

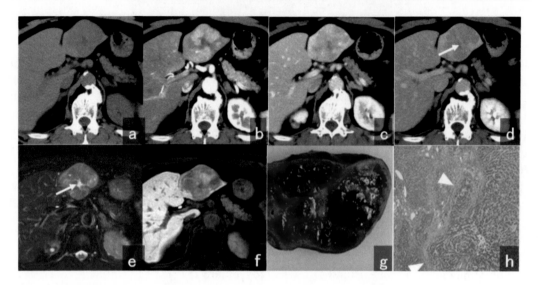

Figure 16. Dynamic CT scan (Figure 16a: precontrast, Figure 16b: arterial-dominant, Figure 16c: portal-dominant, Figure 16d: equilibrium), T2-weighted image (Figure 16e) and hepatobiliary phase image of EOB-MRI (Figure 16f) of a classic HCC in a 65-year-old male (same patient with shown as Figure 12, 14) are shown. This tumor is also typical imaging findings of HCC. Its internal structure is a typical mosaic appearance. When comparison the case shown as Figure 14, the fibrous capsule is unclear and the margin of the tumor is irregular. These findings are consistent with fibrous capsular invasion, and the macroscopic type of this tumor is classified as simple nodular type with extranodular growth or confluent multinodular type. The fibrous septa are visualized as slightly enhancing linear structures on equilibrium phase image of dynamic CT scan and stellate-shaped high signal intensity structures on T2-weighted image (arrows). As shown in Figure 15 or 16, EOB-MRI has a clear weakness to evaluate fibrous tissue as comparison with dynamic CT scan. On the maximum section of the fresh specimen (Figure 16g), thick fibrous septa is clearly seen as pink-colored structure penetrating the center of the tumor. The low magnification of HE stain (Figure 16h), the capsular invasions were clearly seen (arrowheads).

6.2. Mosaic Appearance and Nodule-in-Nodule Appearance

The majority of HCCs have heterogeneous inner structures and contain various histopathological subtypes in both sides of the fibrous septa. These mixed inner structures appear as "mosaic patterns" on CT scan or MRI [47]. This is a pathognomic finding of HCC (Figure 15, 16).

We sometimes encounter small hypervascular foci in the hepatic nodules that do not show arterial enhancement. This finding is called the "nodule-in-nodule appearance", and is considered for visualization of one step of the hepatocarcinogenesis [48] (Figure 17).

6.3. Fat Deposition

Fat deposition or steatotic change is frequently seen in HCCs [33]. It is most sensitively observed in T1-weighted in/opposed-phase imaging, but occasionally visualized in CT scan. In general, the steatotic components of HCCs are frequently pathologically well-differentiated HCCs [49] (Figure 10, 17). However, moderately or poorly-differentiated HCCs often have a well-differentiated component with fatty deposition. Therefore, HCCs with steatotic components do not always mean that the histopathological grades of such HCC are well differentiated [50] (Figure 18).

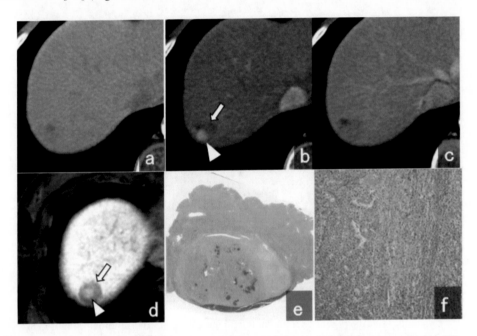

Figure 17. Dynamic CT scan (Figure 17a: precontrast, Figure 17b: arterial-dominant, Figure 17c: equilibrium) and hepatobiliary phase image of EOB-MRI (Figure 17d) of a HCC showing typical nodule-in-nodular appearance in a 65-year-old female is shown. The tumor consists of two different components; the peripheral component which shows fatty deposition and does not show overt arterial enhancement (arrow), and the central component showing arterial enhancement. The hepatobiliary phase image of EOB-MRI also clearly depicts this characteristic structure. This characteristic structure is clearly seen on pathologic specimen (Figure 17e: macroscopic view of HE stain, Fig 17f: low magnification of HE stain). The periphery of the tumor consists of well-differentiated HCC cells with lipid-rich bright cytoplasm (right side of Figure 17f). On the other hand, the center of the tumor shows more prominent hematoxylin stainability and consists of moderately-differentiated HCC cells (left side of Figure 17f).

6.4. Corona Enhancement

HCCs do not have their own draining veins; therefore, the contrast medium pouring in from the hepatic arteries directly excretes into the surrounding hepatic parenchyma and results in corona enhancement [51, 52]. Corona enhancement, named after the corona observed during a solar eclipse, is similar, at a glance, to the visualization of the fibrous capsule but is wider than the fibrous capsule. It is frequently observed on the delayed phase of CTHA, and occasionally depicted in usual dynamic CT/MRI (Figure 1, 4). Corona enhancement was first thought to be a pathognomic finding of HCC; however, it is now regarded as a non-specific finding sometimes observed in various hypervascular hepatic tumors such as focal nodular hyperplasias or perivascular endothelial cell tumors [53, 54]. Repeat multiple scans during the arterial phase with use of MDCT enable the depiction of corona enhancement. However, corona enhancement itself is not an indispensable finding to diagnose HCC when there are various troublesome problems such as increase in radiation exposure or storage of massive imaging data.

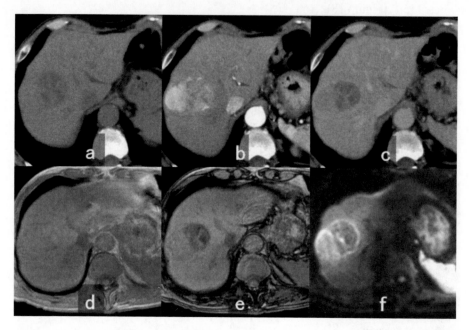

Figure 18. Dynamic CT scan (Figure 18a: precontrast, Figure 18b: arterial-dominant, Figure 18c: equilibrium) and T1-weighted in/opposed phase images (Figure 18d: in-phase, Figure 18e: opposed-phase) and DWI (Figure 18f) of a confluent-multinodular-type HCC of a 65-year-old male is shown. This tumor consists of completely different pathological components. The inner component shows obvious fat-deposition, weak arterial enhancement and is isointense to the surrounding hepatic parenchyma on diffusion weighted image. On the other hand, the outer component does not show fatty deposition, enhances strongly on arterial dominant phase image, and shows hyperintensely on diffusion weighted image. This HCC was treated by transcatheter chemoembolization without pathological examination; therefore, pathological confirmation was not obtained. However, we can easily conjecture that the outer component is more malignant than the inner component and the prognosis of this patient will be determined by the outer component. In this way, the fatty deposition in HCC does not directly mean that the tumor is well-differentiated.

7. Macroscopic Types of HCC

Pathologically, HCCs are classified into five macroscopic types: (i) a small nodular type with indistinct margin, (ii) a simple nodular type, (iii) a simple nodular type with extranodular growth, (iv) a confluent multinodular type, and (v) an infiltrative type [55]. The small nodular type with indistinct margin is a tumor corresponding to early HCC. Types (ii) to (v) correspond to classic HCCs; however, the margin of each tumor becomes unclear as extra-capsular invasion becomes more significant from type (ii) to type (v) (Figure 19).

Eggel's classification can be used for tumors that cannot be classified into the above five types, i.e., nodular type, massive type and diffuse type. This classification is usually indicated for advanced large HCCs [55].

Macroscopic classification of HCCs is undertaken before surgical resection from the imaging findings and after surgical resection from the pathological investigation. However, the preoperative macroscopic classification frequently does not match the final pathological diagnosis. In reality, the preoperatively diagnosed macroscopic type is not of major relevance for decision-making in the treatment strategy. The vascular invasion described in the next section is far more important for deciding the treatment strategy for each HCC patient.

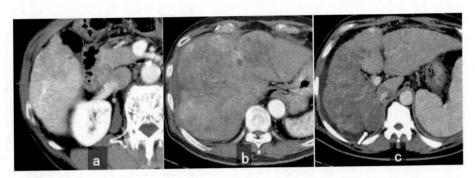

Figure 19. Various macroscopic types of HCCs are shown. HCC shown on Figure 19a is a confluent multinodular type. The large mass replacing whole of the right lobe and medial segment and invading the lateral segment shown in Figure 19b is a massive type of Eggel's classification. The tumor shown in Figure 19c is considered to be an infiltrative type or a diffuse type of Eggel's classification. In the tumor shown on Figure 19c, pathological confirmation is not obtained; therefore, the correct macroscopic type is not obtained. Please pay attention that this tumor directly invades the right adrenal gland (arrow).

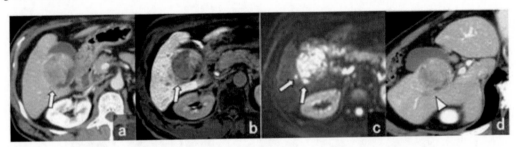

Figure 20. Portal-dominant phase image of dynamic CT scan (Figure 20a), hepatobiliary phase of EOB-MRI (Figure 20b) and DWI (Figure 20c) of the same case presented as Figure 7 and 15 are shown again. The presented slice level in Figure 20 is 1cm below the slice level shown in Figure 15. In this slice level, the tumor looks like showing extracapsular invasion at a glance (arrows); however, the MPR image reconstructed along the posterior branch of the portal vein (Figure 20d) reveals that this findings mimicking extracapsular invasion is a portal venous tumor thrombus (arrowhead). As shown in Figure 7, 15 and 20, both EOB-MRI and MPR-capable dynamic CT scan are indispensable to determine the clinical stage of HCC.

8. Assessment of Vascular Invasion of HCC by Using Multi-Planar Reconstruction of MDCT

The T-category of each HCC patient should be determined on the basis of the number, size, and vascular and/or bile duct invasion [55]. Among these, information about number and size is more precisely provided by EOB-MRI than by dynamic CT scan. On the other hand, vascular and/or biliary duct invasion should not be evaluated in EOB-MRI because the vascular enhancement effect in EOB-MRI decreases rapidly. Multi-planar reconstruction

(MPR) of the portal-dominant phase obtained with MDCT is currently the best modality to evaluate vascular and/or biliary duct invasion of HCC. The source images obtained by MDCT have the same resolution in any orthogonal direction; therefore, MPR images have the same quality as the source images. Proper MPR images obtained from the portal-dominant phase clearly indicate the relationship between the tumors and the vascular structures of the liver (Figure 20).

9. Poorly-Differentiated HCC and Special Types

The majority of classic HCCs are well to moderately differentiated, and their imaging findings are not so varied. On the other hand, the imaging findings of poorly-differentiated HCCs are sometimes atypical and versatile. In general, poorly-differentiated HCCs show more non-homogeneous and/or weaker enhancement effect in the arterial-dominant phase [56]. Poorly-differentiated HCCs far more frequently metastasize to distant organs than well to moderately-differentiated HCCs do (Figure 21). Consequently, liver transplantations are not indicated for patients with poorly-differentiated HCCs when based on the Milan criteria [57, 58]. Additionally, we should add some other imaging examinations such as chest CT or FDG-PET CT that are not routinely indicated for HCC patients when we decide the treatment strategy.

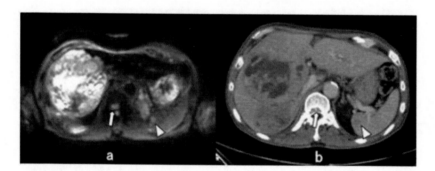

Figure 21. DWI (a) and portal-dominant phase of dynamic CT scan (b) of a massive type poorly-differentiated HCC involving the whole of the right lobe in a 61-year-old male are shown. On diffusion weighted image, metastases in the vertebra (arrow) and the spleen (arrowhead) were clearly depicted. These metastatic lesions can be also pointed out on CT image when we know the MRI findings before the interpretation of CT scan. Please notice that distant metastases are more frequently found in poorly-differentiated HCCs than in well- to moderately-differentiated HCCs.

There are some special types of HCCs. They are rare but often show characteristic imaging findings. If we know the details of their imaging characteristics, we may diagnose them precisely before operation or needle biopsy. In the next part of this section, we list these special types of HCCs and explain their imaging and clinical characteristics.

9.1. Fibrolamellar HCC and Scirrhous HCC

Both fibrolamellar and scirrhous HCCs show similar imaging findings. They are far richer in connective tissue than classic HCCs especially in the center of the tumors, and they usually lack fibrous capsules. Accordingly, they often show delayed enhancement in the central fibrosis in the adjacent liver surfaces. The imaging findings of these two entities are similar; while, the clinical manifestations are completely different. Fibrolamellar HCC occurs in white, young, and non-cirrhotic patients [59]. They are very rare in Asian people including Japanese. Scirrhous HCC had been thought to be a subtype of classic HCCs, and its radiological findings are similar to fibrolamellar HCCs [60]. However, it usually occurs in aged cirrhotic patients, and is sometimes found in Japanese individuals (Figure 22).

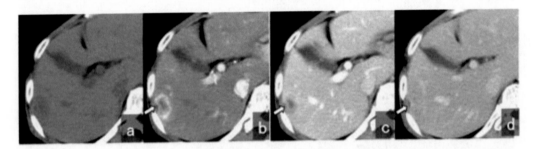

Figure 22. Dynamic CT scan of a hepatic nodule in a 70-year-old cirrhotic male is shown (Fig 22a: precontrast, Fig. 22b: arterial-dominant, Fig. 22c: equilibrium). The ill-demarcated nodule located in the surface of the liver accompanied a dimple in the adjacent hepatic surface (arrow). On arterial-dominant phase image, the nodule showed predominant contrast uptake in its rim and the center of the nodule showed gradual enhancement. There was no fibrous capsule around the tumor. According to these findings, a scirrhous HCC was suspected preoperatively. The pathological examination was performed on the surgically resected specimen. The tumor was a moderately differentiated HCC with rich fibrous connective tissue. However, the proportion of the fibrous connective tissue did not come up to 50% of the tumor. Therefore, pathologists decided that this tumor could not be called a scirrhous HCC, but the imaging findings of this tumor were consistent with a scirrhous HCC.

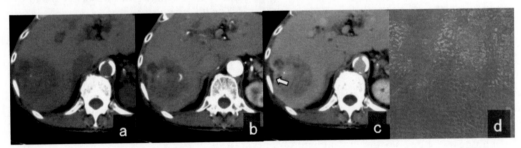

Figure 23. Dynamic CT scan of a hepatic nodule in a 78-year-old cirrhotic male is shown (Figure 23a: precontrast, Figure 23b: arterial-dominant, Figure 23c: equilibrium). The tumor showed poor arterial enhancement and gradual contrast uptake. No fibrous capsule could be pointed out. A dimple which was consistent with a cancer navel was noted in the adjacent hepatic surface (arrow). Surgical excision was performed and the low magnification of HE stain (Figure 23 d) revealed that the tumor was consisted of two distinct components of cholangiocarcinoma (The upper part of Figure 23d) and hepatocellular carcinoma (The lower part of the Figure 23d). According to these pathological characteristics, this tumor was finally diagnosed as a combined type HCC-CC; however, it was difficult to differentiate these components on dynamic CT scan. The imaging findings of this tumor are similar to those of the case shown in Figure 22.

9.2. Combined/Mixed Hepatocellular and Cholangiocarcinoma (HCC-CC)

Sometimes, both hepatocellular carcinoma and cholangiocarcinoma are found in one hepatic tumor. They are called combined or mixed hepatocellular and cholangiocarcinomas (HCC-CC). In "combined" HCC-CC, the parts of HCC and cholangiocarcinoma can be roughly divided pathologically [61]. In "mixed" HCC-CC, both cancer cells are completely mixed, and both cancerous tissues do not show overt regional distribution [62]. In typical cases, their imaging findings well reflect these pathological characteristics. In combined HCC-CC, the HCC portion shows arterial enhancement and delayed washout, and the cholangiocarcinoma portion shows delayed enhancement. Mixed type HCC-CC often show similar findings to those for cholangiocarcinoma (Figure 23). In these tumors, several tumor markers resembling both cancers are often elevated.

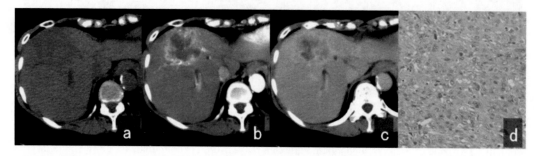

Figure 24. A 60-year-old cirrhotic female who had past history of radio-frequency ablation to a classic HCC complained upper abdominal discomfort and came to our institute. Recurrence of HCC was strongly suspected because AFP and PIVKA-II were high; however, dynamic CT scan (Figure 24a: precontrast, Figure 24b: arterial-dominant, Figure 24c: equilibrium) showed a strange mass in the anterior segment. The margin of the tumor is ill-defined. The tumor showed strong ring enhancement on arterial-dominant phase image and the center of the tumor was supposed to be a necrotic component. The pathological examination to the surgically resected specimen was undergone. The high magnification of HE stain (Figure 24d) revealed that the tumor consisted of spindle cells which were quite different from the cancer cells obtained from the primary HCC before radio-frequency ablation. These clinical course and the findings were typical for HCC with sarcomatoid change.

9.3. Sarcomatoid HCC or HCC with Sarcomatoid Changes

The word "sarcomatoid" means that the tumor includes spindle cells which are dedifferentiated HCC cells. Sarcomatoid HCC is the primary tumor and consists of both HCC and spindle cells. It usually has large necrotic components and is often misdiagnosed as a liver abscess because it often accompanies pyrexia [63].

HCC with sarcomatoid changes is usually found as the recurrence of treated HCC. Preceding treatments such as transcatheter chemoembolization, or local ablation or radiotherapy, are assumed to impair the genes and induce the dedifferentiation of HCC cells to spindle cells [64] (Figure 24). Both tumors are highly malignant and rapidly metastasize to distant organs.

10. Hypovascular HCCs only Visualized in Hepato-Biliary Phase of EOB-MRI

Before the development of EOB-MRI, we often encountered hepatic nodules that did not show overt arterial enhancement and became to show relatively low density/intensity on the equilibrium phase of dynamic CT/MRI in cirrhotic livers [3, 20]. We assumed that they were DNs that did not need to be treated at the time. This diagnostic logic was considered to be appropriate at the time and might not have a bad effect on the prognosis of HCC patients.

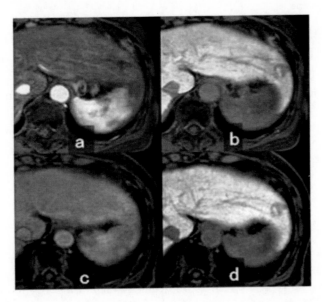

Figure 25. A 64-year-old cirrhotic female who suspected HCC in the lateral segment was examined by EOB-MRI. The tumor did not show overt contrast uptake on arterial-dominant phase image (Figure 25a) and was clearly observed as a well-demarcated nodule on hepatobiliary phase image (Figure 25b). These findings suggested an early HCC and it measured 18 mm in diameter. According to the recent reports, it should be diagnosed as an early HCC having high risk of hypervascularization; however, this lesion was not treated because of poor hepatic function of the patient. The follow-up EOB-MRI (Figure 25c: arterial-dominant, Figure 25d: hepatobiliary) undergone two years later revealed that this hepatic lesion did show overt volume increase or advent of arterial blood supply. In so far as this case, the strategy of no-treatment decided two years ago was considered to be proper for this patient.

Sano et al. reported that the relatively low density/intensity nodules on the equilibrium phase of dynamic CT/MRI could be divided into two groups on hepatobiliary phase images of EOB-MRI [29]. The nodules that were hardly noticeable in dynamic CT or other sequences of MRI but clearly depicted as well-demarcated hypointense nodules in the hepatobiliary phase, were frequently diagnosed as early HCCs in pathological examination. Pathological examination also revealed that in the majority of these nodules, monoclonal hepatic cells with slight cellular atypia invades the Glisson sheath. These characteristics are consistent with early HCCs. On the other hand, they reported that pathologically proven DNs were observed as isointense to hyperintense nodules in the hepatobiliary phase. According to these results, some radiologists have regarded that the hepatobiliary phase of EOB-MRI succeeds in detecting the most important step of hepatocarcinogenesis, which had previously only been visualized by using invasive CTAP/CTHA. However, it is not certain whether the above early

HCCs depicted only in the hepatobiliary phase should be treated positively. Early HCCs do not have metastasizing ability, and probably have hepatic functions. Surgical resections or ablation therapies to these lesions may worsen the hepatic functions, and may not contribute to the prolongation of the prognoses of cirrhotic patients (Figure 25). On the other hand, we cannot neglect early HCCs completely, because some authors have reported that early HCCs measuring more than 10 mm in diameter have high risk of hypervascularization [65]. At the present time, we do not have established concepts for this problem. We are looking forward to future research results regarding this issue.

11. Hepatic Nodular Lesions that Should Be Differentiated from HCCs

Many hepatic lesions that show similar imaging findings to HCCs, and all of them need to be differentiated from HCCs by using imaging modalities. Actually, we can hardly distinguish all of them from HCCs only with imaging modalities. We should take various pieces of clinical information into consideration when we try to diagnose them. We will list representative lesions in the next part of this section.

11.1. Arterioportal Shunts

Arterioportal (AP) shunts are the most frequent lesions that mimic HCC. They are essential conditions in cirrhotic hepatic parenchyma by nature and, moreover, are often induced by treatments for HCCs such as transcatheter chemoembolization or radiofrequency ablation. They are usually seen as well-enhanced, ill-demarcated nodular lesions only on the arterial-dominant phase of dynamic CT/MRI. Occasionally, they are depicted on T2-weighted images as hyperintense lesions because of secondary edema. On hepatobiliary phase images of EOB-MRI, they are usually observed as normal hepatic parenchyma. AP shunts often appear wedge-shaped or polygonal-shaped in either direction of the MPR images of the arterial-dominant phase of dynamic CT [66] (Figure 26).

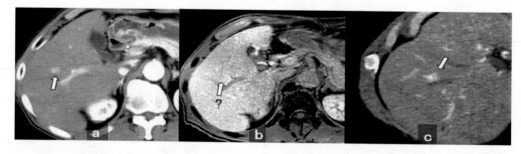

Figure 26. A 77-year-old cirrhotic male was examined by dynamic CT scan for screening of HCC. On arterial dominant-phase image (Figure 26a), an enhancing nodule was depicted in the anterior segment; however it could not be pointed out in other phase of dynamic CT scan and even on hepatobiliary phase image of EOB-MRI (Figure 26b). On the MPR image generated from arterial dominant phase images of dynamic CT scan (Figure 26c), the lesion is not oval but polygonal. These findings were consistent with an arterio-portal shunt.

11.2. Localized Fatty Liver and Adrenal Rest Tumors

The majority of localized fatty livers are segmental and are easily distinguished from steatotic HCCs. However, in some patients, especially in patients with alcoholic liver impairment, we sometimes encounter localized fatty liver that is difficult to differentiate from steatotic HCCs. It usually rapidly disappears after abstinence and hepatic alleviation. Therefore, invasive diagnostic methods such as needle biopsy need not to be hurried.

Adrenal rest tumor is a rare tumor-like hamartomatous lesion that derives from the adrenal tissue remnant in the liver. It always arises in the posterior segment of the liver, facing to the right adrenal gland. It is usually observed as a fat-containing mass, and its radiological findings are similar to steatotic HCC. The location of the lesion and the presence or absence of cirrhosis are important to diagnose adrenal rest tumor [67] (Figure 27).

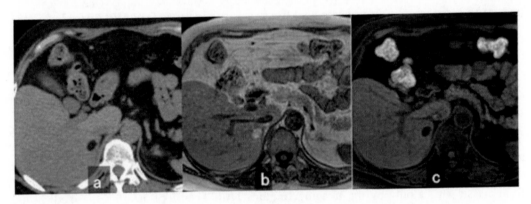

Figure 27. A 63-year-old non-cirrhotic female was examined the upper abdomen by using CT (Figure 27a: precontrast) and MRI (Figure 27b: T1WI, Figure 27c: fat suppressed T1WI) to screen adrenal gland abnormality. A fatty nodule is visualized in the posterior segment. The CT number of the lesion was under zero on precontrast CT image, showed clear high signal on T1-weighted image and its signal intensity turned dark by simultaneous use of fat suppression technique. According to these imaging findings and the location of the lesion, we diagnosed this lesion as an adrenal rest tumor.

11.3. Hyperplastic Nodules

It is well known that various hyperplastic nodules such as focal nodular hyperplasia (FNH), nodular reactive hyperplasia (NRH) and partial nodular transformation (PNT) occur in the liver [68]. Among them, FNH and FNH-like lesions are most frequently found in the clinical setting. They show strong contrast uptake in the arterial-dominant phase and rapid washout in the portal-dominant or equilibrium phase. Therefore, they are often misdiagnosed as classic HCCs. We can differentiate these entities from HCCs on the grounds of some clinical characteristics such as abnormal vessels penetrating the center of the lesions, obstruction or congenital hypoplasia of the portal veins, or history of chemotherapy. Some recent reports mentioned that FNHs and FNH-like lesions often show characteristic ring enhancement in the hepatobiliary phase of EOB-MRI. This imaging finding also assists the differentiation of FNHs or FNH-like lesions from HCCs [69] (Figure 28).

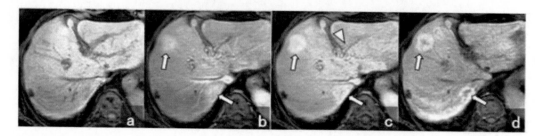

Figure 28. Multiple hepatic nodules in a 78-year-old female were examined by EOB-MRI (Figure 28a: precontrast, Fig, 28b: arterial-dominant, Fig, 28c: portal-dominant, Fig, 28d: hepatobiliary). In this patient, congenital hypoplasia of the portal vein (arrowhead) and dilatation of the hepatic artery were also pointed out. Each hepatic nodules showed slight arterial enhancement on arterial dominant phase image and gradually increasing contrast uptake on portal dominant phase image and demonstrated characteristic ring enhancement on hepatobiliary phase image (arrows). According to these imaging findings, these lesions were diagnosed as FNH like lesions. However, the EOB-MRI findings of FNH or FNH like lesion are various. The findings shown in Figure 28 are not the only characteristic findings for FNH or FNH-like lesions.

11.4. Hepatocellular Adenomas

In the clinical setting, hepatocellular adenomas are usually found in young women who have a history of oral contraceptive use. Glycogen storage disease and anabolic steroid use are also risk factors for this tumor. Hepatocellular adenoma shows arterial enhancement and delayed washout. It usually has fibrotic capsules. Therefore, it can hardly be differentiated from classic HCCs only by the imaging findings [70]. Therefore, hearing the medical and medication histories is exceedingly important to diagnose this tumor (Figure 29). Hepatocellular adenoma is benign but sometimes accompanies intratumoral hemorrhage or rupture. Such cases are considered to be an indication for surgical resection or emergent transcatheter arterial embolization.

11.5. Hypervascular Hepatic Metastases

Various extra-hepatic malignancies make HCC-like hypervascular metastases in the liver. Neuroendocrine tumors such as islet cell tumors or carcinoid tumors are typical. When we find HCC-like hypervascular liver tumors in non-cirrhotic patients, we should consider the possibility of hepatic metastases due to extra-hepatic malignancies (Fig. 30).

11.6. Perivascular Endothelial Cell Tumor (PEComa)

Perivascular endothelial cell tumor (PEComa) is a rare tumor that is considered to be a family of mesenchymal tumors typified by angiomyolipoma [71]. This tumor consists of a fat, vascular structure and smooth muscle in various ratios. When the fat ratio is very low, the imaging finding of this tumor is very similar to classic HCC: strong arterial enhancement and delayed washout. Differently from HCC, PEComa twice as frequently occurs in women and does not have a fibrous capsule. When we see a hypervascular tumor without a fibrous capsule in a non-cirrhotic female patient, we should consider this tumor as a differential diagnosis (Figure 31).

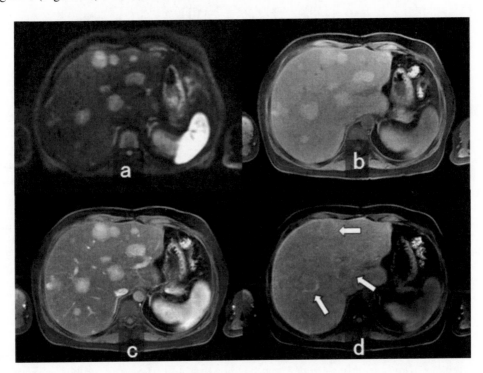

Figure 29. A 23-year-old female having glycogen storage disease type 1a was suspected multiple hepatic nodules. DWI (Figure 29a) and EOB-MRI (Figure 29b: precontrast, Figure 29c: arterial-dominant, Figure 29d: hepatobiliary) revealed multiple hypervascular tumors in the liver. Each tumor was hyperintense on diffusion weighted image. With knowing the past history of this patient, it was easy to diagnose these tumors as hepatocellular adenomas. However, the imaging findings were basically similar to HCCs. Please pay attention that characteristic ring-like enhancement was observed around the tumors on hepatobiliary phase image (arrow).

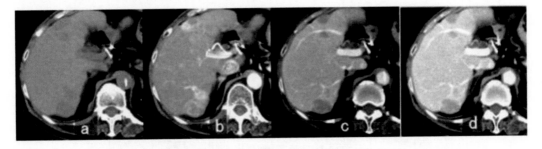

Figure 30. Dynamic CT scan (Figure 30a: precontrast, Figure 30b: arterial-dominant, Figure 30c: portal-dominant, Figure 30d: equilibrium) of multiple hepatic metastases due to neuroendocrine tumor of the rectum in a 78-year-old non-cirrhotic female are shown. Each metastatic tumor showed arterial enhancement on arterial-dominant phase image and rapid washout on portal-dominant phase and equilibrium phase images. This enhancement pattern is characteristic in HCC but not pathognomonic for HCC. All hepatic tumors having similar pathological characteristics (hypervascular and hypercellular) may show the similar findings to HCCs.

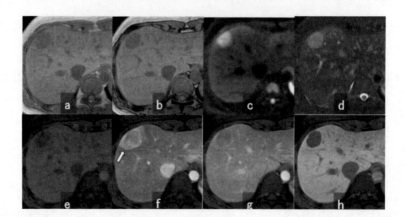

Figure 31. A 35-year-old non-cirrhotic female was suspected a hepatic tumor and examined by MRI including T1-weighted in/opposed phase imaging (Figure 31a: in-phase, Figure 31b: opposed-phase), DWI (Figure 31c), T2WI (Figure 31d) and EOB-MRI (Figure 31e: precontrast, Figure 31f: arterial-dominant, Figure 31g: portal-dominant, Figure 31h: hepatobiliary). The patient did not have any history of hepatitis or administration of pills. MRI findings were very similar to HCC except for no visual-ization of fibrous capsule. Needle biopsy was undergone and a pathological examination revealed that this lesion was a perivascular endothelial cell tumor (PEComa). Please notice that corona enhancement was observed on arterial dominant-phase image (arrow).

11.7. Cholangiolocellular Carcinoma (CoCC)

Cholangiolocellular carcinoma (CoCC) is a rare malignant neoplasm of the liver thought to be derived from a hepatic stem cell that has potential to differentiate to both hepatic cells and bile duct epithelial cells. Reflecting these pathological characteristics, the imaging findings of this tumor are a mixture of the findings of HCC and intrahepatic cholangiocarcinoma. It shows both arterial and persistent enhancement and does not have a fibrous capsule or necrosis (Figure 32). Asayama et al. reported that the Glisson sheath penetrating the tumor is the pathognomic finding of this tumor; however, this finding is not always seen [72].

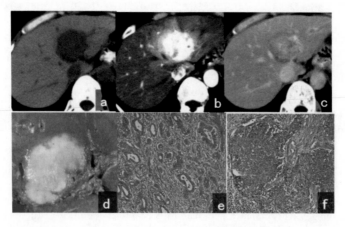

Figure 32. A 63-year-old non-cirrhotic female was suspected a hepatic tumor and examined by dynamic CT scan (Figure 32a: precontrast, Figure 32b: arterial-dominant, Figure 32c: equilibrium). Blood sample test revealed that no tumor markers were elevated in this patient. The tumor in the lateral segment showed marked contrast uptake on arterial-dominant phase image and persistent enhancement

on equilibrium phase image. No fibrous capsule could be pointed out. Surgical resection was undergone. The pathological examination revealed that this lesion was lobulated, had an irregular margin and did not have fibrous capsule at all on the maximum section of the fresh pathological specimen (Figure 32d). The pathological examination revealed that the majority of the tumor consisted of moderately differentiated adenocarcinoma forming ductal structure (Figure 32e). However, some part of the tumor was poorly differentiated carcinoma showing solid pattern resembling HCC (Figure 32f). According to the pathological characteristics, this tumor was finally diagnosed as a cholangiolocellular carcinoma.

Column 4. Classic HCCs Accumulating Gd-EOB-DTPA in Hepatobiliary Phase

Right after the introduction of Gd-EOB-DTPA to the clinical setting, it has been a well-known fact that some classic HCCs accumulate Gd-EOB-DTPA in the hepatobiliary phase (Figure 33). Especially, some authors reported that HCCs in which organ anion transporting polypeptide (OATP) 1B3 are expressed on the surface of cancer cells frequently accumulate Gd-EOB-DTPA in the hepatobiliary phase. However, we should understand that OATP1B3 is a non-specific transporter that is commonly expressed in various malignancies such as breast, gastric and colon cancers, and the uptake of Gd-EOB-DTPA in a hepatic tumor does not directly mean that the tumor is derived from hepatocytes. Actually, some authors have reported that hepatic metastases due to breast cancer or intrahepatic cholangiocarcinoma accumulate Gd-EOB-DTPA in the hepatobiliary phase [73, 74] (Figure 34).

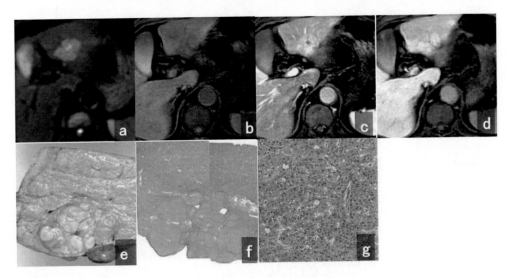

Figure 33. A 67-year-old cirrhotic male was pointed out multiple hepatic tumors and examined by DWI (Figure 33a) and EOB-MRI (Figure 33b: precontrast, Figure 33c: arterial-dominant, Figure 33d: hepatobiliary). Blood sample test revealed elevation of AFP and PIVKA-II. The tumor in the lateral segment showed high signal intensity on diffusion weighted image and arterial enhancement on arterial-dominant phase image. These findings were consistent with a moderately differentiated HCC; however, it became almost isointense to the surrounding hepatic parenchyma on hepatobiliary phase image. The maximum section of undyed surgical specimen revealed that this tumor was slightly green-colored (Figure 33e); however, the low magnification (Figure 33f) and high magnification (Figure 33g) of HE stain revealed that this tumor is an ordinary moderately differentiated HCC and pseudo-glandular components were not prominent. Please notice that the EOB uptake on hepatobiliary phase does not directly mean that the tumor is dominant with pseudo-glandular component.

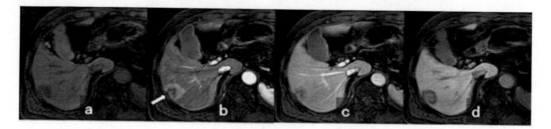

Figure 34. A 71-year-old cirrhotic male was pointed out a hepatic tumor in the posterior segment and examined by EOB-MRI (a: precontrast, b: arterial-dominant, c: portal-dominant, d: hepatobiliary). Blood sample test revealed slight elevation of CEA but AFP and PIVKA-II were within normal limits. There was a dimple in the hepatic surface adjacent to the tumor (arrow). The tumor showed ring enhancement on arterial dominant phase image and gradual contrast uptake on portal dominant phase. Additionally, the center of the tumor showed stronger contrast uptake in hepatobiliary phase image than that in portal dominant phase image. Surgical resection was undergone and the pathological examination revealed that this lesion was an intrahepatic cholangiocarcinoma. Please pay attention that EOB uptake into tumors does not directly mean that the tumor is derived from hepatic cells.

Column 5. Correlation between Gd-EOB-DTPA Uptake into the Hepatic Parenchyma and Hepatic Function

The uptake of Gd-EOB-DTPA into the hepatic parenchyma differs for each patient. Now, many abdominal radiologists assume that the EOB-uptake into the hepatic parenchyma is almost the same as that of indocyanine green (ICG), and quantitative analysis of the hepatic parenchymal enhancement effect in the hepatobiliary phase of EOB-MRI can replace the ICG test when we need to know the hepatic function [75].

On the other hand, the above facts lead to another important assumption: if the hepatic enhancement effect in hepatobiliary phase of EOB-MRI is decreased in patients with poor hepatic function, the detectability for HCCs in such patients may be lower than that in patients with good hepatic function. We have to more carefully evaluate EOB-MRIs of patients showing high ICG-R15 values than those of patients whose ICG-R15 values are within normal limits. Of course, EOB-uptake into hepatic tumors should be evaluated while considering the hepatic parenchymal enhancement effect (30).

Conclusion

Diagnostic imaging for HCC by using CT and MRI has made great strides in the last 20 years. In particular, various problems regarding the diagnosis of classic HCCs have already been roughly resolved. From now on, diagnostic advances for poorly-differentiated HCCs, atypical HCCs, and early HCCs are expected.

The technical developments of CT and MRI are still continuing. Space does not permit to discuss some novel developments of these entities here because there are too many newly developed techniques in these modalities. However, some of them are already being used in the clinical setting and their usefulness has begun to be reported. It may not be a fantasy that CT and MRI will resolve the remaining problems regarding the diagnosing HCC in near future.

Acknowledgment

While writing this chapter, the authors were financially assisted from the health and labor science research grants of the third term comprehensive research for cancer.

References

[1] Llovet JM, Bustamante J, Castells A, et al. Natural history of untreated nonsurgical hepatocellular carcinoma: rationale for the design and evaluation of therapeutic trials. *Hepatology* 1999; 29:62–67.

[2] Cancer statistics in Japan-2013. *Foundation of promotion of cancer research,* http://ganjoho.jp/professional/statistics/backnumber/2013_jp.html.

[3] Kojiro M. Focus on dysplastic nodules and early hepatocellular carcinoma: an eastern point of view. *Liver Transplantation* 2004; 10: pp S3–S8.

[4] International Working Party. Terminology of nodular hepatocellular lesions. *Hepatology* 1995; 22: 983–993.

[5] Wada K, Kondo Y, Kondo F. Large regenerative nodules and dysplastic nodules in cirrhotic livers: A histopathologic study. *Hepatology* 1988; 8;1684-1688..

[6] Kojiro M, Roskams T. Early hepatocellular carcinoma and dysplastic nodules. *Semin Liver Dis* 2005; 25: 133–142.

[7] Hayashi M, Matsui O, Ueda K, et al. Correlation between the blood supply and grade of malignancy of hepatocellular nodules associated with liver cirrhosis: evaluation by CT during intraarterial injection of contrast medium. *AJR* 1999; 172:969–976.

[8] Ueda K, Terada T, Nakanuma Y, Matsui O. Vascular supply in adenomatous hyperplasia of the liver and hepatocellular carcinoma: a morphometric study. *Hum Pathol* 1992; 23:619–626.

[9] Hayashi M, Matui O, Ueda K et al. Progression to hypervascular hepatocellular carcinoma: correlation with intranodular blood supply evaluated with CT during intraarterial injection of contrast material. *Radioloy* 2002; 225:143–149.

[10] Nascimento C, Bottino A, Nogueira C, Pannain V. Analysis of morphological variables and arterialization in the differential diagnosis of hepatic nodules in explanted cirrhotic livers. *Diagnostic Pathology* 2007; 2: 51.

[11] Yao DF, Jiang H, Yao M et al. Quantitative analysis of hepatic hypoxia-inducible factor-1alfa and its abnormal gene expression during the formation of hepatocellular carcinoma. *Hepatobiliary Pancreat Dis Int* 2009; 3: 407-413.

[12] Torimura T, Sato M, Ueno T et al. Increased expression of vascular endothelial growth factor is associated tumor progression in hepatocellular carcinoma. *Hum Pathol* 1998; 29: 986-91.

[13] Matsui O, Kadoya M, Suzuki M et al. Dynamic sequential computed tomography during arterial portography in the detection of hepatic neoplasms. *Radiology* 1983; 146: 721-727.

[14] Taguchi T, Asayama Y, Aishima S et al. Morphologic approach to hepatocellular carcinoma development in man: de novo or the so-called 'dysplastic nodule-carcinoma' sequence? *Oncol Rep* 2002; 9: 737-743.

[15] Foley WD, Berland LL, Lawson TL, Smith DF, Thorsen MK. Contrast enhancement technique for dynamic computed tomography scanning. *Radiology* 1983; 147: 797-803.

[16] Laionde L, Van Beers B, Jamart J, Prinqot J. Capsule and mosaic pattern of hepatocellular carcinoma: correlation between CT and MR imaging. *Gastrointest Radiol* 1992; 17: 241-244.

[17] Lim JH, Kim MJ, Park CK, Kang SS, Lim HK et al. Dysplastic nodules in liver cirrhosis: detection with triple phase helical dynamic CT. *Br J Radiol* 2004; 77: 911-916.

[18] Kim YK, Kim CS, Chung GH et al. Comparison of gadobenate dimeglumine-enhanced dynamic MRI and 16-MDCT for detection of hepatocellular carcinoma. *AJR* 2006; 186:149–157.

[19] Onishi H, Kin T, Imai Y et al. Hypervascular hepatocellular carcinoma: detection with gadoxetate disodium-enhanced MR imaging and multiphase multidetector CT. *Eur Radiol* 2012; 22: 845-854..

[20] Rhee H, Kim MJ, Park YN, Choi JS, Kim KS. Gadoxetic acid-enhanced MRI findings of early hepatocellular carcinoma as defined by new histologic criteria. *JMRI* 2012; 35: 393-398.

[21] Kudo M. Diagnostic imaging of hepatocellular carcinoma: recent progress. *Oncology* 2011; 81: 73-85.

[22] Goldstein EJ, Burnett KR, Hansell JR et al. Gadolinium DTPA (an NMR proton imaging contast agenet): chemical structure, paramagnetic properties and pharmatokinetis. *Physiol Chem Phys med NMR* 1984; 16: 97-104.

[23] Yamashita Y, Mitsuzaki K, Yi T et al. Small hepatocellular carcinoma in patient with chronic liver damage: prospective comparison of detection with dynamic MR imaging and helical CT of the whole liver. *Radiology* 1996; 200: 79-84.

[24] Semelka RC, Shoenut JP, Kroeker MA et al. Focal liver disease: comparison of dynamic contrast-enhanced CT and T2-weighted fat-suppressed, FLASH, and dynamic gadolinium-enhanced MR imaging at 1.5T. *Radiology* 1992; 184: 687-94.

[25] Chenevert TL, Helvie MA, Francis IR et al. Dynamic three-dimensional imaging with partial k-space sampling: initial application for gadolinium-enhanced characterization of breast lesions. *Radiology* 1995; 196: 135-142.

[26] Brasch RC, Weinmann HJ, Wesbey GE Contrast-enhanced NMR imaging: animal studies using gadolinium-DTPA complex. *AJR* 1984; 142: 625-630.

[27] Zech CJ, Herrmann KA, Reiser MF, Schoenberg SO. MR imaging in patients with suspected liver metastases: value of liver-specific contrast agent Gd-EOB-DTPA. *Magn Reson Med Sci.* 2007; 6:43-52..

[28] Weinmann HJ, Schuhmann-Giampieri G, Schmitt-Willich H, Vogler H, Frenzel T, Gries H. A new lipophilic gadolinium chelate as a tissue-specific contrast medium for MRI. *Magn Reson Med.* 1991;22:233-237.

[29] Sano K, Ichikawa T, MOtosugi T et al. Imaging study of early hepatocellular carcinoma: usefulness of gadoxetic acid-enhanced MR imaging. *Radiology* 2011; 261: 834-844.

[30] The Japan society of hepatology. *Guideline on liver cancer examination and treatment.* 2013. Kanehara and co. Ltd, Tokyo.

[31] Merkle EM, Rendon C, Nelson RC. Dual gradient-echo in-phase and opposed phase hepatic MR imaging: a useful tool for evaluating more than fatty infiltration or fatty sparing. *Radiographics* 2006; 26: 1409-1418.

[32] Grossholz M, Terrier F, Rubbia L, et al. Focal sparing in the fatty liver as a sign of an adjacent space-occupying lesion. *AJR* 1998;171: 1391–1395..

[33] Basaran C, Karcaaltincaba M, Akata D, et al. Fatcontaining lesions of the liver: cross-sectional imaging findings with emphasis on MRI. *AJR* 2005; 184: 1103–1110..

[34] Gandon Y, Olivie D, Guyader D et al. Non-invasive assessment of hepatic iron stores by MRI. *Lancet* 2004; 363: 357–362.

[35] Henninger B, Kremser C, Rauch S et al. Evaluation of liver fat in the presence of iron with MRI using T2* correction: a clinical approach. *Eur Radiol.* 2013; 23: 1643-1649.

[36] Albiin N. MRI of focal liver lesions. *Curr Med Imaging Rev.* 2012; 8: 107-116.

[37] Ebara M, Fukuda H, Morimoto N et al. Small hepatocellular carcinoma: relationship of signal intensity to histopathologic findings and metal content of the tumor and surrounding hepatic parenchyma. *Radiology* 1999; 210: 81-88.

[38] Bonekamp S, Corona-Villalobos CP, Kamel IR. Oncologic applications of diffusion-weighted MRI in the body. *JMRI* 2012; 35: 257-279.

[39] Nasu K, Kuroki Y, Tsukamoto T, Nakajima H, Mori K, Minami M. Diffusion-weighted imaging of surgically resected hepatocellular carcinoma: imaging characteristics and relationship among signal intensity, apparent diffusion coefficient and histopathological grade. *AJR* 2009; 193: 438-444.

[40] Nakanishi M, Chuma M, Hige S et al. Relationship between diffusion-weighted magnetic resonance imaging and histological tumor grading of hepatocellular carcinoma. *Ann Surg Oncol* 2012; 19: 1302-1309.

[41] Wu X, Wang H, Chen F et al. Rat model of reperfused partial liver infarction: characterization with multiparametric magnetic resonance imaging, microangiography and histopathology. *Acta Radiol.* 2009; 50: 276-87.

[42] Chiu FY, Jao JC, Chen CY et al. Effect of intraveneous gadolinium-DTPA on diffusion-weighted magnetic resonance images for evaluation of focal hepatic lesions. *JCAT* 2005; 29: 176-180.

[43] Nagasue N, Uchida M, Makino Y et al. Incidence and factors associated with intrahepatic recurrence following resection of hepatocellular carcinoma. *Gastroenterology* 1993; 105: 488-493.

[44] Kadoya M, Matsui O, Takashima T, Nonomura A. Hepatocellular carcinoma: correlation of MR imaging and histopathological findings. *Radiology* 183; 819-825.

[45] Lee S, Kim SH, Park CK, Kim YS, Lee WJ, Lim AK. Comparison between areas with Gd-EOB-DTPA uptake and without in hepatocellular carcinomas on Gd-EOB-DTPA-enhanced hepatobiliary-phase MR imaging: pathological correlation. *JMRI* 2010; 32: 719-725.

[46] Ishizaki M, Ashida K, Higashi T et al. The formation of capsule and septum in human hepatocellular carcinoma. *Virchow Arch.* 2001; 438: 574-58.

[47] Stevens WR, Gulino SP, Batts KP, Stephens DH, Johnson CD. Mosaic pattern of hepatocellular carcinoma: histologic basis for a characteristic CT appearance. *JCAT* 1996; 20: 337-342.

[48] Winter TC 3rd, Takayasu K, Muramatsu Y et al. Early advanced hepatocellular carcinoma: evaluation of CT and MR appearance with pathologic correlation. *Radiology* 1994; 192: 379-387.

[49] Sato M, Watanabe Y, Lee T. et al. well-differentiated hepatocellular carcinoma: clinicopathological features and results of hepatic resection. *Am J Gastroenterol.* 1995; 90: 112-116.

[50] Ishikawa E, Munetomo E. *Surgical pathology* 1999 Bunkodo co. LTD. Tokyo.

[51] Kitao A, Zen Y, Matsui O, Gabata T, Nakamura Y. Hepatocarcinogenesis: multistep changes of drainage vessels at CT during arterial portography and hepatic arteriography-radiologicpathologic correlation. *Radiology* 2009; 252: 605–614.

[52] Ueda K, Matsui O, Kawamori Y et al. Hypervascular hepatocellular carcinoma: evaluation of hemodynamics with dynamic CT during hepatic arteriography. *Radiology* 1998; 206: 161-166.

[53] Kita R, Nakatsuji M, Mishijima N et al. A case of focal nodular hyperplasia presenting corona enhancement on single-level dynamic CT during hepatic arteriography. *Nihon Shokaibyo Gakkai Zashi* 2008; 105: 550-557.

[54] Motoo I, Takahara T, Matsui K et al. Two cases of hepatic angiomyolipoma with difficulty for imaging differential diagnosis with hepatocellular carcinoma. *Kanzo* 2013; 54: 143-151.

[55] Liver cancer study group of Japan. *General rules for the clinical and pathological study of primary liver cancer.* 2010; Kanehara and Co. Ltd., Tokyo.

[56] Lee JH, Lee JM, Kin SJ et al. Enhancement patterns of hepatocellular carcinomas on multiphasic multidetector row CT: comparison with pathological differentiation. *BJR* 2012; 85: e576-583.

[57] Oishi K, Itamoto T, Amano H et al. Clinicopathological features of poorly differentiated hepatocellular carcinoma. *J Surg Oncol.* 2007; 15: 311-316.

[58] Mazzaferro V, Regalia E, Doci R et al. Liver transplantation for the treatment of small hepatocellular carcinomas in patients with cirrhosis. *N Engl J Med* 1996; 334: 693-699..

[59] Ichikawa T, Federle MP, Grazioli L, Madariaga J, Nakesnik M, Marsh W. Fibrolamellar hepatocellular carcinoma: imaging and pathological findings in 31 recent cases. *Radiology* 1999; 213: 352-361.

[60] Kim SH, Lim HK, Lee WJ, Choi D, Park CK. Scirrhous hepatocellular carcinoma: comparison with usual hepatocellular carcinoma based on CT-pathologic features and long-ter results after curative resection. *EJR* 2009; 69: 123-130.

[61] Fukukura Y, Taguchi J, Nakashima O, Wada Y, Kojiro M. Combined hepatocellular and cholangiocarcinoma: correlation between CT findings and clinicopathological features. *JCAT* 1997; 21: 52-58.

[62] Jarnagin WR, Weber S, Tickoo SK et al. Combined hepatocellular and cholangiocarcinoma, demographic, clinical, and pathological factors. *Cancer* 2002; 94: 2040-2046.

[63] Hayashi T, Honda H, Kaneko Y et al. Hepatocellular carcinoma with pyrexia: report of a case. *Radiat Med.* 1995; 13: 133-136.

[64] Koda M, Maeda Y, Matsunaga Y, Mimura K, Murawaki Y, Horie Y. Hepatocellular carcinoma with sarcomatoid change arising after radiofrequency ablation for well-differentiated hepatocellular carcinoma. *Hepatol Res.* 2003; 27: 163-167.

[65]   Takechi M, Tsuda T, Yoshioka S, et al. Risk of hypervascariztion in small hypovascular hepatic nodues showing hypointense on hepatobiliary phase of gadoxetic acid-enhanced MRI in patients with chronic liver disease. *JJR* 2012; 30: 734-751.

[66]   Choi BI, Lee KH, Han JK, Lee JM. Hepatic arterioportal shunts: dynamic CT and MR features. *KJR* 2002; 3: 1-15.

[67]   Prasad SR, Wang H, Rosas H et al. Fat-containing lesions of the liver: radiologic-pathologic correlation. *Radiographics* 2005; 25: 321-331.

[68]   Anderson SW, Kruskal JB, Kane RA. Benign hepatic tumors and iatragenic pseudotumors. *Radiographics* 2009; 29: 211-229.

[69]   Fujiwara H, Sekine S, Onaya H, Shimada K, Mikata R, Arai Y. Ring-like enhancement of focal nodular hyperplasia with hepatobiliary phase Gd-EOB-DTPA-enhanced magnetic resonance imaging: radiological-pathological correlation. *JJR* 2011; 29: 739-743.

[70]   Sakamoto A, Hayashi H, Sakamoto I et al. Multiple hepatocellular adenoma in a patient with glycogen storange disease type I: various enhancement pattern in MRI with Gd-EOB-DTPA. *Abdominal Imaging* 2012; 37: 239-243.

[71]   Tan Y, Xiao EH. Hepatic perivascular epithelioid cell tumor (PEComa): dynamic CT, MRI, ultrasonography, and pathologic features-analysis of 7 cases and review of the literature. *Abdominal Imaging* 2012; 37: 781-787.

[72]   Asayama Y, Tajima T, Okamoto D et al. Imaging of cholangiolocellular carcinoma of the liver. *EJR* 2010; 75: e120-125.

[73]   Ha S, Kee CH, Kim BH et al. Paradoxical uptake of Gd-EOB-DTPA on the hepatobiliary phase in the evaluation of hepatic metastasis from breast cancer: is the "target sign" a common finding? *Mang Reson Imaging* 2012; 30: 1083-190.

[74]   Kang Y, Lee JM, Kim SH, Han JK, Choi BI. Intrahepatic mass-forming cholangiocarcinoma. *Radiology* 2012; 264: 751-760.

[75]   Yamada A, Hara T, Li F et al. Quantitative evaluation of liver function with use of gadoxetate disodium-enhanced MR imaging. *Radiology* 2011; 260: 727-733.

In: Therapy for Hepatocellular Carcinoma
Editor: Nobuhiro Ohkohchi

ISBN: 978-1-63117-929-7
© 2014 Nova Science Publishers, Inc.

Chapter 3

Clinical Staging and Treatment Selection for Hepatocellular Carcinoma: Overview of the Current Status and Perspectives for the Future

Masato Abei, M.D., Ph.D. [*]

Division of Gastroenterology, Faculty of Medicine, University of Tsukuba
Tsukuba, Ibaraki-ken, Japan

Abstract

Hepatocellular carcinoma (HCC) is the most frequent primary liver tumor, and one of the most common malignancies. Owing to recent advances in surgical and other interventional techniques and development of molecular-targeted drugs, a number of treatment options, including surgical resection, liver transplantation, local ablation, transarterial chemoembolization, radiotherapy, and molecular-targeted therapy, are now available. Since HCC is usually associated with chronic liver disease, particularly cirrhosis, its treatment must take into account not only the stage of the tumor itself but also the stage of the underlying liver disease in order to preserve the liver function. A multidisciplinary approach is necessary with a cancer board including hepatologists, liver surgeons, radiologists, and pathologists involved in the choice of the most appropriate treatment for each case. For very early-stage HCC, hepatic resection is usually the first treatment of choice, but it is now being challenged by local ablative therapy, such as radiofrequency ablation (RFA). The relative efficacy and safety of hepatic resection versus RFA awaits the results of further randomized controlled trials (RCTs). For early-stage HCC that meets the Milan criteria, liver transplantation still offers the best long-term survival, since it removes both the tumor and the underlying liver disease to reduce the possibility of recurrence. However, because its application is limited by the scarcity of donor livers, local ablation can be a substitute when transplantation is not feasible. Innovative radiotherapies, such as proton beam therapy, have also recently emerged as alternatives to surgical resection, although performed in a limited number of facilities.

[*] E-mail: m-abei@md.tsukuba.ac.jp.

For intermediate stage HCC, transarterial chemoembolization (TACE) is generally the treatment of choice. For advanced stage HCC, a molecular-targeted drug, sorafenib, is generally recommended, and the role of hepatic infusion chemotherapy (HAIC) needs to be established by RCTs. As future perspectives, the efficacy of other molecular-targeted drugs as well as combination therapies with sorafenib are currently being evaluated. Since recurrence of HCC remains the major obstacle for long-term survival, novel approaches to prevent the recurrence are also being investigated. Furthermore, oncolytic virus-mediated immune-gene therapy has emerged as a novel cancer therapy with great hope for advanced HCC. This review aims to provide a comprehensive overview of the current treatment options and their proper selection based on the clinical stage of HCC. The clinical trials of some promising novel therapeutic approaches are also introduced.

Keywords: Hepatocellular carcinoma, Radiofrequency ablation, Transarterial chemo-embolization, Sorafenib, Hepatic arterial infusion chemotherapy

1. Introduction

Hepatocellular carcinoma (HCC) accounts for nearly 90% of primary liver tumors and is currently the fifth most common cancer and the third leading cause of cancer-related death worldwide [1-3]. A number of treatment options including surgical resection, liver transplantation, local ablation, chemoembolization, radiotherapy, and molecular-targeted therapy are now available for the treatment of HCC. Since HCC is usually associated with chronic liver disease, particularly cirrhosis, its treatment must take into account not only the stage of the tumor itself but also the stage of the underlying liver disease in order to preserve the liver function, which is often already impaired. Therefore, the choice of therapy is based mainly on the stage of HCC, the severity of the underlying liver disease, the availability of treatment resources, and clinical expertise [1-8]. The aim of this chapter is to provide an update which can be useful in clinical practice for determining the most appropriate treatment for individual HCC patients. Several promising novel therapeutic approaches to inhibit the recurrence of HCC or to treat advanced-stage HCC, the efficacy and safety of which are now being evaluated, are also introduced.

2. Clinical Staging and Treatment Guidelines for HCC

Once HCC is diagnosed, evaluation of the clinical stage is essential to assess the resectability of the tumor, predict the prognosis, and select the most appropriate treatment. The severity of chronic liver disease is usually classified by the Child-Pugh Score and the tumor is staged with the TNM system.

Table 1. Recent trials comparing the value of different clinical staging systems for HCC (reference 7)

Author	Year	Treatment	No. of cases	Staging systems	Methods	Systems in favor
Chen [9]	2007	Hepatectomy	382	Okuda, AJCC, CLIP, BCLC, JIS, CUPI, MELD	Retrospective	CLIP: for staging major hepatectomy cases JIS: for staging minor hepatectomy cases
Kondo [10]	2007	Hepatectomy	235	CLIP, BCLC, GETCH, CUPI, JIS, mJIS, Tokyo	Retrospective	JIS: best
Guglielmi [11]	2008	RFA	112	Okuda, TNM, BCLC, CLIP, GETCH, CUPI, JIS,	Prospective	BCLC: superior discriminatory power and prognosis prediction
Cho [12]	2008	TACE	131	Child-Pugh, Okuda, BCLC, CLIP, mCLIP, JIS, mJIS,	Retrospective	CLIP: for palliative settings
Collette [13]	2008	Palliative Tx	538	Okuda, CLIP, BCLC	Randomized	CLIP: best for prognosis
Camma [14]	2008	LT or none	406	BCLC, CLIP, GETCH	Prospective	CLIP: best discriminatory capacity BCLC: best for predicting survival in treated patients
Lu [15]	2008	Curative resection	234	Okuda, CLIP, TNM, CUPI	Retrospective	TNM: best for prognostic strafication and prediction
Chung [16]	2008	Radical Tx	290	JIS, BCLC, Tokyo	Retrospective	JIS: best prognostic stratification
Zhang [17]	2010	Hepatectomy	306	TNM, Okuda, CLIP, BCLC, JIS	Retrospective	BCLC: strongest potential in prognostic evaluation
Huitzil-Melendez [18]	2010	NA	187	BCLC, TNM, CLIP, CUPI, GETCH	Retrospective	CLIP, CUPI, GETCH: survival prediction
Hsu [19]	2010	NA	1713	BCLC, CLIP, JIS, TNM, Tokyo	Prospective	CLIP: best long-term prognostic model
Kawaoka [20]	2011	TACE	214	JIS, mJIS, BCLC, LCSGJ/ TNM, CLIP	Retrospective	mJIS: best discriminatory ability, prognostic predictive power
Chan [21]	2011	NA	595	TNM, CLIP, BCLC, CUPI, JIS, Okuda	Prospective	CUPI for HBV-related HCC; CUPI, CLIP for advanced HCC
Sirivatanauksorn [22]	2011	Hepatectomy	99	TNM, CLIP, BCLC, CUPI, JIS, Okuda,	Retrospective	TNM, Child-Pugh: best for survival prediction
Kim [23]	2012	Multiple Tx	1717	BCLC, JIS, Tokyo, CLIP,	Prospective	BCLC: best for prognosis

RFA; radiofrequency ablation; TACE: transarterial chemoembolization; LT: liver transplantation; Tx: treatment; NA: not available; CLIP: Cancer of the Liver Italian Program score; BCLC: Barcelona Clinic Liver Cancer staging; CUPI: Chinese University Prognostic Index grade; GETCH: Groupe d'Etude et de Traitement du Carcinome Hépatocellulaire classification; JIS: Japan Integrated Staging score; mJIS: modified JIS score.

In addition, numerous staging systems have been proposed and applied in clinical practice, to discriminate HCC patients, estimate their prognosis and allow appropriate treatment selection: they include the Cancer of the Liver Italian Program (CLIP) score, Barcelona Clinic Liver Cancer (BCLC) staging, Groupe d'Etude et de Traitement du Carcinome Hépatocellulaire (GETCH) classification, Chinese University Prognostic Index (CUPI) grade, Japan Integrated Staging (JIS) score, modified JIS (mJIS) score, Okuda staging, and the Tokyo score. A number of recent studies have compared the value of these different staging systems [9-23] and have recently been summarized by Lin et al., [7] (Table 1).

These data do not suggest any consensus and probably reflect the diversity of HCC in the world in terms of etiology, biological behavior, severity of the coexisting liver disease, and local screening and diagnostic methods, which all lead to different stages of the disease. In the setting of liver transplantation, liver function is evaluated by model for end-stage liver disease (MELD) scores and the indication for liver transplantation is based mainly on the Milan criteria [24].

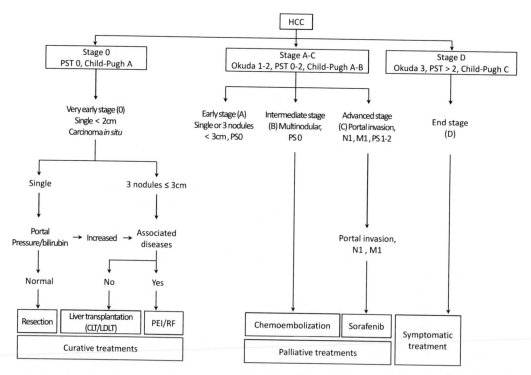

Figure 1. The Barcelona Clinical Liver Cancer (BCLC) staging system and treatment allocation according to the EASL-AASLD guidelines (references 3 and 4). CLD: cadaveric liver transplantation; HCC: hepatocellular carcinoma; LDLT: living donor liver transplantation; PEI: percutaneous ethanol injection; RF: radiofrequency ablation; PST: performance status.

Several treatment guidelines have been proposed for the management of HCC. The European Association for the Study of the Liver (EASL) and the American Association for the Study of Liver Diseases (AASLD) have adopted treatment guidelines based on the BCLC staging system [1, 3, 4] (Figure 1). The Asian-Pacific Association for the Study of the Liver (APASL) has proposed a consensus recommendation [5] and the Japan Society of Hepatology

(JSH) has proposed its own consensus-based treatment algorithm for HCC [6] (Figure 2). However, the basic ideas behind these guidelines do not differ much and take into account the characteristics of the tumor as well as the liver function and the general condition of the patient [3-6] (Figure 1, 2). This is because HCC is a unique cancer with a prognosis that is significantly affected not only by the tumor stage but also by the severity of the coexisting liver disease. In this review, I will describe the treatment selection for HCC based on the EASL-AASLD guidelines with the BCLC staging system, since they are the most commonly used guidelines in the world. The BCLC staging system was developed on the basis of a retrospective analysis of several cohort studies on patients with different stages of HCC. This system identifies patients with very early-stage (stage 0) and early- stage (stage A) HCC who may benefit from curative therapies, those at intermediate (stage B) or advanced (stage C) stages who may benefit from palliative treatments, and those at the terminal stage with a very poor life expectancy (stage D) (Figure 1).

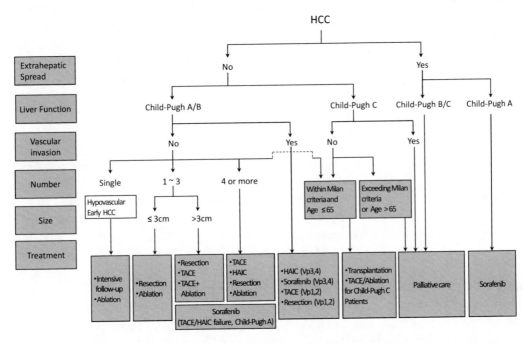

Figure 2. Consensus-based treatment algorithm for HCC proposed by the Japan Society of Hepatology (JSH), revised in 2010 (reference 6). TACE: transarterial chemoembolization; HAIC: hepatic arterial infusion chemotherapy.

3. Therapeutic Strategies Based on Clinical Stage of HCC

3.1. Very Early-Stage HCC

Very early-stage HCC is defined as asymptomatic, small, solitary HCC without macrovascular or extrahepatic invasion. The diameter of HCC should be < 2 cm according to the BCLC staging system [3, 4] and < 3cm according to the APASL [5] or JSH [6] guidelines.

Surgical hepatic resection is recommended for patients with this stage of HCC and Child–Pugh A liver function. The 5-year overall survival (OS) and recurrence rates after hepatic resection of very early-stage HCC are reportedly 70% and 68%, respectively [25]. The presence of satellite nodules and platelet counts < 150,000/μL are independently associated with poor survival, whereas the presence of satellite nodules and cirrhosis and the use of nonanatomic resection are independently associated with tumor recurrence [25]. Percutaneous local ablation, particularly radiofrequency ablation (RFA) [26-29], can also achieve an excellent outcome, such as 5-year disease-free survival (DFS) of 62% and OS of 78%, for very early-stage HCC [29]. Some reports suggest that RFA should be considered as the first-line therapy for very early-stage HCC, even when resection is possible, because it is associated with fewer side effects and lower morbidity [30]. The question of whether surgical resection is superior to RFA remains controversial. Wang et al., [31] suggested that although surgical resection was equivalent to RFA in terms of overall OS, it achieved better DFS. Markov model analysis also indicated that surgical resection was preferable to RFA in terms of OS [32]. However, Peng et al., [33] reported that RFA was associated with better OS when compared with surgical resection. A randomized controlled trial (RCT) that includes only very early-stage HCC has not been conducted and such trial is necessary to elucidate the relative effectiveness of RFA and surgical resection for this stage of HCC.

3.2. Early-Stage HCC

Early-stage HCC is defined according to the Milan criteria as a single tumor nodule ≤ 5 cm in diameter or ≤ 3 nodules of ≤ 3 cm in diameter without macrovascular or extrahepatic invasion [24]. Very early- and early-stage HCC represents 62% of newly diagnosed HCC in Japan, whereas they represent only 30% of those in Western countries [34]. Early-stage HCC is an indication for liver transplantation or RFA according to the EASL-AASLD guidelines [3, 4]. The 4- and 5-year OS of patients who meet the Milan criteria and subsequently undergo liver transplantation are 85% and 70%, respectively [24, 35]. For patients with early-stage HCC, liver transplantation reportedly offers the best chances for long-term survival, when compared with surgical resection, RFA, percutaneous ethanol injection (PEI), and transarterial chemoembolization (TACE) [36]. On the other hand, in Japan, liver transplantation is much less frequently performed than in many other countries, because of the scarcity of donor livers. Thus, the Japanese treatment guidelines recommend liver transplantation for later-stage patients with poor liver function who have few treatment options [6]. However, even in Europe and North America, a shortage of donor livers and tumor progression during the waiting period sometimes inevitably leads patients to drop out of the waiting list, despite the excellent efficacy of liver transplantation for early-stage HCC. The monthly drop-out rate has been reported to be approximately 4% [35, 37].

Therefore, although liver transplantation is the optimal approach, hepatic resection or local ablation is a substitute when liver transplantation is not feasible. Liver resection should be considered when patients present with a solitary tumor and preserved liver function. Local ablation therapies, primarily RFA, have also been performed as alternative treatments for early-stage HCC that meet the Milan criteria. Currently, 4 RCTs [38-41] are available comparing hepatic resection and local ablative therapy for early-stage HCC; they are summarized in Table 2. Chen et al., [38], Feng et al., [39] and Fang et al., [40] have observed no difference in OS and DFS, whereas RFA was associated with lower morbidity and mortality in early-stage HCC that meets the Milan criteria. By contrast, Huang et al., [41] observed significantly higher OS and DFS in the surgical resection group than in the RFA group for early-stage HCC (Table 2). The difference in tumor size (< 3 cm or 3-5 cm), leading to different incidence of "satellite lesion", might account for the different results. On the other hand, 4 recent meta analysis [42-45] supported the superiority of resection for the treatment of early-stage HCC, but this should be interpreted with caution since most data in 3 [42-44] of the 4 meta-analysis are from retrospective non-RCTs. It should be noted that the patients receiving RFA generally include not only operable patients but also inoperable patients who have poorer liver function and thus poorer estimated prognosis than do operable patients. Inclusion of these patients could have significantly worsened the outcome of the RFA group in the non-RCTs. Conversely, the recent meta-analysis by Qi et al., [45], which excluded these non-RCTs, analyzed only 3 RCTs including a small total number of cases (289 cases). Furthermore, the reason for the inconsistencies in the results of the RCTs and meta-analysis are potentially related to the issue of "satellite lesion", which can be resected by surgery but cannot be treated with RFA. These studies include HCCs larger than 3 cm, which often have the "satellite lesions" around the main tumor, in different proportions, and this could have caused the variable results. In addition, a sufficient "safety ablative margin" around the tumor is known to play a significant role in preventing local recurrence after RFA, and variation in the "ablative margin" may account for the different outcomes [46]. To summarize, therefore the superiority of surgical resection remains controversial. More RCTs, particularly paying attention to the size of HCC (≤ 3 cm or 3-5 cm) and sufficient ablative margin, are necessary to clarify whether RFA and surgical resection have equivalent efficacy for the treatment of very early-stage and early-stage HCCs.

Table 2. Results of RCTs comparing the efficacy of local ablative therapies versus hepatic resection for early-stage HCC

Studies	Treatments	No. of Patients	No. of HCC	Size (cm) of HCC	OS	RFS	DFS
Chen et al. [38]	LAT	90	1	≤ 3	NS	NS	NA
	HR	90					
Feng et al. [39]	RFA	84	≤ 2	≤ 4	NS	NS	NA
	HR	84					
Fang et al. [40]	RFA	60	≤ 3	≤ 3	NS	NS	NS
	HR	60					
Huang et al. [41]	RFA	115	≤ 3	≤ 5	RFA < HR	RFA < HR	NA
	HR	115					

OS: overall survival; RFS: recurrence-free survival; DFS: disease-free survival; LAT: local ablative therapies; HR: hepatic resection; RFA: radiofrequency ablation; NS: not significant; NA: not assessed.

On the other hand, innovative radiotherapies, such as proton beam therapy (PBT), which can focus potent radiation to the target tumor to achieve "radiological radical hepatic ablation", have emerged as an alternative option to surgical resection. Although PBT can be performed only at a very limited number of facilities, it can treat solitary HCC, large or small, effectively and safely as surgical resection [47, 48]. It is an excellent option, particularly for aged patients [49] or patients with limited treatment options, because of non-hepatic complications [50] or poor liver function [51].

3.3. Intermediate-Stage HCC

HCC patients with Child–Pugh A or B liver function who present with a large or multifocal tumor mass without macrovascular invasion, extrahepatic metastasis, or cancer-related symptoms are diagnosed as having intermediate-stage HCC. Approximately 20% to 30% of HCC patients are diagnosed as intermediate-stage HCC. Transarterial therapy, especially transarterial chemoembolization (TACE) [52, 53], is recommended. The survival benefit of TACE was the subject of a few RCTs, which have provided inconsistent results [54-60] (Table 3).

Table 3. Results of RCTs comparing TACE or TAE with conservative management or suboptimal therapies for treatment of intermediate-stage HCC (reference 52)

Studies	Treatments	No. of cases	OS (%)		
			1 year	2 year	P value
Lin et al. [54]	TAE (Gelfoarm + Ivalon)	21	42	25	NS
	TAE + IV 5-fluorouracil	21	20	20	
	IV 5-fluorouracil	21	13	13	
Pelletier et al. [55]	TACE (doxorubicin, Gelfoarm)	21	24	NA	NS
	Conservative management	21	33	NA	
GETCH *[56]	TACE (cisplatin, Gelfoarm)	50	62	38	NS
	Conservative management	46	43	26	
Bruix et al. [57]	TAE (Gelfoarm + coil)	40	70	49	NS
	Conservative management	40	72	50	
Pelletier et al. [58]	TACE (cisplatin, Gelfoarm) + tamoxifen	37	51	24	NS
	Tamoxifen	36	55	26	
Lo et al. [59]	TACE (cisplatin, Gelfoarm)	40	57	31	0.002
	Conservative management	39	32	11	
Llovet et al. [60]	TACE (doxorubicin, Gelfoarm)	40	82	63	0.009
	TAE (Gelfoarm)	37	75	50	
	Conservative management	35	63	27	

A meta-analysis of these trials identified a distinct survival benefit for TACE as compared with the control [61].
IV: intravenous; NA: not available; NS: not significant; * Groupe d'Etude et de Traitement du Carcinome Hépatocellulaire classification; ** Chemoembolization vs conservative management (TAE vs conservative management: NS; TACE vs. TAE: NS); OS: overall survival.

However, a cumulative meta-analysis of these trials clearly demonstrated that the survival of patients treated with transarterial embolization (TAE) or TACE is improved, when compared with conservative management [61]. As a result of this analysis, TACE has become established as the standard of care for patients with intermediate-stage HCC. However, more trials are required to further elucidate the efficacy of transarterial therapy [62].

Patients with intermediate-stage HCC are generally not suitable for RFA, but surgical resection is indicated in Japan, even for large, solitary HCC, if liver function permits. Some have reported the benefit of surgery, when they observed that the 3-year OS of patients who underwent surgery was 56% compared to 13% of those who did not [63]. Others, however, reported that surgical resection was associated with poor long-term survival [64]. The value of liver transplantation for intermediate-stage HCC (beyond the Millan criteria) has also been much debated. The role of sorafenib, in combination with TACE, is also currently being investigated. These issues will be discussed later.

3.4. Advanced-Stage HCC

HCC patients with either vascular invasion, extrahepatic spread, no response to TACE or no indication for TACE are considered to be in the advanced stage. Advanced-stage and terminal stage HCC represent only 6% of newly diagnosed HCC cases in Japan, while they represent 50% of those in Western countries [34]. Patients with advanced-stage HCC cannot benefit from curative therapies (such as hepatic resection, local ablation or transplantation) or TACE. The emergence of sorafenib highlights the treatment for advanced-stage HCC. Two prospective RCTs, the SHARP trial [65] and the Asian-Pacific trial [66], have clearly demonstrated the survival benefit of advanced stage HCC patients taking sorafenib over those not taking the drug. Sorafenib is the first-line treatment of choice for advanced-stage HCC patients with Child A liver function [3, 5, 6]. The major side effects of sorafenib are hand-foot skin reaction, diarrhea, fatigue, anorexia, nausea, vomiting, hypertension, and weight loss. Despite improvements in OS after oral sorafenib treatment, the prognosis for patients with advanced-stage HCC is still poor, with a median OS of 6.5 to 10.7 months [65, 66]. No second-line treatment options currently exist for patients who are resistant or refractory to and/or intolerant of sorafenib.

Hepatic arterial infusion chemotherapy (HAIC) is also often performed for advanced-stage HCC in many institutes in Japan [67]. On the basis of the Japanese HCC management guideline [6], HAIC is indicted and recommended for treating multiple liver cancer with 4 or more lesions or HCC with major vascular invasion (Figure 2). In Japan, combinations of interferon plus 5-fluorouracil (5-FU), or cisplatin plus low dose 5-FU, are used as the regimens for HAIC to treat advanced-stage HCC and favorable outcomes have been obtained. Although HAIC was developed in Japan, it is not appreciated in Western countries because no RCT has been conducted and its use is based only on empirical data. Indeed, the AASLD clinical practice guidelines [3, 4] strongly recommend not to use HAIC as the standard of care. Since the effectiveness of HAIC has been widely accepted by Japanese hepatologists, RCTs have not been conducted owing to ethical concerns. However, to demonstrate the clear efficacy of HAIC and establish its role, there is a strong need to conduct RCTs of HAIC for advanced-stage HCC. Innovated radiotherapy, such as proton beam therapy (PBT) [68] or stereotactic radiotherapy (SBRT) [69] has recently emerged as another approach to treat advanced-stage HCC with portal vein tumor thrombus (PVTT).

3.5. Terminal-Stage HCC

Terminal-stage HCC includes severe deterioration of physical capacity and symptoms related to liver failure, vascular invasion, or extrahepatic spread. At this stage, only symptomatic treatments are available, and the median survival is less than 3 months.

4. Therapeutic Approaches for HCC

Next, each of the different therapeutic approaches for HCC including surgical resection, liver transplantation, local ablative therapy, transarterial chemoembolization (TACE), radiotherapy, and systemic chemotherapy and molecular-targeted therapy will be briefly described. For the details of these different therapeutic approaches, please visit other chapters of this book, including "Hepatic Resection" by Dr. Fukunaga et al., (Chapter IV), "Transplantation for HCC" by Dr. Kawagishi, (Chapter V), "Transcatheter Arterial Chemoembolization" by Dr. Miyayama (Chapter VI), and "Proton Beam Therapy for HCC" by Dr. Sakurai et al., (Chapter VII).

4.1. Hepatic Resection

Surgical hepatic resection has been considered as a potentially curative treatment with an acceptable outcome for selected patients with HCC. Refined surgical techniques and introduction of staging systems have allowed the 5-year survival rates after surgical resection to be approximately 50% to 70% [70–74]. As described above, the best candidates for hepatic resection are patients with very early- or early-stage HCC, although hepatic resection in more advanced stages has been reported with acceptable outcomes [64, 75, 76]. Tumor size, tumor nodules, liver function, and portal pressure have been identified as prognostic indicators after hepatic resection [72, 77, 78]. Although liver transplantation offers a better outcome than hepatic resection, the shortage of donor livers limits its application, even in Europe and North America where donor livers are relatively more available. Thus, hepatic resection seems to remain as the major treatment option for the very early- and early-stage HCCs. To reduce the risk of local recurrence, complete resection (R0) is required, while an adequate residual liver volume is necessary to avoid postoperative liver failure [79]. Since the functional reserve of the normal liver is generally large, major hepatic resection of up to 70% is feasible for a noncirrhotic liver. However, residual liver volume after resection must be considerably increased in cirrhotic livers [80]. When the estimated volume of the remnant liver following surgical resection is expected to be insufficient, preoperative portal vein embolization (PVE) is recommended [81, 82]. The prognosis of HCC patients after liver resection is mainly influenced by the recurrence of HCC, either a *de novo* recurrence in a cirrhotic liver or growth of minute metastatic lesions [83, 84]. In concept, the intrahepatic spread of primary HCC is responsible for early recurrence (within 2 years of resection of HCC), while *de novo* carcinogenesis in the remnant liver after resection may cause later recurrence [85]. Re-resection, RFA, and salvage liver transplantation are potential therapeutic approaches to intrahepatic recurrence [86, 87].

4.2. Liver Transplantation

Liver transplantation offers a better outcome than surgical resection because it not only removes all malignant lesions within the liver but also cures the underlying liver disease. Early results of liver transplantation for HCC were poor with 5-year OS of 15% to 40% [88-

90]. However, the 5-year OS of liver transplantation for HCC increased to 70% to 80% [91-93] after the establishment of the Milan criteria [24]. The Milan criteria was identified as an independent prognostic factor after liver transplantation in a recent systematic review of 90 studies that followed 17,780 cases over 15 years [92]. There is a tendency to expand the Milan criteria for liver transplantation, but such an expansion increases the incidence of HCC recurrence and reduces the length of survival [93, 94]. Down-staging of HCC by RFA or TACE before transplantation to within the Milan criteria is possible with acceptable survivals [95–97]. The scarcity of donor livers remains the main obstacle and increases the waiting time for transplantation. The progression of HCC during the waiting period leads patients to drop out of the waiting list [32, 35]. A current strategy to inhibit tumor progression during the waiting time for transplantation is to use RFA or TACE as bridging therapy [97-99]. Alternatively, living donor liver transplantation (LDLT) [100, 101], which is now performed worldwide, has become an alternative for deceased donor liver transplantation (DDLT) [102]. Outcomes for LDLT are similar to those for DDLT in terms of OS and recurrence rates, but the waiting time for LDLT is lower than that for DDLT [102]. The patient allocation system is also important in decreasing the waiting time and drop-outs. The Model for End-Stage Liver Disease (MELD) is a widely accepted allocation system and has served to decrease the waiting time and drop-out rates [103]. A new allocation system, the BAR system, has recently been proposed as an alternative to MELD, which predicts survival better than does MELD [104].

4.3. Local Ablation Therapy before RFA

Local ablation techniques can be performed either through a percutaneous approach or less commonly, through laparoscopy [26, 27]. These include chemical ablation methods, such as percutaneous ethanol injection (PEI) and percutaneous acetic acid injection (PAI), and thermal ablation methods, such as radiofrequency ablation (RFA), microwave ablation (MWA), cryoablation, and laser ablation [27]. Among these, I will discuss on PEI, PAI, RFA and MWA. The evaluation of responses to the locoregional treatments and molecular-targeted therapies of HCC is currently based on modified RECIST (mRECIST) criteria, which measure the diameter of the viable tumor component of the target lesions [105].

4.3.1. Percutaneous Ethanol Injection (PEI)

The first percutaneous treatment was PEI, which induces coagulation necrosis of the tumor as a result of cellular dehydration, protein denaturation and chemical occlusion of the small tumor vessels by the injected absolute alcohol. PEI is a well-established technique for the treatment of nodular-type HCC. Injected ethanol diffused within the tumor easily and selectively. The standard PEI protocol includes 4-6 sessions performed under ultrasound guidance by using fine needles. In patients with early-stage HCC and Child A cirrhosis, treatment with PEI has been shown to result in 5-year OS rates of 47% to 53%. The major limitation of PEI is the high local recurrence rate, which may reach 33% in tumors ≤ 3 cm and 43% in tumors > 3 cm [27]. The injected ethanol does not always achieve complete tumor ablation because of its inhomogeneous distribution within the lesion, especially in the presence of intratumoral septa, and the limited effect on extracapsular cancerous spread [27].

4.3.2. Percutaneous Acetic Acid Injection (PAI)

Percutaneous acetic acid injection (PAI) was proposed as a viable alternative to PEI for chemical ablation of HCC. Although the first RCT showed favorable results of PAI in comparison with PEI [106], subsequent RCTs [107, 108] and meta-analysis [109] have concluded that its efficacy does not differ significantly from PEI in terms of OS, recurrence-free survival, and local recurrence rate, although PAI required lesser treatment sessions.

4.3.3. Microwave Ablation

Microwave ablation (MWA) is another potentially curative ablation procedure that has been proven to be safe in percutaneous and intraoperative settings [27, 110-112]. MWA creates an electromagnetic field in the tissues surrounding the ablation antenna with an extension of several centimeters, without flow of the electrical current. Tissue within the MWA field heats rapidly to temperatures over 100°C without the detrimental effects of tissue impedance, allowing a more rapid and consistent ablation. MWA can be a valuable alternative to RFA for thermal ablation of HCC. A RCT comparing the efficacy of MWA with that of RFA has shown no statistically significant difference on the efficacy of these two procedures with a tendency favoring RFA for local recurrence and complication rates [113]. An important advantage of MWA over RFA might be that the treatment outcome of MWA is not affected by vessels located in the proximity of the tumor [27].

4.4. Radiofrequency Ablation (RFA)

4.4.1. Emergence of RFA

Percutaneous RFA is a treatment method causing coagulation necrosis of the liver tumors by dielectric heating with radio waves (460 ± 5 Hz) around an electrode inserted into a lesion. RFA has mostly replaced PEI, PAI and MWA, and it is currently the most frequently performed local ablation method for HCC [26, 27]. RFA can be performed percutaneously under imaging guidance (ultrasound (US), CT or MRI) or during surgery guided by intraoperative US. It allows selective destruction of the tumor, sparing the surrounding parenchyma with "safety ablative margins" around the tumor, and can be easily repeated. Complete ablation of very early-stage HCC (≤ 2 cm) is possible in more than 90% of cases with a local recurrence rate of less than 1% [30]. The effectiveness of RFA has been proven for very-early or early stage HCCs: the 5-year OS rates are as high as 51% to 76% in patients with early-stage HCC and Child-Pugh A liver function [114-117]. Five RCTs [118-122] have compared RFA versus PEI for the treatment of early-stage HCC (Table 4). These RCTs have consistently demonstrated that RFA has stronger antitumor effects than PEI, leading to a higher rate of complete necrosis and local control of tumor, while requiring fewer treatment sessions (Table 4). The impact of RFA on OS was more controversial. While the 3 RCTs performed in Asia [108, 119, 120] have demonstrated survival benefit, the 2 RCTs [118, 121] in Europe failed to show significant difference in OS between patients who received RFA and those received PEI, despite the trend favoring RFA (Table 4). Nevertheless, 3 meta-analysis [28, 109, 122] including these 5 RCTs have confirmed that RFA has a survival benefit compared with PEI, particularly for HCC > 2 cm, and thus RFA was established as the standard of percutaneous ablation methods. However, the efficacy of RFA was not significantly better than PEI for HCC ≤ 2 cm in diameter and the adverse events were more frequent with RFA.

Table 4. Results of RCTs comparing the efficacy of RFA versus PEI for early-stage HCC (reference 27)

| Studies | Treatments | No. of Patients | Initial CR (%) | Treatment failure (%)* | OS (%) | | |
					1-year	3-year	P value
Lencioni et al. [118]	RFA	52	91	8	88	81	NS
	PEI	50	82	34	96	73	
Lin et al. [119]	RFA	52	96	17	82	74	0.014
	PEI	52	88	45	61	50	
Shiina et al. [120]	RFA	118	100	2	90	80	0.02
	PEI	114	100	11	82	63	
Lin et al. [108]	RFA	62	97	16	88	74	0.031
	PEI	62	89	42	96	51	
Brunello et al. [121]	RFA	70	96	34	88	59	NS
	PEI	69	66	64	96	57	

Three meta-analysis of these trials identified a distinct survival benefit for RFA compared with PEI [28, 109, 122]; * Includes initial treatment failure (incomplete response) and late failure (local recurrence).
CR: complete response; NS: not significant; PEI: percutaneous ethanol injection; OS: overall survival; RFA: radiofrequency ablation.

RFA is especially recommended for patients with a few (3 or less), small (< 3 cm) HCCs which are unresectable because of compromised (Child B) liver function or other complications. In addition, RFA has been proposed as an alternative to surgical hepatic resection, but its superiority to surgical resection remains controversial. Four RCTs [38-41] are available for this issue. Three of the 4 RCTs have found no difference in OS and DFS between local ablation and hepatic resection. Briefly, Chen et al., [38] have found in a RCT for small (≤ 3 cm) solitary HCC, no difference in OS and DFS, whereas ablative therapy was associated with lower morbidity (4% vs 56%, $P < 0.05$) and mortality (0% vs 1%). Feng et al., [39] have also reported no difference in OS and DFS by resection or RFA in a RCT for early-stage HCC. Furthermore, Fang et al., [40] have also recently provided evidence supporting these data. By contrast, Huang et al., [41] have observed significantly higher OS and DFS in the resection group than in the RFA group in their RCT for early-stage HCC (Table 2). In addition, 4 meta-analysis [42-45] have recently been published. They indicate that surgical resection is superior to RFA in terms of low recurrence rate and longer OS and DFS, whereas RFA was associated with fewer complications and shorter hospital stay. However, these conclusions should be interpreted with caution because 9 of the 10 studies, 6 of the 8 studies, and 10 of the 12 studies included in the meta-analysis by Zhou et al., [42], Li et al., [43], and Duan et al., [44], respectively, were non-RCTs.

Several limitations exist for RFA. First, complete necrosis is rarely obtained when the tumor diameter is > 3 cm or when the tumor is adjacent to a major blood vessel owing to the cooling effect of the blood flow. For patients with single tumors > 3 cm in diameter, surgery is significantly more effective than RFA: the 3-year OS rates were 66% after surgery vs 37% after RFA ($P = 0.004$) and the 3-year DFS rates were 44% after surgery vs 19% after RFA ($P = 0.001$) [123]. This observation was confirmed by other studies [124, 125]. Second, some areas of the liver parenchyma cannot be reached percutaneously. Third, RFA at subcapsular lesions can cause their rupture in the peritoneum. Forth, RFA for tumors near the gallbladder can cause gallbladder injury. Therefore, RFA and hepatic resection are effective therapeutic options that can be chosen based on the severity of chronic liver disease as well as the size and location of the tumor.

4.4.2. Recent Technical Refinements and Expansion of Indication of RFA

As described above, RFA could not be applied to all HCCs and there were locations of HCC which were difficult to be treated with RFA. Recently, attempts have been made to expand the indication of RFA to many of the previously contraindicated lesions by introducing various techniques. These include large HCCs (> 3 cm), HCCs located at right subdiaphragmatic lesion or on the intra-abdominal free surfaces, HCCs unclear on B-mode US, locally recurrent HCCs, and HCCs proximal to the hepatic portal glisson's capsule [26]. In the case of large HCC (> 3 cm), lipiodol TACE-preceded RFA has been actively performed for such lesions, aiming at treating satellite nodules and microscopic vascular invasion [126-130]. Yamakado et al., [127] reported that lipiodol TACE-preceded RFA demonstrated almost equivalent OS to surgical resection for large HCC cases. HCCs which are located at right sub-diaphragmatic lesion or on the intra-abdominal free surface have the high-risk for complications, such as perforation of diaphragm, intestine or gallbladder, and it was previously considered hard to treat them by RFA. These problems were overcome by RFA in the presence of "artificial pleural effusion" [131-134], or "artificial ascites" [135-137], which are induced by infusing normal saline or 5% glucose solution into the intrapleural or intraperitoneal cavity, respectively. On the other hand, recent introduction of real-time virtual sonography, which synchronized US and CT, allowed RFA treatment guided by this virtual image for HCCs which had been unclear on the conventional B-mode US [137-139]. Furthermore, recent introduction of a new contrast media, Sonazoid, allowed clearer visualization of HCC and more accurate pinpoint guidance for RFA treatment on Kupffer-phase and on subsequent defect reperfusion image following reinjection of the contrast media [140-147]. Defect reperfusion image with Sonazoid is especially useful in localizing and treating the local recurrence of HCC [140, 141]. Bile duct injury and its associated complications, such as biloma or abscess, are major complications of RFA, especially when treating HCC located near the hepatic portal Glisson's capsular region. Insertion of endoscopic nasobiliary (ENB) tube and cooling of the bile duct by the perfusion of ice-cold water through the tube was found to be a good solution for this problem [148,149].

The concept of a "safety ablative margin" is considered important in order to prevent the local recurrence following RFA. It has been reported that intrahepatic metastatic lesions are present in 66.7% and 11.1% at a site within 2 mm and 5 mm, respectively, from the primary lesion [150]. Thus, intrahepatic metastatic lesions can be included in the treatment area by setting a safety margin of 5 mm. Others have also reported that "satellite nodules" were present in 19% of 194 resected HCC of 3-cm or smaller, and 33% of these were present within 5 mm from the main tumor [151]. The local recurrence rates after 4 years were reportedly 2.6% and 20.8% in cases with 5-mm or wider safety ablative margin and in cases with the margin narrower than 5 mm, respectively, with a significant statistical difference [152]. It was also reported that the local recurrence rate was significantly different between cases with HCC of $\leq$ 2.3 cm and those with HCC of > 2.3 cm in diameter, and it was significantly lower in cases with a sufficient safety ablative margin than those without it

[153]. In addition, a sufficient safety ablative margin was the sole predictor of the local recurrence rate on multivariate analysis [154]. Therefore, evaluation of precise "safety ablative margin" following RFA is important in predicting the local recurrence and evaluating the necessity for additional treatments. Currently, contrast-enhanced ultrasonography is often used for this purpose [155-157], but the safety ablative margin can be identified in only 50-60% of cases [26]. Mori, et al., [158], our colleagues at Tsukuba University Hospital, have recently developed a MR imaging method with ferucarbotran, which can clearly visualize and distinguish non-ablated and ablated HCC tissues as well as ablated surrounding normal tissues and allow precise assessment of the "safety ablative margin". A study analyzing the clinical efficacy of this new method is currently underway.

4.5. Transarterial Chemoembilization (TACE)

TACE is the most commonly used initial treatment for patients with the intermediate-stage HCC of the BCLC staging system who are not suitable candidates for curative treatment options but present with multinodular HCC and relatively preserved liver function and without cancer-related symptoms, vascular invasion, or extrahepatic metastasis [51, 52]. The rationale behind TACE is the well-characterized hypervascular nature of advanced HCC as a result of its angiogenic activity. This technique depends on the intraarterial infusion of a cytotoxic chemotherapeutic agent emulsioned with Lipiodol followed by embolization of the feeding vessels through a transarterial catheter [159]. Several RCTs for TACE have provided inconsistent results [54-60] (Table 3). However, a meta-analysis [61] of these trials, which clearly demonstrated the survival benefit for patients treated with TAE or TACE, as compared with those receiving only conservative managements, has established the role of TACE as the standard of care for patients with intermediate-stage HCC. In addition, TACE may be considered as a neoadjuvant treatment that can be used before hepatic resection or RFA ablation to reduce tumor volume and possibly target satellite micrometastases or as a bridging therapy before liver transplantation. Furthermore, drug-eluting beads [160, 161], such as doxorubicin-eluting beads, have recently been introduced in clinical practice and are considered as improvements over conventional TACE. Contraindications for TACE are decompensated cirrhosis (Child-Pugh B $\geq$ 8, including jaundice, clinical encephalopathy, or refractory ascites), extensive tumor with massive replacement of both lobes in their entirety, portal vein occlusion, or impaired renal function [162].

4.6. Radiation Therapy

Until the late 1980's, radiation therapy (RT) for HCC was not successful, because only insufficient doses (< 30 Gy) could be applied to the cirrhotic liver to avoid fetal radiation-induced liver disease (RILD). RT is generally not considered an option in HCC consensus documents or national guidelines, primarily because of the lack of evidence of survival benefit in RCTs [69, 163-165]. However, recently experience with conformal RT [166-179], intensity-modulated RT, stereotactic body RT [180-192] and particle beam therapy [47-51, 193-205] is rapidly increasing. RT should be considered as a treatment option in patients unsuitable for other established local therapies [69, 163-165]. RT has also been safely combined with locoregional therapies such as TACE or used as a bridge to liver transplant.

4.6.1. 3D-Conformal Radiotherapy

There are a number of reports on 3D-conformal RT (3D-CRT), especially from Asian-pacific regions. These reports have shown that high dose photon (40-60 Gy) can be irradiated safely to HCC by the 3D-CRT technology [167-179]. It is often combined with TACE [167-170] or used after failed TACE [171]. Furthermore, it has been applied for treating portal vein tumor thrombus [173-176]. However, 3D-CRT still sometimes induces radiation-induced liver disease and worsens the Child-Pugh scores, and when this happens the OS of the patients can even be shortened [177-179]. This is the limitation of this approach as well as the lack of RCT and poor long-term survival because it is mostly used as a palliative treatment.

4.6.2. Stereotactic Body Radiotherapy (SBRT)

Stereotactic body radiotherapy (SBRT) is a high-precision conformal external beam radiation technique that ablates the target with hypofractionated high-dose radiation while sparing the surrounding normal tissues. Recently, reports of SBRT for HCC is increasing [180-192]. Since this method allows more potent hypofractionated radiation, it gave good local tumor control. However, liver function damage, as indicated by the increase in Child-Pugh score, is often associated with this approach, especially in cases with Child B liver function, large HCC, or when treated by aggressive hypofraction [183, 184, 189]. Thus, it is not indicated for Child C or even B cases. Long-term survival remains unknown and RCT is lacking.

4.6.3. Particle Beam Radiotherapy

Proton beam, unlike conventional X-ray, forms a unique Bragg peak ionization that enables "potent tumor-targeted irradiation" [193]. On the basis of this unique property, we have introduced proton beam therapy (PBT) for HCC since 1983, in collaboration with the High Energy Accelerator Research Organization at Tsukuba, and demonstrated the first evidence of curative yet safe radiotherapy for HCC [194]. Subsequently, we observed an excellent 5-year local tumor control rate of 87% and a 5-year OS of 24% in the first 168 HCC patients treated with PBT [47]. Patients with solitary HCC and Child-Pugh A liver function were associated with a good 5-year OS of 53.5% [47], which was comparable to the results obtained by surgical resection [195]. We then opened an in-house PBT facility at Tsukuba University Hospital in 2001, and could demonstrate its excellent local tumor control rate (83%) and a further improved 5-year OS (44.6%) in HCC patients [48]. Since PBT is safe and has limited effects on liver function [196], we especially recommend it for elderly HCC patients [49] who prefer not to undergo the risk of surgery or to patients with limited treatment options due to various extrahepatic complications [50] or poor liver function [51]. We have also reported on its excellent efficacy for large HCC (> 5 cm) [197], HCC with PVTT [68], or HCC adjacent to the porta hepatis [198] or alimentary tract [199]. In addition, PBT can be further intensified by hypofractionation [200] and can be repeated safely [201]. The limitation of PBT includes the high treatment cost (approximately 250 million yen or 25 thousand US dollar) for patients, and the lack of RCT comparing with other treatment modalities. Following these preceding clinical data of ours, a high efficacy of PBT for HCC has been confirmed by other PBT facilities in the world [202-205]. The recent increase in PBT facilities worldwide may indicate that more HCC patients, especially elderly patients or those with complications, will be treated by PBT in the near future.

4.7. Systemic Chemotherapy, Sorafenib, and Hepatic Arterial Infusion Chemotherapy (HAIC)

4.7.1. Conventional Chemotherapy

Systemic chemotherapy for HCC has been very limited. Doxorubicin, gemcitabine, or combined regimens for palliative care has shown only limited efficacy in advanced HCC patients [206-210]. A prospective RCT revealed that doxorubicin monotherapy provided only a 3-week increase in MST as compared without chemotherapy, while it caused severe complications such as septicemia and cardiotoxicity [210]. Gemcitabine also showed only marginal antitumor effects in a phase II study in patients with advanced HCC [207, 208]. A randomized phase III study comparing the combination of cisplatin, interferon, doxorubicin, and fluorouracil (PIAF) with doxorubicin alone resulted in no significant difference in the MST, while the PIAF regimen significantly increased the incidence of complications [209]. The drug resistance of HCC, both intrinsic and acquired, was considered to be mainly responsible for the failure of the chemotherapies [210]. These results indicate that conventional chemotherapy is ineffective for HCC.

4.7.2. Emergence of Sorafenib

Sorafenib is a tyrosine kinase inhibitor of Raf serine/threonine kinases, vascular endothelial growth factor receptor (VEGFR-1, VEGFR-2, VEGFR-3), and platelet-derived growth factor receptor-h (PDGFR-h) tyrosine kinases [211]. A global prospective phase III trial conducted in the West (the SHARP study) for patients with advanced HCC and Child-Pugh A liver function has demonstrated that the median OS significantly improved in patients treated with oral sorafenib when compared with those treated with placebo (10.7 vs. 7.9 months, respectively; hazard ratio (HR): 0.69, $P < 0.001$) [65]. The 1 year OS rate (33% vs. 44%, respectively) and the median time to progression (TTP; 5.5 vs. 2.8 months, respectively; HR: 0.58, $P < 0.001$) also improved in the sorafenib group when compared with the placebo group [65]. An Asian-Pacific RCT conducted by Cheng et al., [66] further confirmed these results: the median OS significantly improved in the sorafenib group compared with the placebo group (6.5 vs. 4.2 months, respectively; HR: 0.68, $P = 0.014$) and the TTP (2.8 vs. 1.4 months, respectively; HR: 0.57, $P = 0.0005$) as well. From these results, sorafenib has become the first-line treatment of choice for advanced-stage HCC patients with preserved liver function [3, 5, 6]. The major side effects of sorafenib are hand-foot syndrome, diarrhea, anorexia, nausea, vomiting, hypertension, and weight loss. A subanalysis of the SHARP trial revealed that sorafenib is beneficial in patients with alcohol-related, hepatitis B-related or hepatitis C-related HCC [212].

4.7.3. Hepatic Arterial Infusion Chemotherapy (HAIC)

Hepatic arterial infusion chemotherapy (HAIC) has been performed for advanced stage HCC. HAIC is indicted for treating multiple HCCs with 4 or more lesions or HCC with major vascular invasion [67] (Figure 2). According to a nationwide survey of HCC in Japan [123], combinations of either interferon plus 5-fluorouracil (5-FU), low dose 5-FU plus cisplatin (CDDP), or CDDP monotherapy regimens account for 49%, 30%, and 11% of patients, respectively. The favorable results have been obtained with a good response rate (complete response [CR] plus partial response [PR]; 45.9%) and a disease control rate (76.5%). Ueshima et al., [213] have demonstrated a median survival time (MST) of 15.9 months and a median TTP of 4.1 months by HAIC. They have also reported that responders to HAIC (CR + PR) showed significantly better survival (MST, 40.7 months), than did nonresponders (MST, 6.8 months). It is a great advantage of HAIC that the responders and the nonresponders to the treatment can be distinguished in less than 1 month [67]. However, HAIC is not currently accepted by the Western hepatologists as the standard of care for advanced HCC, owing to the lack of a RCT. Whether HAIC can improve the survival of advanced HCC patients needs to be uncovered by RCTs [67].

5. Multidisciplinary Management of HCC

As described above, no treatment modality should be applied to all patients with HCC and treatment selection should be individualized. Therefore, which treatment modality is the most appropriate for each patient with HCC should be decided by a multidisciplinary cancer board composed of hepatologists, hepatobiliary surgeons, transplant surgeons, radiologists, and pathologists [214]. In the management of HCC, the presence and degree of the underlying chronic liver disease will influence the choice of the treatment and must be precisely evaluated. Liver resection can be offered to patients with well-preserved liver function. In cases with impaired liver function, nonsurgical procedures or liver transplantation should be offered. In this setting, the number, size and location of the nodules determine the choice of treatment. Surgical resection, transplantation and ablation are the treatments that offer the highest rates of complete response and are therefore considered as curative treatment [4]. No RCT have been conducted comparing the efficacy of these 3 approaches, and all evidence is based on the empirical data reported in different series.

6. Future Perspectives

The future perspectives for the treatment of HCC are many. Among them, I will focus on the new treatments for advanced-stage HCC, since the prognosis for this stage is still very poor and further advances in this area are necessary. In addition, attempts to prevent the recurrence of the disease are introduced, since they are also necessary to extend the survival of patients with HCC.

6.1. Clinical Trials of Combination Therapy with Sorafenib

Despite the positive effect of sorafenib on the survival of patients with advanced HCC, the response to sorafenib remains low and the median OS has been extended by merely 2.3 to

2.8 months [65, 66]. To further extend the benefits of sorafenib, combination therapies of sorafenib plus conventional chemotherapy or TACE have been investigated.

A RCT that compared the combination of sorafenib plus doxorubicin with doxorubicin alone found a median TTP of 6.4 vs. 2.8 months, median OS of 13.7 vs. 6.5 months, and median PFS of 6.0 vs. 2.7 months, respectively [212]. These results did not support that the superiority of the combination of sorafenib plus doxorubicin to sorafenib alone.

The efficacy of sequential sorafenib treatment following TACE has been evaluated. It was reported that HCC patients who respond to TACE did not benefit from sorafenib treatment [215]. However, another RCT conversely found a significantly longer TTP in patients receiving conventional TACE followed by sorafenib [216]. On the basis of these controversial results, further trials with a larger number of patients are required to elucidate the effects of sequential sorafenib treatment after TACE.

Simultaneous therapy of sorafenib and TACE has also been retrospectively analyzed, and the median OS for the combination group was found to be 27 months as compared with 17 months for the TACE-alone group [217]. A phase III clinical study evaluating sorafenib and TACE versus TACE alone is ongoing [218]. Further trials are needed to validate the efficacy of the combination therapy.

6.2. Clinical Trials of Other Molecular-Targeted Drugs

Recently, the efficacy of a variety of other molecular-targeted drugs, including sunitinib, brivanib, linifanib, erlotinib, lipatinib, everolimus, have been investigated either as an alternative to sorafenib as the first-line therapy, or as the second-line therapy following failure or intolerance to sorafenib or as the combination with sorafenib [219, 220]. Results of the recent clinical trails for these drugs are summarized in Table 5 [221-237].

Several phase III trials for these drugs have been completed. Briefly, sunitinib is the most studied multikinase inhibitor targeting VEGFR-1 and VEGFR-2 and also displays inhibitory activities against other receptor tyrosine kinases, including PDGFR-a/b, c-KIT, FLT3, and RET kinases. The drug is currently indicated for the treatment of renal cell carcinoma and gastrointestinal stromal tumors. However, sunitinib was recently found, by a phase III RCT, not to be superior or equivalent but to be significantly inferior to sorafenib as a first-line therapy for advanced HCC [222].

Brivanib is a dual inhibitor of vascular endothelial growth factor receptor (VEGFR) and fibroblast growth factor receptor (FGFR) signaling pathways. A phase III (BRISK-FL) RCT comparing the efficacy of brivanib with sorafenib as first-line therapy for advanced HCC did not meet its primary endpoint of OS noninferiority for brivanib versus sorafenib [225]. A phase III (BRISK-PS) RCT aiming to elucidate the role of brivanib as second-line therapy following failure or intolerance to sorafenib also did not show improvement in the OS [226].

Erlotinib is a potent and reversible inhibitor of EGFR tyrosine kinase. Erlotinib has been shown to inhibit the RAF/MEK/ERK signaling pathway and to block the signal transducer and activator of transcription-mediated signaling. The phase III placebo-controlled, double-blind SEARCH trial was conducted comparing sorafenib plus erlotinib and sorafenib plus placebo in patients with advanced HCC. However, no significant differences were observed in OS or TTP between the 2 arms and it was concluded that erlotinib, when added to sorafenib, does not prolong the OS of advanced HCC [231].

Table 5. Summary of recent clinical trials of molecular-targeted drugs for advanced-stage HCC (reference 220)

Target pathway / Agents	Phase	Efficacy	References
VEGF / VEGFR pathway			
Sorafenib	Phase III (SHARP) (sorafenib vs placebo)	Median OS: 10.7 m vs. 7.9 m	[65]
	Phase III (Asian-Pacific) (sorafenib vs placebo)	Median OS: 6.5 m vs. 4.2 m	[66]
Sunitinib	Phase II	Median OS: 9.8 m; median PFS: 3.9 m	[221]
	First-line, randomized phase II (sunitinib vs sorafenib)	Median OS: 7.9 m vs. 10.2 m	[222]
Brivanib	First-line, phase II	Median OS: 10 m; median PFS: 2.8 m	[223]
	Second-line, phase II	Median OS: 9.8 m; median PFS: 2.7 m	[224]
	First-line, phase III (BRISK-FL) (brivanib vs placebo)	Median OS: 9.5 m vs. 9.9 m TTP: 4.2 m vs. 4.1 m	[225]
	Second-line, Phase III (BRISK-PS) (brivanib vs placebo)	Median OS: 9.4 m vs. 8.3 m TTP: 4.2 m vs. 2.7 m	[226]
Vatalanib (PTK787)	Phase I/II combined with doxorubicin	Median OS: 7.3 m; median PFS: 5.4 m	[227]
Linifanib (ABT-869)	Phase II	Median OS: 9.7 m; TTP: 3.7 m	[228]
Cediranib (AZD2171)	Phase II	Median OS: 5.8 m; TTP: 2.8 m	[229]
EGF /EGFR pathway			
Cetuximab	Phase II	Median OS: 9.6 m; median PFS: 1.4 m	[230]
Erlotinib	Phase III (SEARCH) (sorafenib+erlotinib vs orafenib+placebo)	Median OS: 9.5 m vs. 8.5 m TTP: 3.2 m vs. 4.0 m	[231]
Lapatinib	Phase II	Median OS: 6.2 m; TTP: 2.3 m	[232]
	Phase III (lapatinib vs sorafenib)	Median OS: 9.1 m vs. 9.8 m	
IGF /IGFR pathway			
Cituxumumab	Phase II	Median OS: 8.0 m	[233]
Ras/ Raf / MEK/ ERK pathway			
Selumetinib (AZD6244)	Phase I/II	11 cases enrolled (PD in 3, SD in 6, PD in 2)	[234]
PI3K/Akt/mTOR pathway			
Everolimus	Phase I / II	Median OS: 8.4 m; median PFS: 3.8 m	[235]
Sirolimus	Phase II	Median OS: 26.4 wk; median PFS: 15.3 wk	[236]
MET pathway			
Tivantinib	Randomized phase II (tivantinib vs placebo)	Median OS: 6.6 wk vs 6.2 wk; Median TTP: 6.9 wk vs 6.0 wk	[237]

OS: overall survival; PD: progressive disease; PFS: progression-free survival; PR: partial response; SD: stable disease; TTP: time to progression; VEGF: vascular endothelial growth factor; VEGFR: vascular endothelial growth factor receptor; mTOR: mammalian target of rapamycin; PI3K: phosphatidylinositol-3-kinase; MET: met protooncogene; EGFR: epidermal growth factor receptor

In summary, unfortunately, no drug has demonstrated superior efficacy to sorafenib as the first-line therapy nor has shown efficacy as the second-line therapy or combined efficacy with sorafenib. However, further multiple clinical trials are ongoing to explore the efficacy of the various new molecular-targeted drugs for HCC that are listed in Table 5.

6.3. Clinical Trials for Preventing the Recurrence of HCC

HCC is a cancer with a very high incidence of recurrence, owing to frequent intrahepatic metastasis and *de novo* carcinogenesis, and thus remains one of the most difficult cancers to cure. Among all of the current therapeutic modalities, only liver transplantation can inhibit the recurrence of HCC.

6.3.1. STORM Study

Ongoing clinical trials aimed at preventing recurrence include the Sorafenib as Adjuvant Treatment in the Prevention of Recurrence of HCC (STORM) study of sorafenib and another study of peretinoin (NIK333), an acyclic retinoid. The STORM study is a global trial to evaluate the preventive effect of sorafenib on recurrence in patients who have undergone RFA or resection. Patient enrollment has been completed, and the study is currently in the follow-up period.

6.3.2. Peretinoin

NIK333 (peretinoin) is an oral acyclic retinoid developed in Japan, which has a vitamin A-like structure and primarily targets the nuclear receptors of retinoid, namely retinoic acid receptor (RAR) and retinoid X receptor (RXR). Peretinoin exerts transcriptional activation- and differentiation-inducing effects via RAR and RXR and is expected to prevent carcinogenesis through HCC precursor removal by apoptosis and differentiation induction [238]. A phase III clinical trial to establish the superiority of peretinoin 600 mg over placebo is currently underway.

6.3.3. In Situ Immunotherapy

Another option under investigation for preventing recurrence is tumor immunotherapy. Our collaborators, Dr. Ohno and his colleagues, have successfully demonstrated that autologous formalin-fixed tumor vaccine made from surgically resected HCC tissues significantly inhibited the recurrence of HCC and improved both OS and event-free survivals following surgery in a phase II RCT [239]. However, this method requires a certain volume of autologous cancer tissue to produce the vaccine and thus the treatment availability is limited. To overcome this limitation, we postulated that using *in vivo* tumor tissue following local treatment, such as RFA or radiation, would enable us to induce a systemic immune response against the tumor. According to this idea, we have recently conducted a phase I clinical trial testing the efficacy of an "*in situ* vaccination" approach using CalTUMP, a hydroxyapatite immune adjuvant, injected into HCC tissues pretreated with the potent proton beam radiotherapy (PBT). The results showed that intratumoral injection of CalTUMP following PBT was feasible and safe in patients with heavily pretreated HCC patients [240]. Further clinical studies to evaluate the efficacy of this *in situ* tumor vaccination are warranted.

6.4. Clinical Trials of Oncolytic Virus-Mediated Immune-Gene Therapy

Recent clinical trials have demonstrated the promising clinical efficacy and safety of several oncolytic viruses, which can selectively replicate in and lyse cancer cells, and oncolytic virus therapy is now considered as a new platform for cancer gene therapy [241-244]. Vaccinia virus, especially, has several ideal biological properties, including broad tumor infectivity, rapid replication, high oncolytic potency, resistance to serum neutralization antibody, and efficient spreading through the blood to distant tumors. Pexa-Vec (JX-594) is a thymidine kinase gene-deleted (TK⁻), granulocyte macrophage colony stimulating factor gene-armed (GM-CSF⁺) oncolytic vaccinia virus developed by SillaJen / Jennerex Biotherapeutics [245]. In preclinical studies, Pexa-Vec exhibited multiple modes of anticancer effects, such as potent oncolytic effects, shut-down of tumor blood supply, and enhancement of antitumor immunity [245-248]. A phase I clinical trial of intratumoral Pexa-Vec injections for liver cancers carried out in Korea showed excellent efficacy and safety [249, 250]. A subsequent randomized phase II trial conducted in Korea, the U.S.A. and Canada, comparing 3 intratumoral injections of high-dose (1×10^9 pfu) versus low-dose (1×10^8 pfu) Pexa-Vec in patients (n = 30) with advanced HCC, exhibited excellent antitumor efficacy and safety with significantly better survival in the high-dose group (median OS, 14.1 vs. 6.7 months, hazard ratio: 0.39, $P = 0.02$) [251]. Furthermore, a phase I clinical trial of dose-escalating single intravenous Pexa-Vec infusion was performed in 23 patients with various advanced cancers [252]. In this trial, potent and specific transgene expression in the tumor tissues was successfully achieved in patients receiving intravenous Pexa-Vec (3×10^7 pfu/kg or 1×10^9 pfu) without any severe side effects. Since this was the first demonstration of specific gene delivery to yet potent gene expression in tumors through intravenous injection, it was regarded as a breakthrough in the history of cancer gene therapy [252]. Further clinical trials for HCC and colorectal cancers are now ongoing in the U.S.A., Canada, Korea, Hong Kong, and Taiwan with a plan for a global phase III trial. This virus is expected to open a new era of potent oncolytic virus-mediated cancer gene therapy for advanced HCC and other intractable malignancies.

Conclusion

The treatment of HCC has much advanced during the past several decades, with significant progress in surgical resection and transplantation techniques, local ablative techniques, interventional radiology, innovative radiotherapy, and molecular-targeted drugs, as well as in multidisciplinary approaches to properly select these therapeutic options. Improved management of underlying liver disease has also contributed to the extension of patients' survival. Establishment of clinical staging systems and treatment guidelines based on them has made meaningful international comparisons easier on the efficacy of different modalities on these improved results. Currently, early diagnosis followed by liver transplantation provides HCC patients with the best chance for long-term survival. In Japan, unfortunately, only a small portion of HCC can be treated with liver transplantation owing to a scarcity of deceased liver donors, but still the current nationwide 5-year OS of 43% is the highest in the world. The nationwide surveillance system in Japan has contributed much to this, allowing 62% of HCC to be diagnosed at very early- or early- stages and to be treated with curative therapies, while only 30% of HCC are currently diagnosed at these early stages in Western countries [34]. This indicates that to achieve excellent survival of HCC as in Japan, the progress of treatments for HCC in other countries must be accompanied by establishment of a quality system for surveillance and early diagnosis of HCC as in Japan. To further improve the prognosis of HCC, new methods to prevent the recurrence and innovative approaches to extend the survival of patients with advanced-stage HCC also need to be explored further.

References

[1]   El-Serag HB. Hepatocellular carcinoma. *N. Engl. J. Med.* 2011; 365: 1118-1127.

[2]   Cabrera R, Nelson DR. Review article: the management of hepatocellular carcinoma. *Aliment. Pharmacol. Ther.* 2010; 31: 461–476.

[3]   Bruix J, Sherman M. Management of hepatocellular carcinoma: an update. *Hepatology* 2011; 53: 1020–1022.

[4]   Bruix J, Sherman M. Management of hepatocellular carcinoma. *Hepatology* 2005; 42: 1208–1236.

[5]   Omata M, Lesmana LA, Tateishi R, Chen PJ, Lin S-M, Yoshida H, et al., Asian Pacific Association for the Study of the Liver consensus recommendations on hepatocellular carcinoma. *Hepatol. Int.* 2010; 4: 439–474.

[6]   Kudo M, Izumi N, Kokudo N, Matsui O, Sakamoto M, Nakashima O, et al., Management hepatocellular carcinoma in Japan: Consensus-based clinical practice guidelines proposed by the Japan Society of Hepatology (JSH) 2010 uptdated version. *Dig. Dis.* 2011; 29: 339-364.

[7]   Lin S, Hoffmann K, Schemmer P. Treatment of hepatocellular carcinoma: A systematic review. *Liver Cancer* 2012; 1: 144-158.

[8]   Vivarelli M, Nontalti R, Risaliti A. Multimodal treatment of hepatocellular carcinoma: An update. *World J. Gastroenterol.* 2013; 19(42): 7316-7326.

[9]   Chen TW, Chu CM, Yu JC, Chen CJ, Chan DC, Liu YC, et al., Comparison of clinical staging systems in predicting survival of hepatocellular carcinoma patients receiving major or minor hepatectomy. *Eur. J. Surg. Oncol.* 2007; 33: 480–487.

[10]   Kondo K, Chijiiwa K, Nagano M, Hiyoshi M, Kai M, Maehara N, et al., Comparison of seven prognostic staging systems in patients who undergo hepatectomy for hepatocellular carcinoma. *Hepatogastroenterology* 2007; 54: 1534–1538.

[11]   Guglielmi A, Ruzzenente A, Pachera S, Valdegamberi A, Sandri M, D'Onofrio M, et al., Comparison of seven staging systems in cirrhotic patients with hepatocellular carcinoma in a cohort of patients who underwent radiofrequency ablation with complete response. *Am. J. Gastroenterol.* 2008; 103: 597–604.

[12]   Cho YK, Chung JW, Kim JK, Ahn YS, Kim MY, Park YO, et al., Comparison of 7 staging systems for patients with hepatocellular carcinoma undergoing transarterial embolization. *Cancer* 2008; 112: 352-361.

[13]   Collette S, Bonnetain F, Paoletti X, Doffoel M, Bouché O, Raoul JL, et al., Prognosis of advanced hepatocellular carcinoma: comparison of three staging systems in two French clinical trials. *Ann. Oncol.* 2008; 19: 1117–1126.

[14]   Cammà C, Di Marco V, Cabibbo G, Latteri F, Sandonato L, Parisi P, et al., Survival of patients with hepatocellular carcinoma in cirrhosis: a comparison of BCLC, CLIP and GRETCH staging systems. *Aliment Pharmacol. Ther.* 2008; 28: 62–75.

[15]   Lu W, Dong J, Huang Z, Guo D, Liu Y, Shi S. Comparison of four current staging systems for Chinese patients with hepatocellular carcinoma undergoing curative resection: Okuda, CLIP, TNM and CUPI. *J. Gastroenterol. Hepatol.* 2008; 23: 1874–1878.

[16]   Chung H, Kudo M, Takahashi S, Hagiwara S, Sakaguchi Y, Inoue T, et al., Comparison of three current staging systems for hepatocellular carcinoma: Japan integrated staging

score, new Barcelona Clinic Liver Cancer staging classification, and Tokyo score. *J. Gastroenterol. Hepatol.* 2008; 23: 445–452.

[17] Zhang XF, Qi X, Meng B, Liu C, Yu L, Wang B, et al., Prognosis evaluation in alpha-fetoprotein negative hepatocellular carcinoma after hepatectomy: comparison of five staging systems. *Eur. J. Surg. Oncol.* 2010; 36: 718–724.

[18] Huitzil-Melendez FD, Capanu M, O'Reilly EM, Duffy A, Gansukh B, Saltz LL, et al., Advanced hepatocellular carcinoma: which staging systems best predict prognosis? *J. Clin. Oncol.* 2010; 28: 2889–2895.

[19] Hsu CY, Hsia CY, Huang YH, Su CW, Lin HC, Lee PC, et al., Selecting an optimal staging system for hepatocellular carcinoma: comparison of 5 currently used prognostic models. *Cancer* 2010; 116: 3006–3014.

[20] Kawaoka T, Aikata H, Takaki S, Hashimoto Y, Katamura Y, Hiramatsu A, et al., Transcatheter chemoembolization for unresectable hepatocellular carcinoma and comparison of five staging systems. *Hepatol. Res.* 2010; 40: 1082–1091.

[21] Chan SL, Mo FK, Johnson PJ, Liem GS, Chan TC, Poon MC, et al., Prospective validation of the Chinese University Prognostic Index and comparison with other staging systems for hepatocellular carcinoma in an Asian population. *J. Gastroenterol. Hepatol.* 2011; 26: 340–347.

[22] Sirivatanauksorn Y, Tovikkai C. Comparison of staging systems of hepatocellular carcinoma. *HPB Surg.* 2011; 2011: 818217.

[23] Kim BK, Kim SU, Park JY, Kim do Y, Ahn SH, Park MS, et al., Applicability of BCLC stage for prognostic stratification in comparison with other staging systems: single centre experience from long-term clinical outcomes of 1717 treatment-naive patients with hepatocellular carcinoma. *Liver Int.* 2012; 32: 1120–1127.

[24] Mazzaferro V, Regalia E, Doci R, Andreola S, Pulvirenti A, Bozzetti F, et al., Liver transplantation for the treatment of small hepatocellular carcinomas in patients with cirrhosis. *N. Engl. J. Med.* 1996; 334: 693-699.

[25] Roayaie S, Obeidat K, Sposito C, Mariani L, Bhoori S, Pellegrinelli A, et al., Resection of hepatocellular cancer <= 2 cm: results from two western centers. *Hepatology* 2013; 57(4): 1426-1435.

[26] Kudo M. Radiofrequency ablation for hepatocellular carcinoma: updated review in 2010. *Oncology* 2010; 78(suppl 1): 113-124.

[27] Lencioni R. Loco-regional treatment of hepatocellular carcinoma. *Hepatology* 2010; 52: 762-773.

[28] Cho YK, Kim JK, Rhim H, Han JK. Systemic review of randomized trials for hepatocellular carcinoma treated with percutaneous ablation techniques. *Hepatology* 2009; 49: 453-459.

[29] Kuang M, Xie XY, Huang C, Wang Y, Lin MX, Xu ZF, et al., Long-term outcome of percutaneous ablation in very early-stage hepatocellular carcinoma. *J. Gastrointest. Surg.* 2011; 15: 2165–2171.

[30] Livraghi T, Meloni F, Di Stasi M, Rolle E, Solbiati L, Tinelli C, et al., Sustained complete response and complications rates after radiofrequency ablation of very early hepatocellular carcinoma in cirrhosis: Is resection still the treatment of choice? *Hepatology* 2008; 47: 82–89.

[31] Wang JH, Wang CC, Hung CH, Chen CL, Lu SN. Survival comparison between surgical resection and radiofrequency ablation for patients in BCLC very early/early stage hepatocellular carcinoma. *J. Hepatol.* 2012; 56: 412–418.

[32] Cho YK, Kim JK, Kim WT, Chung JW. Hepatic resection versus radiofrequency ablation for very early stage hepatocellular carcinoma: a Markov model analysis. *Hepatology* 2010; 51: 1284–1290.

[33] Peng ZW, Lin XJ, Zhang YJ, Liang HH, Guo RP, Shi M, et al., Radiofrequency ablation versus hepatic resection for the treatment of hepatocellular carcinomas 2 cm or smaller: a retrospective comparative study. *Radiology* 2012; 262: 1022-1033.

[34] Kudo M. Japan's successful model of nationwide hepatocellular carcinoma surveillance highlighting the urgent need for global surveillance. *Liver Cancer* 2012; 1: 141-143.

[35] Sarasin FP, Majno PE, Llovet JM, Bruix J, Mentha G, Hadengue A. Living donor liver transplantation for early hepatocellular carcinoma: A life-expectancy and cost-effectiveness perspective. *Hepatology* 2001; 33: 1073–1079.

[36] Farinati F, Sergio A, Baldan A, Giacomin A, Di Nolfo MA, Del Poggio P, et al., Early and very early hepatocellular carcinoma: when and how much do staging and choice of treatment really matter ? A multi-center study. *BMC Cancer* 2009; 9: 33 doi:10.1186/1471-2407-9-33.

[37] Llovet JM, Schwartz M, Mazzaferro V. Resection and liver transplantation for hepatocellular carcinoma. *Semin Liver Dis* 2005; 25: 181–200.

[38] Chen MS, Li JQ, Zheng Y, Guo RP, Liang HH, Zhang YQ, et al., A prospective randomized trial comparing percutaneous local ablative therapy and partial hepatectomy for small hepatocellular carcinoma. *Ann. Surg.* 2006; 243: 321-328.

[39] Feng K, Yan J, Li X, Xia F, Ma K, Wang S, Bie P, Dong J. A randomized controlled trial of radiofrequency ablation and surgical resection in the treatment of small hepatocellular carcinoma. *J. Hepatol.* 2012: 57(4):794-802.

[40] Fang Y, Chen W, Liang X, Li D, Lou H, Chen R, Wang K, Pan H. Comparison of long-term effectiveness and complications of radiofrequency ablation with hepatectomy for small hepatocellular carcinoma. *J. Gastroenterol. Hepatol.* 2014; 29(1): 193-200.

[41] Huang J, Yan L, Cheng Z, Wu H, Du L, Wang J, et al., A randomized trial comparing radiofrequency ablation and surgical resection for HCC conforming to the Milan criteria. *Ann. Surg.* 2010; 252: 903-912.

[42] Zhou Y, Xhao Y, Xu D, Yin Z, Xie F, Yang J. Meta-analysis of radiofrequency ablation versus hepatic resection for small hepatocellular carcinoma. *BMC Gastroenterology.* 2010; 10:78.

[43] Li L, Zhang J, Liu X, Li X, Jiao B, Kang T. Clinical outcomes of radiofrequency ablation and surgical resection for small hepatocellular carcinoma: a meta-analysis. *J. Gastroenterol. Hepatol* 2012; 27: 51–58.

[44] Duan C, Liu M, Zhang Z, Ma K, Bie P. Radiofrequency ablation versus hepatic resection for the treatment of early-stage hepatocellular carcinoma meeting Milan criteria: a systematic review and meta-analysis. *World J. Surg. Oncol.* 2013; 11: 190.

[45] Qi X, Tang Y, An D, Bai M, Shi X, Wang J, Han G, Fan D. Radiofrequency ablation versus hepatic resection for small hepatocellular Carcinoma: A meta-analysis of randomized controlled trials. *J. Clin. Gastroenterol.* 2013 Oct 28. [Epub ahead of print].

[46] Cho YK, Rhim H, Noh S. Radiofrequency ablation versus surgical resection as primary treatment of hepatocellular carcinoma meeting Milan criteria: a systematic review. *J. Gastroenterol. Hepatol* 2011; 26: 1354-1360.

[47] Chiba T, Tokuuye K, Matsuzaki Y, Sugahara S, Chuganji Y, Kagei K, et al., Proton beam therapy for hepatocellular carcinoma: a retrospective review of 162 patients. *Clin. Cancer Res.* 2005; 11: 3799–3805.

[48] Nakayama H, Sugahara S, Tokita M, Fukuda K, Mizumoto M, Abei M, et al., Proton beam therapy for hepatocellular carcinoma: the university of Tsukuba experience. *Cancer* 2009; 115: 5499–5506.

[49] Hata M, Tokuuye K, Sugahara S, Tohno E, Nakayama H, Fukumitsu N, et al., Proton beam therapy for aged patients with hepatocellular carcinoma. *Int. J. Rad. Oncol. Biol. Phys.* 2007; 69: 805–812.

[50] Hata M, Tokuuye K, Sugahara S, Fukumitsu N, Hashimoto T, Ohnishi K, et al., Proton beam therapy for hepatocellular carcinoma with limited treatment options. *Cancer* 2006; 107: 591–598.

[51] Hata M, Tokuuye K, Sugahara S, Fukumitsu N, Hashimoto T, Ohnishi K, et al., Proton beam therapy for hepatocellular carcinoma patients with severe cirrhosis. *Strahlenther Onko* 2006; 182: 713–720.

[52] Lencioni R. Chemoembolization in patients with hepatocellular carcinoma. *Liver Cancer* 2012; 1: 41-50.

[53] Takayasu K, Arii S, Ikai I, Omata M, Okita K, Ichida T, et al., Prospective cohort study of transarterial chemoembolization for unresectable hepatocellular carcinoma in 8510 patients. *Gastroenterology* 2006; 131: 461-469.

[54] Lin DY, Liaw YF, Lee TY, Lai CM. Hepatic arterial embolization in patients with unresectable hepatocellular catcinoma- a randomized of controlled trial. *Gastroenterology* 1988; 94: 453-456.

[55] Pelletier G, Roche A, Ink O, Anciaux ML, Derhy S, Rougier P, et al., A randomized trial of hepatic arterial embilization in patients with unresectable hepatocellular carcinoma. *J. Hepatol.* 1990; 11: 181-184.

[56] Groue d'TEtude et de Traitement du Carcinome Hepatocellulaire. A comparison of lipiodol chemoembolization and conservative treatment for unresectable hepatocellular carcinoma. *N. Engl. J. Med.* 1995; 332: 1256-1261.

[57] Bruix J, Llovet JM, Castells A, Montañá X, Brú C, Ayuso MC, et al., Transarterial embolization versus symptomatic treatment in patients with advanced hepatocellular carcinoma: results of a randomized controlled trial in a single institution. *Hepatology* 1998; 27: 1578-1583.

[58] Pelletier G, Ducreux M, Gay F, et al., Treatment with lipiodol chemoembilization: a multicenter randomized trial. *J. Hepatol.* 1998; 29: 129-134.

[59] Lo CM, Ngan H, Tso WK, Liu CL, Lam CM, Poon RT, et al., Randomized controlled trial of transarterial lipiodol chemoembolization for unresectable hepatocellular carcinoma. *Hepatology* 2002; 35: 1164–1171.

[60] Llovet JM, Real MI, Montaña X, Planas R, Coll S, Aponte J, et al., Arterial embolisation or chemoembolisation versus symptomatic treatment in patients with unresectable hepatocellular carcinoma: a randomised controlled trial. *Lancet* 2002; 359: 1734-1739.

[61] Llovet JM, Bruix J. Systematic review of randomized trials for unresectable hepatocellular carcinioma: chemoembolization improves survival. *Hepatology* 2002; 35: 1164–1171.

[62] Kudo M, Han KH, Kokudo N, Cheng AL, Choi BI, Furuse J, et al., Liver Cancer Working Group report. *Jpn J. Clin. Oncol.* 2010; 40(Suppl 1): i19–i27.

[63] Vitale A, Saracino E, Boccagni P, Brolese A, D'Amico F, Gringeri E, et al., Validation of the BCLC prognostic system in surgical hepatocellular cancer patients. *Transplant Proc.* 2009; 41: 1260–1263.

[64] Chen XP, Qiu FZ, Wu ZD, Zhang BX. Hepatectomy for huge hepatocellular carcinoma in 634 cases. *World J. Gastroenterol.* 2006; 12: 4652–4655.

[65] Llovet JM, Ricci S, Mazzaferro V, Hilgard P, Gane E, Blanc JF, et al., Sorafenib in advanced hepatocellular carcinoma. *N. Engl. J. Med.* 2008; 359: 378–390.

[66] Cheng AL, Kang YK, Chen Z, Tsao CJ, Qin S, Kim JS, et al., Efficacy and safety of sorafenib in patients in the Asia-Pacific region with advanced hepatocellular carcinoma: a phase III randomised, double-blind, placebo-controlled trial. *Lancet Oncol.* 2009; 10: 25–34.

[67] Kudo M. Treatment of advanced hepatocellular carcinoma with emphasis on hepatic arterial infusion chemotherapy and molecular targeted therapy. *Liver Cancer* 2012; 1 : 62-70.

[68] Sugahara S, Nakayama H, Fukuda K, Mizumoto M, Tokita M, Abei M, et al., Proton-beam therapy for hepatocellular carcinoma associated with portal vein tumor thrombosis. *Strahlenther Onkol.* 2009; 185: 782–788.

[69] Klein J, Dawson LA. Hepatocellular carcinoma radiation therapy: review of evidence and future opportunities. *Int. J. Radiat. Oncol. Biol. Phys.* 2013; 87: 22-32.

[70] Taura K, Ikai I, Hatano E, Yasuchika K, Nakajima A, Tada M, et al., Influence of coexisting cirrhosis on outcomes after partial hepatic resection for hepatocellular carcinoma fulfilling the Milan criteria: an analysis of 293 patients. *Surgery* 2007; 142: 685–694.

[71] Young AL, Adair R, Prasad KR, Toogood GJ, Lodge JP. Hepatocellular carcinoma within a noncirrhotic, nonfibrotic, seronegative liver: surgical approaches and outcomes. *J. Am. Coll. Surg.* 2012;214:174–183.

[72] Zhou XD, Tang ZY, Yang BH, Lin ZY, Ma ZC, Ye SL, et al., Experience of 1000 patients who underwent hepatectomy for small hepatocellular carcinoma. *Cancer* 2001;91:1479–1486.

[73] Poon RT, Fan ST, Lo CM, et al., Long-term survival and pattern of recurrence after resection of small hepatocellular carcinoma in patients with preserved liver function: implications for a strategy of salvage transplantation. *Ann. Surg.* 2002;235:373–382.

[74] Lee KK, Kim DG, Moon IS, Lee MD, Park JH. Liver transplantation versus liver resection for the treatment of hepatocellular carcinoma. *J. Surg. Oncol.* 2010;101:47–53.

[75] Fukuda S, Okuda K, Imamura M, Imamura I, Eriguchi N, Aoyagi S. Surgical resection combined with chemotherapy for advanced hepatocellular carcinoma with tumor thrombus: report of 19 cases. *Surgery* 2002;131:300–310.

[76] Yang T, Lin C, Zhai J, Shi S, Zhu M, Zhu N, et al., Surgical resection for advanced hepatocellular carcinoma according to Barcelona Clinic Liver Cancer (BCLC) staging. *J. Cancer Res. Clin. Oncol.* 2012; 138: 1121–1129.

[77] Ishizawa T, Hasegawa K, Aoki T, Takahashi M, Inoue Y, Sano K, et al., Neither multiple tumors nor portal hypertension are surgical contraindications for hepatocellular carcinoma. *Gastroenterology* 2008; 134: 1908–1916.

[78] Ng KK, Vauthey JN, Pawlik TM, Lauwers GY, Regimbeau JM, Belghiti J, et al., Is hepatic resection for large or multinodular hepatocellular carcinoma justified? Results from a multi-institutional database. *Ann. Surg. Oncol.* 2005; 12: 364–373.

[79] Jarnagin WR. Management of small hepatocellular carcinoma: a review of transplantation, resection, and ablation. *Ann. Surg. Oncol.* 2010; 17: 1226–1233.

[80] Breitenstein S, Apestegui C, Petrowsky H, Clavien PA. "State of the art" in liver resection and living donor liver transplantation: a worldwide survey of 100 liver centers. *World J. Surg.* 2009; 33: 797–803.

[81] Thakrar PD, Madoff DC. Preoperative portal vein embolization: an approach to improve the safety of major hepatic resection. *Semin. Roentgenol.* 2011; 46: 142–153.

[82] Farges O, Belghiti J, Kianmanesh R, Regimbeau JM, Santoro R, Vilgrain V, et al., Portal vein embolization before right hepatectomy: prospective clinical trial. *Ann. Surg.* 2003; 237: 208–217.

[83] Hanazaki K, Kajikawa S, Shimozawa N, Mihara M, Shimada K, Hiraguri M, et al., Survival and recurrence after hepatic resection of 386 consecutive patients with hepatocellular carcinoma. *J. Am. Coll. Surg.* 2000; 191: 381–388.

[84] Portolani N, Coniglio A, Ghidoni S, Giovanelli M, Benetti A, Tiberio GA, et al., Early and late recurrence after liver resection for hepatocellular carcinoma: prognostic and therapeutic implications. *Ann. Surg.* 2006; 243: 229–235.

[85] Kudo M. Adjuvant therapy after curative treatment for hepatocellular carcinoma. *Oncology* 2011; 81(Suppl 1):50–55.

[86] Chan AC, Poon RT, Cheung TT, Chok KS, Chan SC, Fan ST, et al., Survival analysis of re-resection versus radiofrequency ablation for intrahepatic recurrence after hepatectomy for hepatocellular carcinoma. *World J. Surg.* 2012;36:151–156.

[87] Del Gaudio M, Ercolani G, Ravaioli M, Cescon M, Lauro A, Vivarelli M, et al., Liver transplantation for recurrent hepatocellular carcinoma on cirrhosis after liver resection: University of Bologna experience. *Am. J. Transplant* 2008; 8: 1177–1185.

[88] Yokoyama I, Sheahan DG, Carr B, Kakizoe S, Selby R, Tzakis AG, et al., Clinicopathologic factors affecting patient survival and tumor recurrence after orthotopic liver transplantation for hepatocellular carcinoma. *Transplant Proc.* 1991; 23: 2194–2196.

[89] Ringe B, Pichlmayr R, Wittekind C, Tusch G. Surgical treatment of hepatocellular carcinoma: experience with liver resection and transplantation in 198 patients. *World J. Surg.* 1991; 15: 270–285.

[90] Iwatsuki S, Starzl TE, Sheahan DG, Yokoyama I, Demetris AJ, Todo S, et al., Hepatic resection versus transplantation for hepatocellular carcinoma. *Ann. Surg.* 1991; 214: 221–228, discussion 228–229.

[91] Poon RT, Fan ST, Lo CM, Liu CL, Wong J. Difference in tumor invasiveness in cirrhotic patients with hepatocellular carcinoma fulfilling the Milan criteria treated by resection and transplantation: impact on long-term survival. *Ann. Surg.* 2007; 245: 51–58.

[92] Mazzaferro V, Bhoori S, Sposito C, Bongini M, Langer M, Miceli R, Mariani L. Millan criteria in liver transplantation for hepatocellular carcinoma: an evidence-based analysis of 15 years of experience. *Liver Transpl.* 2011; 17: Supple 2: S44-S57.

[93] Mazzaferro V, Llovet JM, Miceli R, Bhoori S, Schiavo M, Mariani L, et al., Predicting survival after liver transplantation in patients with hepatocellular carcinoma beyond the Milan criteria: a retrospective, exploratory analysis. *Lancet Oncol.* 2009; 10: 35–43.

[94] Sauer P, Kraus TW, Schemmer P, Mehrabi A, Stremmel W, Buechler MW, et al., Liver transplantation for hepatocellular carcinoma: is there evidence for expanding the selection criteria ? *Transplantation* 2005; 80: S105–S108.

[95] Yao FY, Kerlan RK Jr, Hirose R, Davern TJ 3rd, Bass NM, Feng S, et al., Excellent outcome following down-staging of hepatocellular carcinoma prior to liver transplantation: an intention-to-treat analysis. *Hepatology* 2008; 48: 819–827.

[96] Chapman WC, Majella Doyle MB, Stuart JE, Vachharajani N, Crippin JS, Anderson CD, et al., Outcomes of neoadjuvant transarterial chemoembolization to downstage hepatocellular carcinoma before liver transplantation. *Ann. Surg.* 2008; 248: 617–625.

[97] Heckman JT, Devera MB, Marsh JW, Fontes P, Amesur NB, Holloway SE, et al., Bridging locoregional therapy for hepatocellular carcinoma prior to liver transplantation. *Ann. Surg. Oncol.* 2008;15:3169–3177.

[98] Llovet JM, Mas X, Aponte JJ, Fuster J, Navasa M, Christensen E, et al., Cost effectiveness of adjuvant therapy for hepatocellular carcinoma during the waiting list for liver transplantation. *Gut* 2002; 50: 123–128.

[99] DuBay DA, Sandroussi C, Kachura JR, Ho CS, Beecroft JR, Vollmer CM, et al., Radiofrequency ablation of hepatocellular carcinoma as a bridge to liver transplantation. *HPB (Oxford)* 2011; 13: 24–32.

[100] Hashikura Y, Makuuchi M, Kawasaki S, Matsunami H, Ikegami T, Nakazawa Y, et al., Successful living-related partial liver transplantation to an adult patient. *Lancet* 1994; 343: 1233–1234.

[101] Sugawara Y, Makuuchi M. Living donor liver transplantation: present status and recent advances. *Br. Med. Bull.* 2005; 75–76: 15–28.

[102] Sandhu L, Sandroussi C, Guba M, Selzner M, Ghanekar A, Cattral MS, et al., Living donor liver transplantation versus deceased donor liver transplantation for hepatocellular carcinoma: comparable survival and recurrence. *Liver Transpl.* 2012;18:315– 322.

[103] Wiesner RH, Freeman RB, Mulligan DC. Liver transplantation for hepatocellular cancer: the impact of the MELD allocation policy. *Gastroenterology* 2004; 127: S261–S267.

[104] Dutkowski P, Oberkofler CE, Slankamenac K, Puhan MA, Schadde E, Müllhaupt B, et al., Are there better guidelines for allocation in liver transplantation? A novel score targeting justice and utility in the model for end-stage liver disease era. *Ann. Surg.* 2011; 254: 745–753.

[105] Lencioni R, Llovet JM. Modified RECIST (mRECIST) assessment for hepatocellular carcinoma. *Semin. Liver Dis.* 2010; 30:52-60.

[106] Ohnishi K, Yoshioka H, Ito S, Fujiwara K. Prospective randomized controlled trial comparing percutaneous acetic acid injection and percutaneous ethanol injection for small hepatocellular carcinoma. *Hepatology* 1998; 27: 67-72.

[107] Huo TI, Huang YH, Wu JC, Lee PC, Chang FY, Lee SD. Comparison of percutaneous acetic acid injection and percutaneous ethanol injection for hepatocellular carcinoma in cirrhotic patients: a prospective study. *Scand. J. Gastroenterol.* 2003; 38: 770-778.

[108] Lin SM, Lin CJ, Lin CC, Hsu CW, Chen YC. Randomised controlled trial comparing percutaneous radiofrequency thermal ablation, percutaneous ethanol injection, and percutaneous acetic acid injection to treat hepatocellular carcinoma of 3 cm or less. *Gut* 2005; 54: 1151-1156.

[109] Germani G, Pleguezuelo M, Gurusamy K, Meyer T, Isgrò G, Burroughs AK. Clinical outcomes of radiofrequency ablation, percutaneous alcohol and acetic acid injection for hepatocelullar carcinoma: a meta-analysis. *J. Hepatol.* 2010; 52(3): 380-388.

[110] Simon CJ, Dupuy DE, Mayo-Smith WW. Microwave ablation: principles and applications. *Radiographics* 2005; 25 Suppl 1: S69-S83.

[111] Bertot LC, Sato M, Tateishi R, Yoshida H, Koike K. Mortality and complication rates of percutaneous ablative techniques for the treatment of liver tumors: a systematic review. *Eur. Radiol.* 2011; 21: 2584-2596.

[112] Liang P, Wang Y, Yu X, Dong B. Malignant liver tumors: treatment with percutaneous microwave ablation - complications among cohort of 1136 patients. *Radiology* 2009; 251: 933-940.

[113] Shibata T, Iimuro Y, Yamamoto Y, Maetani Y, Ametani F, Itoh K, et al., Small hepatocellular carcinoma: cpmparison of radio-frequency ablation and perqutaneous microwave coagulation therapy. *Radiology* 2002; 223: 331-337.

[114] Lencioni R, Cioni D, Crocetti L, Franchini C, Pina CD, Lera J, et al., Early-stage hepatocellular carcinoma in patients with cirrhosis: long-term results of percutaneous image-guided radiofrequency ablation. *Radiology* 2005; 234: 961-967.

[115] Tateishi R, Shiina S, Teratani T, Obi S, Sato S, Koike Y, et al., Percutaneous radiofrequency ablation for hepatocellular carcinoma. *Cancer* 2005; 103: 1201-1209.

[116] Choi D, Lim HK, Rhim H, Kim YS, Lee WJ, Paik SW, et al., Percutaneous radiofrequency ablation for early-stage hepatocellular carcinoma as a first-line treatment: long-term results and prognostic factors in a larger single-institution series. *Eur. Radiol.* 2007; 17: 684-692.

[117] N'Kontchou G, Mahamoudi A, Aout M, Ganne-Carrie N, zGrando V, Coderc E, et al., Radiofrequency ablation of hepatocellular carcinoma: long-term results and prognostic factors in 235 Western patients with cirrhosis. *Hepatology* 2009; 50: 1475-1483.

[118] Lencioni R, Allgaier HP, Cioni D, Olschewski M, Deibert P, Crocetti L, et al., Small hepatocellular carcinoma in cirrhosis: randomized comparison of radiofrequency thermal ablation versus percutaneous ethanol injection. *Radiology* 2003; 228: 235-240.

[119] Lin SM, Lin CJ, Lin CC, Hsu CW, Chen YC. Radiofrequency ablation improves prognosis compared with ethanol injection for hepatocellular carcinoma < or 4 cm. *Gastroenterology* 2004; 127: 1714-1723.

[120] Shiina S, Teratani T, Obi S, Sato S, Tateishi R, Fujishima T, et al., A randomized controlled trial of radiofrequency ablation versus ethanol injection for small hepatocellular carcinoma. *Gastroenterology* 2005; 129: 122-130.

[121] Brunello F, Veltri A, Carucci P, Pagano E, Ciccone G, Moretto P, et al., Radiofrequency ablation versus ethanol injection for early hepatocellular carcinoma: a randomized controlled trial. *Scand. J. Gastroenterol.* 2008; 43: 727-735.

[122] Orlando A, Leandro G, Olivo M, Andriulli A, Cottone M. Radiofrequency thermal ablation vs. percutaneous ethanol injection for small hepatocellular carcinoma in cirrhosis: meta-analysis of randomized controlled trials. *Am. J. Gastroenterol.* 2009; 104: 514–524.

[123] Vivarelli M, Guglielmi A, Ruzzenente A, Cucchetti A, Bellusci R, Cordiano C, et al., Surgical resection versus percutaneous radiofrequency ablation in the treatment of hepatocellular carcinoma on cirrhotic liver. *Ann. Surg.* 2004; 240: 102-107.

[124] Imai K, Beppu T, Chikamoto A, Doi K, Okabe H, Hayashi H, et al., Comparison between hepatic resection and radiofrequency ablation as first-line treatment for solitary small-sized hepatocellular carcinoma of 3 cm or less. *Hepatol. Res.* 2013; 43: 853-864.

[125] Parisi A, Desiderio J, Trastulli S, Castellani E, Pasquale R, Cirocchi R, et al., Liver resection versus radiofrequency ablation in the treatment of cirrhotic patients with hepatocellular carcinoma. *Hepatobiliary Pancreat Dis. Int.* 2013; 12: 270-277.

[126] Kitamoto M, Imagawa M, Yamada H, Watanabe C, Sumioka M, Satoh O, et al., Radiofrequency ablation in the treatment of small hepatocellular carcinomas: comparison of the radiofrequency effect with and without chemoembolization. *Am. J. Roentgenol.* 2003; 181: 997–1003.

[127] Yamakado K, Nakatsuka A, Takaki H, Yokoi H, Usui M, Sakurai H, et al., Early-stage hepatocellular carcinoma: radiofrequency ablation combined with chemoembolization versus hepatectomy. *Radiology* 2008; 247: 260–266.

[128] Takaki H, Yamakado K, Uraki J, Nakatsuka A, Fuke H, Yamamoto N, et al., Radiofrequency ablation combined with chemoembolization for the treatment of hepatocellular carcinomas larger than 5 cm. *J. Vasc. Interv. Radiol.* 2009; 20: 217–224.

[129] Kirikoshi H, Saito S, Yoneda M, Fujita K, Mawatari H, Uchiyama T, et al., Outcome of transarterial chemoembolization monotherapy, and in combination with percutaneous ethanol injection, or radiofrequency ablation therapy for hepatocellular carcinoma. *Hepatol. Res.* 2009; 39: 553–562.

[130] Peng ZW, Chen MS, Liang HH, Gao HJ, Zhang YJ, Li JQ, et al., A case control study comparing percutaneous radiofrequency ablation alone or combined with transcatheter arterial chemoembolization for hepatocellular carcinoma. *Eur. J. Surg. Oncol.* 2010; 36: 257–263.

[131] Minami Y, Kudo M, Kawasaki T, Chung H, Ogawa C, Shiozaki H. Percutaneous radiofrequency ablation guided by contrast-enhanced harmonic sonography with artificial pleural effusion for hepatocellular carcinoma in the hepatic dome. *Am. J. Roentgenol* 2004; 182: 1224–1226.

[132] Lee MW, Kim YJ, Park SW, Jeon HJ, Yi JG, Choe WH, et al., Percutaneous radiofrequency ablation of liver dome hepatocellular carcinoma invisible on ultrasonography: a new targeting strategy. *Br. J. Radiol.* 2008; 81: e130–e134.

[133] Wang ZY, Sun WB, Li MY, Zhang XX, Ding XM. Percutaneous extrapulmonary radiofrequency ablation for tumors in the hepatic dome. *Hepatogastroenterology* 2008; 55: 1164–1166.

[134] Rhim H, Lim HK, Kim YS, Choi D. Percutaneous radiofrequency ablation with artificial ascites for hepatocellular carcinoma in the hepatic dome: initial experience. *Am. J. Roentgenol* 2008; 190: 91–98.

[135] Kondo Y, Yoshida H, Tateishi R, Shiina S, Kawabe T, Omata M. Percutaneous radiofrequency ablation of liver cancer in the hepatic dome using the intrapleural fluid infusion technique. *Br. J. Surg* 2008; 95: 996–1004.

[136] Park SY, Tak WY, Jeon SW, Cho CM, Kweon YO, Kim SK, et al., The efficacy of intraperitoneal saline infusion for percutaneous radiofrequency ablation for hepatocellular carcinoma. *Eur. J. Radiol.* 2010; 74: 536–540.

[137] Song I, Rhim H, Lim HK, Kim YS, Choi D. Percutaneous radiofrequency ablation of hepatocellular carcinoma abutting the diaphragm and gastrointestinal tracts with the use of artificial ascites: safety and technical efficacy in 143 patients. *Eur. Radiol.* 2009.

[138] Nakai M, Sato M, Sahara S, Takasaka I, Kawai N, Minamiguchi H, et al., Radiofrequency ablation assisted by real-time virtual sonography and CT for hepatocellular carcinoma undetectable by conventional sonography. *Cardiovasc Intervent Radiol.* 2009; 32: 62–69.

[139] Minami Y, Chung H, Kudo M, Kitai S, Takahashi S, Inoue T, et al., Radiofrequency ablation of hepatocellular carcinoma: value of virtual CT sonography with magnetic navigation. *Am. J. Roentgenol.* 2008; 190:W335–W341.

[140] Minami Y, Kudo M, Chung H, Inoue T, Takahashi S, Hatanaka K, et al., Percutaneous radiofrequency ablation of sonographically unidentifiable liver tumors. Feasibility and usefulness of a novel guiding technique with an integrated system of computed tomography and sonographic images. *Oncology* 2007; 72(suppl 1): 111–116.

[141] Kudo M, Hatanaka K, Maekawa K. Sonazoid-enhanced ultrasound in the diagnosis and treatment of hepatic tumors. *J. Med. Ultrasound* 2008; 16: 130–139.

[142] Kudo M, Hatanaka K, Maekawa K. Defect reperfusion imaging, a newly developed novel technology using Sonazoid in the treatment of hepatocellular carcinoma. *J. Med. Ultrasound* 2008; 16: 169–175.

[143] Minami Y, Kudo M, Chung H, Kawasaki T, Yagyu Y, Shimono T, Shiozaki H. Contrast harmonic sonography-guided radiofrequency ablation therapy versus B-mode sonography in hepatocellular carcinoma: prospective randomized controlled trial. *Am. J. Roentgenol.* 2007; 188: 489–494.

[144] Maruyama H, Takahashi M, Ishibashi H, Okugawa H, Okabe S, Yoshikawa M, Yokosuka O. Ultrasound-guided treatments under low acoustic power contrast harmonic imaging for hepatocellular carcinomas undetected by B-mode ultrasonography. *Liver Int.* 2009; 29: 708–714.

[145] Miyamoto N, Hiramatsu K, Tsuchiya K, Sato Y, Terae S, Shirato H. Sonazoid-enhanced sonography for guiding radiofrequency ablation for hepatocellular carcinoma: better tumor visualization by Kupffer-phase imaging and vascular-phase imaging after reinjection. *Jpn J. Radiol.* 2009; 27: 185–193.

[146] Minami Y, Kudo M, Kawasaki T, Chung H, Ogawa C, Shiozaki H. Treatment of hepatocellular carcinoma with percutaneous radiofrequency ablation: usefulness of contrast harmonic sonography for lesions poorly defined with B-mode sonography. *Am. J. Roentgenol.* 2004; 183: 153–156.

[147] Miyamoto N, Hiramatsu K, Tsuchiya K, Sato Y. Carbon dioxide microbubbles-enhanced sonographically guided radiofrequency ablation: treatment of patients with local progression of hepatocellular carcinoma. *Radiat. Med.* 2008; 26: 92–97.

[148] Lam VW, Ng KK, Chok KS, Cheung TT, Wat J, Fan ST, Poon RT. Safety and efficacy of radiofrequency ablation for periductal hepatocellular carcinoma with intraductal cooling of the central bile duct. *J. Am. Coll. Surg.* 2008; 207:e1–e5.

[149] Ohnishi T, Yasuda I, Nishigaki Y, Hayashi H, Otsuji K, Mukai T, et al., Intraductal chilled saline perfusion to prevent bile duct injury during percutaneous radiofrequency ablation for hepatocellular carcinoma. *J. Gastroenterol. Hepatol.* 2008; 23:e410–e415.

[150] Nakashima Y, Nakashima O, Tanaka M, Okuda K, Nakashima M, Kojiro M. Portal vein invasion and intrahepatic micrometastasis in small hepatocellular carcinoma by gross type. *Hepatol. Res.* 2003; 26: 142–147.

[151] Okusaka T, Okada S, Ueno H, Ikeda M, Shimada K, Yamamoto J, et al., Satellite lesions in patients with small hepatocellular carcinoma with reference to clinicopathologic features. *Cancer* 2002; 95: 1931–1937.

[152] Kudo M. Local ablation therapy for hepatocellular carcinoma: current status and future perspectives. *J. Gastroenterol.* 2004; 39: 205–214.

[153] Zytoon AA, Ishii H, Murakami K, El-Kholy MR, Furuse J, El-Dorry A, El-Malah A. Recurrence- free survival after radiofrequency ablation of hepatocellular carcinoma. A registry report of the impact of risk factors on outcome. *Jpn J. Clin. Oncol.* 2007; 37: 658–672.

[154] Takahashi S, Kudo M, Chung H, Inoue T, Ishikawa E, Kitai S, et al., Initial treatment response is essential to improve survival in patients with hepatocellular carcinoma who underwent curative radiofrequency ablation therapy. *Oncology* 2007; 72(suppl 1):98–103.

[155] Wen YL, Kudo M, Zheng RQ, Minami Y, Chung H, Suetomi Y, et al., Radiofrequency ablation of hepatocellular carcinoma: therapeutic response using contrast-enhanced coded phase-inversion harmonic sonography. *Am. J. Roentgenol.* 2003; 181: 57–63.

[156] Bartolotta TV, Taibbi A, Midiri M, De Maria M. Hepatocellular cancer response to radiofrequency tumor ablation: contrast-enhanced ultrasound. *Abdom. Imaging* 2008; 33: 501–511.

[157] Zhou P, Kudo M, Minami Y, Chung H, Inoue T, Fukunaga T, et al., What is the best time to evaluate treatment response after radiofrequency ablation of hepatocellular carcinoma using contrast-enhanced sonography ? *Oncology* 2007; 72(suppl 1):92–97.

[158] Mori K, Fukuda K, Asaoka H, Ueda T, Kunimatsu A, Okamoto Y, et al., Radiofrequency ablation of the liver: determination of ablative margin at MR imaging with impaired clearance of ferucarbotran – feasibility study. *Radiology* 2009; 251: 557–565.

[159] Goldberg SN, Grassi CJ, Cardella JF, Charboneau JW, Dodd GD, Dupuy DE, et al., Image guided tumor ablation: standardization of terminology and reporting criteria. *J. Vasc. Interv. Radiol.* 2009; 20: S377-S390.

[160] Varela M, Real MI, Burrel M, Forner A, Sala M, Brunet M, et al., Chemoembolization of hepatocellular carcinoma with drug eluting beads: efficacy and doxorubicin pharmacokinetics. *J. Hepatol.* 2007; 46: 474-481.

[161] Burrel M, Reig M, Forner A, Barrufet M, de Lope CR, Tremosini S, et al., Survival of patients with hepatocellular carcinoma treated by transarterial chemoembolisation (TACE) using Drug Eluting Beads. Implications for clinical practice and trial design. *J. Hepatol.* 2012; 56: 1330-1335.

[162] Raoul JL, Sangro B, Forner A, Mazzaferro V, Piscaglia F, Bolondi L, et al., Evolving strategies for the management of intermediate-stage hepatocellular carcinoma: available evidence and expert opinion on the use of transarterial chemoembolization. *Cancer Treat Rev.* 2011; 37: 212-220.

[163] Hawkins MA, Dawson LA. Radiation therapy for hepatocellular carcinoma: from palliation to cure. *Cancer* 2006; 106: 1653-1663.

[164] Merle P, Mornex F, Trepo C. Innovative therapy for hepatocellulaer carcinoma: three-dimensional high-dose photon radiotherapy. *Cancer Letters* 2009; 286: 129-133.

[165] Bujold A, Dawson LA. Stereotsctic radiation therapy and selective internal radiation therapy for hepatocellular carcinoma. *Cancer Radiotherapie* 2011; 54-63.

[166] Park HC, Seong J, Han KH, Chon CY, Moon YM, Suh CO. Dose-response relationship in local radiotherapy for hepatocellular carcinoma. *Int. J. Radiat. Oncol. Biol. Phys..* 2002 Sep 1;54(1):150-5.

[167] Yamada K, Izaki K, Sugimoto K, Mayahara H, Morita Y, Yoden E, et al., Prospective trial of combined transcatheter arterial chemoembolization and three-dimensional conformal radiotherapy for portal vein tumor thrombus in patients with unresectable hepatocellular carcinoma. *Int. J. Radiat. Oncol. Biol. Phys..* 2003; 57: 113-119.

[168] Seong J, Park HC, Han KH, Chon CY, Chu SS, Kim GE, et al., Clinical results of 3-dimensional conformal radiotherapy combined with transarterial chemoembolization for hepatocellular carcinoma in the cirrhotic patients. *Hepatol. Res.* 2003; 27: 30-35.

[169] Li B, Yu J, Wang L, Li C, Zhou T, Zhai L, Xing L. Study of local three-dimensional conformal radiotherapy combined with transcatheter arterial chemoembolization for patients with stage III hepatocellular carcinoma. *Am. J. Clin. Oncol* 2003; 26: e92-9.

[170] Wu DH, Liu L, Chen LH. Therapeutic effects and prognostic factors in three-dimensional conformal radiotherapy combined with transcatheter arterial chemoembolization for hepatocellular carcinoma. *World J. Gastroenterol.* 2004; 10: 2184-2189.

[171] Liu MT, Li SH, Chu TC, Hsieh CY, Wang AY, Chang TH, et al., Three-dimensional conformal radiation therapy for unresectable hepatocellular carcinoma patients who had failed with or were unsuited for transcatheter arterial chemoembolization. *Jpn J. Clin. Oncol* 2004; 34: 532-539.

[172] Ben-Josef E, Normolle D, Ensminger WD, Walker S, Tatro D, Ten Haken RK, Knol J, et al., Phase II trial of high-dose conformal radiation therapy with concurrent hepatic artery floxuridine for unresectable intrahepatic malignancies. *J. Clin. Oncol.* 2005; 23: 8739-8747.

[173] Kim JY, Chung SM, Choi BO, Kay CS. Hepatocellular carcinoma with portal vein tumor thrombosis: Improved treatment outcomes with external beam radiation therapy. *Hepatol. Res.* 2011; 41: 813-824.

[174] Yoon SM, Lim YS, Won HJ, Kim JH, Kim KM, Lee HC, et al., Radiotherapy plus transarterial chemoembolization for hepatocellular carcinoma invading the portal vein: long-term patient outcomes. *Int. J. Radiat. Oncol. Biol. Phys..* 2012; 82: 2004-2011.

[175] Hou JZ, Zeng ZC, Zhang JY, Fan J, Zhou J, Zeng MS. Influence of tumor thrombus location on the outcome of external-beam radiation therapy in advanced hepatocellular carcinoma with macrovascular invasion. *Int. J. Radiat. Oncol. Biol. Phys.* 2012; 84: 362-368.

[176] Murakami E, Aikata H, Miyaki D, Nagaoki Y, Katamura Y, Kawaoka T, et al., Hepatic arterial infusion chemotherapy using 5-fluorouracil and systemic interferon-α for advanced hepatocellular carcinoma in combination with or without three-dimensional conformal radiotherapy to venous tumor thrombosis in hepatic vein or inferior vena cava. *Hepatol. Res.* 2012; 42: 442-453.

[177] Liang SX, Zhu XD, Xu ZY, Zhu J, Zhao JD, Lu HJ, et al., Radiation-induced liver disease in three-dimensional conformal radiation therapy for primary liver carcinoma: the risk factors and hepatic radiation tolerance. *Int. J. Radiat. Oncol. Biol. Phys.* 2006; 65: 426-434.

[178] Mornex F, Girard N, Beziat C, Kubas A, Khodri M, Trepo C, Merle P. Feasibility and efficacy of high-dose three-dimensional-conformal radiotherapy in cirrhotic patients with small-size hepatocellular carcinoma non-eligible for curative therapies--mature results of the French Phase II RTF-1 trial. *Int. J. Radiat. Oncol. Biol. Phys.* 2006; 66: 1152-1158.

[179] Kim TH, Kim DY, Park JW, Kim SH, Choi JI, Kim HB, et al., Dose-volumetric parameters predicting radiation-induced hepatic toxicity in unresectable hepatocellular carcinoma patients treated with three-dimensional conformal radiotherapy. *Int. J. Radiat. Oncol. Biol. Phys.* 2007; 67: 225-231.

[180] Méndez Romero A, Wunderink W, Hussain SM, De Pooter JA, Heijmen BJ, Nowak PC, et al., Stereotactic body radiation therapy for primary and metastatic liver tumors: A single institution phase i-ii study. *Acta Oncol.* 2006; 45: 831-837.

[181] Choi BO, Jang HS, Kang KM, Lee SW, Kang YN, Chai GY, et al., Fractionated stereotactic radiotherapy in patients with primary hepatocellular carcinoma. *Jpn J. Clin. Oncol.* 2006; 36: 154-158.

[182] Wulf J, Guckenberger M, Haedinger U, Oppitz U, Mueller G, Baier K, et al., Stereotactic radiotherapy of primary liver cancer and hepatic metastases. *Acta Oncol.* 2006; 45: 838-847.

[183] Takeda A, Takahashi M, Kunieda E, Takeda T, Sanuki N, Koike Y, et al., Hypofractionated stereotactic radiotherapy with and without transarterial chemoembolization for small hepatocellular carcinoma not eligible for other ablation therapies: Preliminary results for efficacy and toxicity. *Hepatol. Res.* 2008; 38: 60-69.

[184] Tse RV, Hawkins M, Lockwood G, Kim JJ, Cummings B, Knox J, et al., Phase I study of individualized stereotactic body radiotherapy for hepatocellular carcinoma and intrahepatic cholangiocarcinoma. *J. Clin. Oncol.* 2008; 26: 657-64. [Erratum in: J. Clin. Oncol. 2008; 26: 3911-3912].

[185] Louis C, Dewas S, Mirabel X, Lacornerie T, Adenis A, Bonodeau F, Lartigau E. Stereotactic radiotherapy of hepatocellular carcinoma: preliminary results. Preliminary result of stereotactic body radiotherapy as a local salvage treatment for inoperable hepatocellular carcinoma. *Technol Cancer Res. Treat.* 2010; 9: 479-487.

[186] Seo YS, Kim MS, Yoo SY, Cho CK, Choi CW, Kim JH, Han CJ, Park SC, Lee BH, Kim YH, Lee DH. Preliminary result of stereotactic body radiotherapy as a local salvage treatment for inoperable hepatocellular carcinoma. *J. Surg. Oncol.* 2010; 102: 209-214.

[187] Cárdenes HR, Price TR, Perkins SM, Maluccio M, Kwo P, Breen TE, Henderson MA, Schefter TE, Tudor K, Deluca J, Johnstone PA. Phase I feasibility trial of stereotactic

body radiation therapy for primary hepatocellular carcinoma. *Clin. Transl. Oncol.* 2010 ;12: 218-225.

[188] Kwon JH, Bae SH, Kim JY, Choi BO, Jang HS, Jang JW, et al., Long-term effect of stereotactic body radiation therapy for primary hepatocellular carcinoma ineligible for local ablation therapy or surgical resection. Stereotactic radiotherapy for liver cancer. *BMC Cancer.* 2010; 10: 475.

[189] Andolino DL, Johnson CS, Maluccio M, Kwo P, Tector AJ, Zook J, et al., Stereotactic body radiotherapy for primary hepatocellular carcinoma. *Int. J. Radiat. Oncol. Biol. Phys..* 2011; 81: e447-453.

[190] Bujold A, Massey CA, Kim JJ, Brierley J, Cho C, Wong RK, et al., Sequential phase I and II trials of stereotactic body radiotherapy for locally advanced hepatocellular carcinoma. *J. Clin. Oncol.* 2013; 31: 1631-1639.

[191] Kang JK, Kim MS, Cho CK, Yang KM, Yoo HJ, Kim JH, et al., Stereotactic body radiation therapy for inoperable hepatocellular carcinoma as a local salvage treatment after incomplete transarterial chemoembolization. *Cancer* 2012; 118: 5424-5431.

[192] Choi BO, Choi IB, Jang HS, Kang YN, Jang JS, Bae SH, et al., Stereotactic body radiation therapy with or without transarterial chemoembolization for patients with primary hepatocellular carcinoma: preliminary analysis. *BMC Cancer.* 2008; 8: 351.

[193] Schulz-Ertner D, Tsujii H. Particle radiation therapy using proton and heavier beams. *J. Clin. Oncol.* 2007; 25: 953–964.

[194] Matsuzaki Y, Osuga T, Saito Y, Chuganji Y, Tanaka N, Shoda J, et al., A new, effective, and safe therapeutic option using proton irradiation for hepatocellular carcinoma. *Gastroenterology* 1994; 106: 1032–1041.

[195] Ikai I, Kudo M, Arii S, Omata M, Kojiro M, Sakamoto M, et al., Report of the 18th follow-up survey of primary liver cancer in Japan. *Hepatol. Res.* 2010; 40: 1043-1059.

[196] Mizumoto M, Okumura T, Hashimoto T, Fukuda K, Oshiro Y, Fukumitsu N, et al., Evaluation of liver function after proton beam therapy for hepatocellular carcinoma. *Int. J. Radiat. Oncol. Biol. Phys.* 2012; 82: e529–e535.

[197] Sugahara S, Oshiro Y, Nakayama H, Fukuda K, Mizumoto M, Abei M, et al., Proton beam therapy for large hepatocellular carcinoma. *Int. J. Rad. Oncol. Biol. Phys.* 2010; 76: 460–466.

[198] Mizumoto M, Tokuuye K, Sugahara S, Nakayama H, Fukumitsu N, Ohara K, et al., Proton beam therapy for hepatocellular carcinoma adjacent to the porta hepatis. *Int. J. Radiat. Oncol. Biol. Phys.* 2008; 71: 462–467.

[199] Nakayama H, Sugahara S, Fukuda K, Abei M, Shoda J, Sakurai H, et al., Proton beam therapy for hepatocellular carcinoma located adjacent to the alimentary tract. *Int. J. Rad. Oncol. Biol. Phys.* 2011; 80: 992–995.

[200] Fukumitsu N, Sugahara S, Nakayama H, Fukuda K, Mizumoto M, Abei M, et al., A prospective study of hypofractionated proton beam therapy for patients with hepatocellular carcinoma. *Int. J. Radiat. Oncol. Biol. Phys.* 2009; 74: 831–836.

[201] Hashimoto T, Tokuuye K, Fukumitsu N, Igaki H, Hata M, Kagei K, et al., Repeated proton beam therapy for hepatocellular carcinoma. *Int. J. Radiat. Oncol. Biol. Phys.* 2006; 65: 196–202.

[202] Kawashima M, Furuse J, Nishio T, Konishi M, Ishii H, Kinoshita T, et al., Phase II study of radiotherapy employing proton beam for hepatocellular carcinoma. *J. Clin. Oncol* 2005; 23: 1839–1846.

[203] Bush DA, Hillebrand DJ, Slater JM, Slater JD. High-dose proton beam radiotherapy for hepatocellular carcinoma: preliminary results of a phase II trial. *Gastroenterology* 2004; 127: S189–S193.

[204] Bush DA, Kayali Z, Grove R, Slater JD. The safety and efficacy of high-dose proton beam radiotherapy for hepatocellular carcinoma: a phase 2 prospective trial. *Cancer* 2011; 117: 3053–3059.

[205] Komatsu S, Fukumoto T, Demizu Y, Miyawaki D, Terashima K, Sasaki R, et al., Clinical results and risk factors of proton and carbon ion therapy for hepatocellular carcinoma. *Cancer* 2011; 117: 4890–4904.

[206] Lai CL, Wu PC, Chan GC, Lok AS, Lin HJ. Doxorubicin versus no antitumor therapy in inoperable hepatocellular carcinoma. A prospective randomized trial. *Cancer* 1988; 62: 479–483.

[207] Yang TS, Lin YC, Chen JS, Wang HM, Wang CH. Phase II study of gemcitabine in patients with advanced hepatocellular carcinoma. *Cancer* 2000; 89: 750–756.

[208] Fuchs CS, Clark JW, Ryan DP, Kulke MH, Kim H, Earle CC, et al., A phase II trial of gemcitabine in patients with advanced hepatocellular carcinoma. *Cancer* 2002; 94: 3186–3191.

[209] Yeo W, Mok TS, Zee B, Leung TW, Lai PB, Lau WY, et al., A randomized phase III study of doxorubicin versus cisplatin/interferon alpha-2b/doxorubicin/fluorouracil (PIAF) combination chemotherapy for unresectable hepatocellular carcinoma. *J. Natl. Cancer Inst.* 2005; 97: 1532–1538.

[210] Thomas MB, O'Beirne JP, Furuse J, Chan AT, Abou-Alfa G, Johnson P. Systemic therapy for hepatocellular carcinoma: cytotoxic chemotherapy, targeted therapy and immunotherapy. *Ann. Surg. Oncol.* 2008; 15: 1008–1014.

[211] Wilhelm SM, Adnane L, Newell P, Villanueva A, Llovet JM, Lynch M. Preclinical overview of sorafenib, a multikinase inhibitor that targets both Raf and VEGF and PDGF receptor tyrosine kinase signaling. *Mol. Cancer Ther.* 2008; 7: 3129–3140.

[212] Bruix J, Raoul JL, Sherman M, Mazzaferro V, Bolondi L, Craxi A, et al., Efficacy and safety of sorafenib in patients with advanced hepatocellular carcinoma: subanalyses of a phase III trial. *J. Hepatol.* 2012; 57: 821-829.

[213] Ueshima K, Kudo M, Takita M, Nagai T, Tatsumi C, Ueda T, et al., Hepatic arterial infusin chemotherapy using low-dose 5-fluorouracil and cisplatin for advanced hepatocellular carcinoma. *Oncology* 2010; 78: S148-S153.

[214] Gish RG, Lencioni R, Di Bisceglie AM, Raoul JL, Mazzaferro V. Role of the multidisciplinary team in the diagnosis and treatment of hepatocellular carcinoma. *Expert Rev Gastroenterol Hepatol* 2012; 6: 173-185.

[215] Kudo M, Imanaka K, Chida N, Nakachi K, Tak WY, Takayama T, et al., Phase III study of sorafenib after transarterial chemoembolisation in Japanese and Korean patients with unresectable hepatocellular carcinoma. *Eur. J. Cancer* 2011; 47: 2117–2127.

[216] Sansonno D, Lauletta G, Russi S, Conteduca V, Sansonno L, Dammacco F. Transarterial chemoembolization plus sorafenib: a sequential therapeutic scheme for HCV-related intermediate-stage hepatocellular carcinoma: a randomized clinical trial. *Oncologist* 2012; 17: 359–366.

[217] Qu XD, Chen C, Wang J, Yan ZP, Chen JM, Gong GQ, et al., The efficacy of TACE combined sorafenib in advanced stages hepatocellullar carcinoma. *BMC Cancer* 2012; 12: 263.

[218] Hoffmann K, Glimm H, Radeleff B, Richter G, Heining C, Schenkel I, et al., Prospective, randomized, double-blind, multi-center, Phase III clinical study on transarterial chemoembolization (TACE) combined with Sorafenib versus TACE plus placebo in patients with hepatocellular cancer before liver transplantation – HeiLivCa [ISRCTN24081794]. *BMC Cancer 2008*; 8: 349.

[219] Kudo M. Signaling pathway/molecular targets and new targeted agents under development in hepatocellular carcinoma. *World J. Gastroenterol.* 2012; 18(42): 6005-6017.

[220] Shin JW, Chung Y-H. Molecular targeted therapy for hepatocellular carcinoma. *World J. Gastroenterol.* 2013;19: 6144-6155.

[221] Faivre S, Raymond E, Boucher E, Douillard J, Lim HY, Kim JS, et al., Safety and efficacy of sunitinib in patients with advanced hepatocellular carcinoma: an open-label, multicentre, phase II study. *Lancet Oncol.* 2009; 10: 794-800.

[222] Cheng AL, Kang YK, Lin DY, Park JW, Kudo M, Qin S, et al., Sunitinib versus sorafenib in advanced hepatocellular cancer: results of a randomized phase II trial. *J. Clin. Oncol.* 2013; 31: 4067-4075.

[223] Park JW, Finn RS, Kim JS, Karwal M, Li RK, Ismail F, et al., Phase II, open-label study of brivanib as first-line therapy in patients with advanced hepatocellular carcinoma. *Clin. Cancer Res.* 2011; 17: 1973-1983.

[224] Finn RS, Kang YK, Mulcahy M, Polite BN, Lim HY, Walters I, et al., Phase II, open-label study of brivanib as second-line therapy in patients with advanced hepatocellular carcinoma. *Clin. Cancer Res.* 2012; 18: 2090-2098.

[225] Johnson PJ, Qin S, Park JW, Poon RT, Raol JL, Philip PA, et al., Brivanib versus sorafenib as first-line therapy in patients in patients with unresectable, advanced hepatocellular carcinoma: results from the randomized phase III BRISK-FL study. *J. Clin. Oncol.* 2013; 31: 3517-3524.

[226] Llovet JM, Decaens T, Raoul JL, Boucher E, Kudo M, Chang C, et al., Brivanib in patients with advanced hepatocellular carcinoma who were intolerant to sorafenib or for whom sorafenib failed: results from the randomized phase III BRISK-PS study. *J. Clin. Oncol* 2013; 31(28): 3509-3516.

[227] Yau T, Chan P, Pang R, Ng K, Fan ST, Poon RT. Phase 1-2 trial of PTK787/ZK222584 combined with intravenous doxorubicin for treatment of patients with advanced hepatocellular carcinoma: implication for antiangiogenic approach to hepatocellular carcinoma. *Cancer* 2010; 116: 5022-5029.

[228] Toh HC, Chen PJ, Carr BI, Knox JJ, Gill S, Ansell P, et al., Phase 2 trial of linifanib (ABT-869) in patients with unresectable or metastatic hepatocellular carcinoma. *Cancer* 2013; 119: 380-387.

[229] Alberts SR, Fitch TR, Kim GP, Morlan BW, Dakhil SR, Gross HM, et al., Cediranib (AZD2171) in patients with advanced hepatocellular carcinoma: a phase II North Central Cancer Treatment Group Clinical Trial. *Am. J. Clin. Oncol.* 2012; 35: 329-333.

[230] Zhu AX, Stuart K, Blaszkowsky LS, Muzikansky A, Reitberg DP, Clark JW, et al., Phase 2 study of cetuximab in patients with advanced hepatocellular carcinoma. *Cancer* 2007; 110: 581-589.

[231] Zhu AX, Rosmorduc O, Evans J, Ross P, Santoro A, Carrilho FJ, et al., SEARCH: a phase III, randomized, double-blind, placebo-controlled trial of sorafenib plus erlotinib in patients with hepatocellular carcinoma (HCC). *Ann. Oncol.* 2012; 23: Abstract LBA2.

[232] Ramanathan RK, Belani CP, Singh DA, Tanaka M, Lenz HJ, Yen Y, et al., A phase II study of lapatinib in patients with advanced biliary tree and hepatocellular cancer. *Cancer Chemother Pharmacol.* 2009; 64: 777-783.

[233] Abou-Alfa GK, Gansukh B, Chou JF, Shia J, Capanu M, Kalin M, et al., Phase II study of Cixutumumab (IMC-A12, NSC742460; C) in hepatocellular carcinoma. *J. Clin. Oncol.* 2011; 29: Abstract 4043.

[234] Choo S, Ng Q, Chen W, Tham C, Yong W, Wang L, et al., A phase I/II study of AZD6244 in combination with sorafenib in advanced hepatocellular carcinoma. *J. Clin. Oncol.* 2012; 30: A4100.

[235] Zhu AX, Abrams TA, Miksad R, Blaszkowsky LS, Meyerhardt JA, Zheng H, et al., Phase 1/2 study of everolimus in advanced hepatocellular carcinoma. *Cancer* 2011; 117: 5094-5102.

[236] Decaens T, Luciani A, Itti E, Hulin A, Roudot-Thoraval F, Laurent A, et al., Phase II study of sirolimus in treatment-naive patients with advanced hepatocellular carcinoma. *Dig. Liver Dis.* 2012; 44: 610-616.

[237] Santoro A, Rimassa L, Borbath I, Daniele B, Salvagni S, Van Laethem JL, et al., Tivantinib for second-line treatment of advanced hepatocellular carcinoma: a randomized placebo-controlled phase 2 study. *Lancet Oncol.* 2013; 14: 55-63.

[238] Okita K, Matsui O, Kumada H, Tanaka K, Kaneko S, Moriwaki H, et al., Effect of peretinoin on recurrence of hepatocellular carcinoma (HCC): Results of a phse II/III randomized placebo-controlled trial. (Abstract #4024), ASCO, June, 2010.

[239] Kuang M, Peng BG, Lu MD, Liang LJ, Huang JF, He Q, et al., Phase II randomized trial of autologous formalin-fixed tumor vaccine for postsurgical recurrence of hepatocellular carcinoma. *Clin. Cancer Res.* 2004; 10:1574–1579.

[240] Abei M, Okumura T, Fukuda K, Hashimoto T, Araki M, Ishige K, et al., A phase I study on combined therapy with proton-beam radiotherapy and in situ tumor vaccination for locally advanced recurrent hepatocellular carcinoma. *Radiat. Oncol.* 2013; 8 : 239.

[241] Liu T-C, Galanis E, Kirn D. Clinical trial results with oncolytic virotherapy: a century of promise, a decade of progress. *Nat. Clin. Pract. Oncol.* 2007; 4: 101-117.

[242] Parato KA, Senger D, Forsyth PA, Bell JC. Recent progresss in the battle between oncolytic viruses and tumors. *Nat. Rev. Cancer* 2005; 5: 965-976.

[243] Russell SJ, Peng KW, Bell JC. Oncolytic virotherapy. *Nat. Biotechnol.* 2012; 30: 658-670.

[244] Bourke MG, Salwa S, Harrington KJ, Kucharczyk MJ, Forde PF, de Kruijf M, et al., The emerging role of viruses in the treatment of solid tumors. *Cancer Treat. Rev.* 2011; 37: 618-632.

[245] Kirn DH, Thorne SH. Targeted and armed oncolytic poxviruses: a novel multi-mechanistic therapeutic class for cancer. *Nature Rev Cancer* 2009; 9: 64-71.

[246] Kim JH, Oh JY, Park BH, Lee DE, Kim JS, Park HE, et al., Systemic armed oncolytic and immunologic therapy for cancer with JX-594, a targeted poxviruss expressing GM-CSF. *Mol. Ther.* 2006; 14: 361-370.

[247] Lee J-H, Roh M-S, Lee Y-K, Kim MK, Han JY, Park BH, et al., Oncolytic and immuneostimulatory efficacy of a targeted oncolytic poxviruss expressing human GM-CSF following intravenous administration in a rabbit model. *Cancer Gene Ther.* 2010; 17: 73-79.

[248] Prato KA, Breitbach CJ, Le Boeuf F, Wang J, Storbeck C, Ilkow C, et al., The oncolytic poxvirus JX-594 selectively replicates in and destroys cancer cells driven by genetic pathways commonly activated in cancers. *Mol. Ther.* 2011; 20: 749-758.

[249] Park BH, Hwang T, Liu TC, Sze DY, Kim JS, Kwon HC, et al., Use of a targeted oncolytic poxvirus, JX-594, in patients refractory primary or metastatic liver cancer: a phase I clinical trial. *Lancet Oncol.* 2008; 9: 533-542.

[250] Heo J, Breitbach CJ, Moon A, Kim CW, Patt R, Kim MK, et al., Sequential therapy with JX-594, a targeted oncolytic poxviruss, followed by sorafenib in hepatocellular carcinoma: Preclinical and clinical demonstration of combination efficacy. *Mol. Ther.* 2011; 19: 1170-1179.

[251] Heo J, Reid T, Ruo L, Breitbach CJ, Rose S, Bloomston M, et al., Randomized dose-finding clinical trial of oncolytic immunotherapeutic vaccinia JX-594 in liver cancer. *Nature Med.* 2013; 19: 329-336.

[252] Breitbach CJ, Burke J, Jonker D, Stephenson J, Haas AR, Chow LQ, et al., Intravenous delivery of a multi-mechanistic cancer-targeted oncolytic poxvirus in humans. *Nature* 2011; 477: 99-102.

In: Therapy for Hepatocellular Carcinoma
Editor: Nobuhiro Ohkohchi

ISBN: 978-1-63117-929-7
© 2014 Nova Science Publishers, Inc.

Chapter 4

Hepatic Resection for Hepatocellular Carcinoma

Kiyoshi Fukunaga, Keisuke Kohno
and Nobuhiro Ohkohchi, M.D., Ph.D.[*]
Department of Surgery, Faculty of Medicine, University of Tsukuba

Abstract

Hepatic resection is a potentially curative treatment for patients with early-stage HCC who are eligible to undergo the procedure. Preoperative assessment, especially liver functional reserve along with the HCC characteristics is an important factor because most HCC patients have underlying chronic liver disease. According to clinical practice guidelines produced in different regions of the world, hepatic resection is unanimously indicated for solitary tumors without vascular invasion of Child-Pugh class A cirrhotic patients. The indocyanine green clearance test has also been reported to be useful for reducing mortality and morbidity. Another critical preoperative assessment is estimate of the postoperative future liver remnant volume. Recently, three-dimensional image-processing software has enabled planning of hepatic resection and measurement of accurate liver volume. Technical improvements have been introduced for decreasing blood loss during hepatic resection, including surgical technique, i.e., hepatic inflow and outflow controls, various surgical devices for liver parenchymal transection, such as ultrasonic dissector and anesthetic techniques. These improvements have reduced the postoperative mortality to 5% and under. Hepatic resection can achieve a 5-year survival rate of approximately 70% for selected patients with preserved liver function and early stage HCC.

[*] Corresponding author: Nobuhiro Ohkohchi; Department of Surgery, Faculty of Medicine, University of Tsukuba; 1-1-1 Tennodai, Tsukuba, Ibaraki 305-8575, Japan; Tel: +81-29-853-3221; Fax:+81-29-853-3222; e-mail: nokochi3@md.tsukuba.ac.jp.

1. Introduction

Hepatic resection is the main modality of curative treatment for hepatocellular carcinoma (HCC) and achieves good outcome in well-selected patients. Risks associated with hepatic resection for patients with HCC mainly come from the underlying chronic liver disease. Therefore, careful patient selection, based on the liver function and estimate of postoperative future liver remnant (FLR), in addition to patient and HCC characteristics, is essential. Recently, HCC resection in cirrhotic patients can be performed with an acceptable perioperative mortality rate, because the patient selection, surgical technique, and immediate postoperative management have been refined. In this chapter, we show the indications for and surgical procedures and outcomes of hepatic resection for HCC mainly in Japan.

2. Preoperative Assessment (Table 1)

An important aspect of the morbidity, mortality, and long-term outcome of hepatic resection for HCC relates to patient selection. Because most patients with HCC have associated underlying chronic liver disease, hepatic resection carries a higher risk as a result of the removal of functioning liver parenchyma. Therefore, indication for hepatic resection depends primarily on the liver functional reserve, as well as on the HCC characteristics.

Table 1. Clinical practice guidelines for hepatocellular carcinoma

Guideline	Year	Resection for first-line treatment		Additional indication
		HCC characteristics	Liver functional reserve	
Japan	2013	Solitary tumor without vascular invasion	Liver damage of class A-B	-Tumors ≤ 3 and liver damage A-B -Vascular invasion and liver damage A
EASL-EORTC	2012	Solitary tumor without vascular invasion	-ECOG performance status 0 -Child-Pugh A-B -Very well-preserved liver function, defined as normal bilirubin with either hepatic venous pressure gradient ≤ 10 mmHg or platelet count ≥ 100,000	Multifocal tumors meeting Milan criteria (≤3 nodules ≤3 cm) or with mild portal hypertension not suitable for liver transplantation
NCCN	2009	Solitary tumor without major vascular invasion	-Operable by performance status or comorbidity -Child-Pugh A with mild or moderate portal hypertension (e.g., varices, splenomegaly, thrombocytopenia) -Adequate future liver remnant (at least 20% without cirrhosis and at least 30%-40% with Child-Pugh A cirrhosis)	-Multifocal tumors meeting Milan criteria (≤3 nodules ≤3 cm) if transplantation not feasible -Major vascular invasion -In highly selected Child-Pugh B patients with limited resection

According to the NCCN guidelines [1], hepatic resection is indicated as a potentially curative option in the following circumstances: (1) adequate liver function (generally Child-Pugh class A cirrhosis with mild or moderate portal hypertension [PHT]); (2) solitary mass without major vascular invasion; (3) Adequate FLR (at least 20% without cirrhosis and at least 30%-40% with Child-Pugh A cirrhosis). Besides, in highly selected cases, patients with Child-Pugh B cirrhosis may be considered for limited hepatic resection, particularly if the liver function tests are normal and clinical signs of PHT are absent. Hepatic resection is controversial in patients with multifocal disease or major vascular invasion, but can be considered. In the EASL-EORTC clinical practice guidelines [2], resection is the treatment option for patients with solitary tumor and very well-preserved liver function, ie, normal bilirubin with either a hepatic venous pressure gradient ≤10 mmHg or a platelet count ≥100,000 /mm^3. For additional indications for patients with multifocal tumors or with mild PHT, solid evidence is lacking.

On the other hand, in the evidence-based guidelines for HCC in Japan [3], PHT is not described in the surgical indications, because the social situation is different from that of Western countries, where liver transplantations from deceased donors are common treatments for patients with HCC and PHT. The indication for hepatic resection has spread to patients with concomitant PHT and can provide survival benefits even for patients with PHT [4].

2.1. General Condition and Comorbidity

Assessments of patient performance status must be considered. The presence of comorbidity has been shown to be an independent predictor of perioperative mortality [5]. These included diabetes mellitus, cardiovascular disease, peripheral vascular disease, chronic renal dysfunction, and chronic pulmonary disease. In patients with severe pulmonary dysfunction (1-second forced expiratory volume <1L), we consider tracheotomy at the same time as hepatic resection.

In guidelines for perioperative cardiovascular evaluation for noncardiac surgery, intraperitoneal surgery is classified as intermediate-risk surgery [6]. The initial history, physical examination, and electrocardiographic assessment should focus on identification of potentially serious cardiac disorders, including coronary artery disease (eg, prior myocardial infarction, angina pectoris), congestive heart failure, and electrical instability (eg, symptomatic arrhythmias). In addition to identifying the presence of preexisting manifested heart disease, it is essential to define the disease severity, stability, and prior treatment. Other factors that help determine cardiac risk include functional capacity, age, and comorbidity. Functional capacity can be expressed in metabolic equivalent (MET) levels. Perioperative cardiac risk is increased in patients unable to meet a 4-MET demand during most normal daily activities. Clinical predictors of perioperative cardiac risk are presence of prior myocardial infarction by history or electrocardiogram, angina pectoris, compensated or prior congestive heart failure, and/or diabetes mellitus. Noncardiac surgery is generally safe for patients without predictor of clinical risk and moderate or excellent functional capacity (4 METs or greater). Patients with predictor of clinical risk and moderate or excellent functional capacity can generally undergo intermediate-risk surgery with little likelihood of perioperative death or myocardial infarction.

2.2. HCC Characteristics

The assessment of the tumor extent is the first step for determining resectability. The number, size, and vascular invasion of the HCC are important factors for considering hepatic resection. The largest multicenter study conducted by the Liver Cancer Study Group of Japan showed that the treatment results following hepatic resection were better than those following percutaneous ablation in patients with class A or B liver damage who had a solitary tumor regardless of the tumor size. In patients who had no more than 3 tumors (≤3cm) and class A or B liver damage, there were no significant differences between hepatic resection and percutaneous ablation [7, 8].

A treatment algorithm in the Japanese HCC guidelines is made on the basis of these articles (Figure 1). If only one HCC is present, hepatic resection is recommended, irrespective of the diameter of the tumor. Ablation therapy may also be selected if the diameter of the HCC is no more than 3 cm. If 2 to 3 HCCs with diameters of no more than 3 cm are present, hepatic resection or ablation therapy is recommended. If 2 to 3 HCCs with diameters of 3 cm or more are present, hepatic resection or TACE is recommended. For patients with class A liver damage accompanied by vascular invasion, hepatic resection might be selected.

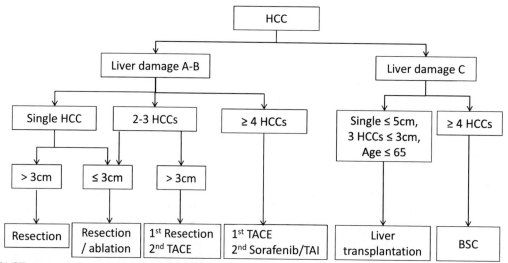

TACE, transcatheter arterial chemoembolization.
TAI, transcatheter arterial infusion chemotherapy.
BSC, best supportive care.

Figure 1. Treatment algorithm for hepatocellular carcinoma (HCC) in Japan.

2.3. Liver Functional Reserve

The management of patients with HCC is complicated by the presence of underlying chronic liver disease. An accurate evaluation of the liver functional reserve is crucial to avoid postoperative hepatic insufficiency and mortality. Hepatic resection is recommended only in the setting of preserved liver function. The Child-Pugh classification was originally developed to estimate the risk of patients with cirrhosis undergoing operations for portal hypertension. It is the oldest and most widely used classification to evaluate preoperative liver functional reserve [9, 10]. In addition to this conventional classification, liver functional reserve is usually evaluated using the indocyanine green (ICG) test before hepatic resection, especially in Asian countries [11-16]. The ICG is an injectable organic anion that binds to albumin. Its hepatocyte uptake is followed by its biliary excretion without enterohepatic circulation. The ICG clearance test (plasma retention at 15 minutes; ICGR15) has been reported to be useful for the assessment of liver functional reserve. ICG clearance is a reflection of liver function, hepatic energy status, and cardiac and arterioportal blood flows. In Japanese evidence-based guidelines for the treatment of HCC, liver functional reserve is estimated by liver damage classification, which consists of ascites, serum bilirubin, serum albumin prothrombin activity, and ICGR15 [17] (Table 2). In patients with mild or moderate liver damage classification, categorized as class A or B, hepatic resection is recommended.

Another important factor in surgical risk assessment is the presence of underlying hepatitis. Preoperative increase in serum aspartate transaminase more than twice the normal upper range was associated with a significant increase in death from liver failure in patients with cirrhosis after major hepatectomy [18]. Therefore, elevated transaminase needs to be treated by intravenous administration of a glycyrrhizin-containing preparation (Stronger Neo-Minophagen C). Portal hypertension can be suspected in cases of splenomegaly, esophageal varices, or hypersplenism. Esophageal varices should be treated endoscopically before hepatic resection.

Table 2. Liver damage classification

	Class A	Class B	Class C
Ascites	None	Controlled	Not controlled
Serum bilirubin (mg/dL)	< 2.0	$2.0 \leq, \leq 3.0$	3.0 <
Serum albumin (g/dL)	> 3.5	$3.0 \leq, \leq 3.5$	3.0 >
ICGR15[*] (%)	< 15	$15 \leq, \leq 40$	40 <
Prothrombin activity (%)	> 80	$50 \leq, \leq 80$	50 >

The patient is classified into a class in which 2 or more factors are met.
* ICGR15, indocyanine green clearance test (plasma retention at 15 minutes).

2.4. Safety Limits for Hepatic Resection

In Japan, a safety decision tree developed by Makuuchi et al., is more commonly used for deciding the safe limits for hepatic resection [13]. The decision tree is determined by a criterion based on 3 variables: the presence or absence of ascites, the total bilirubin level, and the ICGR15. In patients without ascites and with a normal bilirubin level, the ICGR15 becomes the main determinant of resectability. For example, right hemihepatectomy can be tolerated if the ICGR15 is less than 10%. For patients with an ICGR15 of 10% to 19%, one third of the liver parenchyma can be resected, which corresponds to left hemihepatectomy and right-sided paramedian or lateral sectoriectomy. When the ICGR15 ranges from 20% to 29%, approximately one sixth of the liver parenchyma can be resected. This resection is roughly equivalent to Couinaud's segmentectomy. Limited resection is indicated in patients whose ICGR15 is 30% or more. In addition, Okamoto et al., reported a multiple regression equation for prediction of the safety limits for hepatectomy using the ICGR15 and the patient's age [19, 20]. Takasaki et al., also reported a predictive formula using the ICGR15 of the upper limit for safe hepatic resection [21]. Indeed, patient selection by these criteria using the ICG clearance test has greatly reduced the mortality rate. Some centers have reported zero perioperative mortality [11, 22].

2.5. Estimate of FLR Volume

Another critical preoperative assessment is estimation of the postoperative FLR volume as an indicator of postoperative liver function. In earlier years, two-dimensional CT was used to calculate the volume of the FLR with the intended resection line manually determined [23] (Figure 2). Recent developments in image-based computer assistance allow patient's individual liver anatomy to be computed and provides detailed volumetric analyses based on the portal perfusion. This image-based computer assistance is very useful and important because the portal venous and hepatic venous distributions and the size of the independent portal segments show great variations among patients. Virtual hepatic resection systems enable operation planning using 3D image-processing software and calculate the FLR, which have both a portal venous blood supply and hepatic venous drainage [24]. The total liver volume and the FLR were calculated, and the ratio of the FLR to the total liver volume after subtracting the tumor volume was determined.

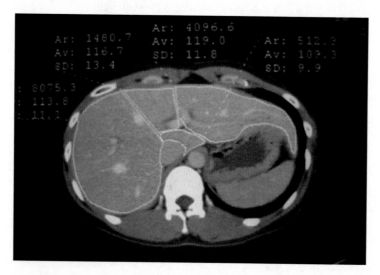

Figure 2. Manually calculated liver volume.

We use the Synapse Vincent medical imaging system (Fujifilm Medical, Tokyo), which was developed specifically for 3D visualization and virtual resection of the liver. This software offers standardized computation of the liver's anatomical functions and volumetric risk analysis based on two-dimensional CT imaging. The structures of the liver, portal vein, hepatic artery, hepatic vein, and tumor are extracted from multidetector-row computed tomography scan data. These images can be rotated (Figure 3).

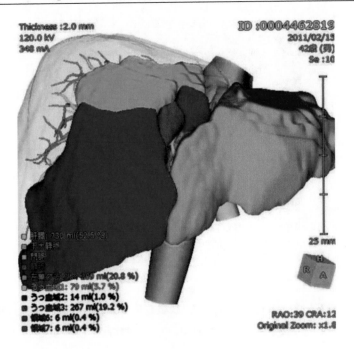

Figure 3. Calculated liver volume by Synapse Vincent.

2.6. Preoperative Portal Vein Embolization (PVE)

PVE induces atrophy of the embolized portion of the liver and compensatory hypertrophy of the FLR by redirecting the portal blood flow toward the portion of the liver that will remain after surgery. According to the NCCN guidelines, preoperative PVE should be considered for patients with chronic liver disease being considered for major resection. This approach is associated with a complication rate of 10 to 20% and occurrence of severe portal hypertension in 1% of cirrhotic patients [25]. However, the effectiveness of PVE for HCC in cirrhosis has yet to be properly tested in large controlled studies. In Japan, if the scheduled operation corresponded to the removal of more than 70% of the total hepatic volume in patients with a normal liver, eg, right trisegmentectomy, preoperative PVE was performed to induce compensatory hypertrophy of the liver remnant to reduce the risk of postoperative hepatic insufficiency [26, 27] (Figure 4). In Western countries, if the calculated standardized FLR volume was inadequate (≤20% of the total liver volume in patients with a normal liver, ≤30% in patients with fibrosis or liver injury, or ≤40% in patients with cirrhosis), preoperative PVE was performed [28-30].

PVE is usually performed either through a percutaneous ipsilateral transhepatic approach or through a transileocolic vein approach by laparotomy. Various embolic materials have been used such as iodized oil (Lipiodol Ultrafluid), absorbable gelatin sponge powder (Gelfoam), 99.5% absolute alcohol, and metallic coil. A specific technique of PVE procedure is required for selective injection of the embolic material into the segmental branches to reduce the risk of embolic agent migration into the FLR.

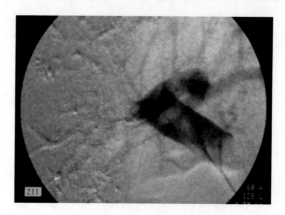

Figure 4. Portal vein embolization (PVE). The right branch of the portal vein is not imaged by angiography after PVE (lower) when compared with before PVE (upper). It is performed by the transileocolic vein approach. The catheter tip is placed in the main trunk of the portal vein.

3. Anesthetic Techniques for Reduction of Intraoperative Blood Loss

Blood loss during hepatic resection is one of the factors affecting the postoperative complications and long-term survival of patients [31-33]. Various surgical techniques have been attempted to reduce the blood loss during hepatic resection. However, the indications for these techniques are limited because they have a profound influence on systemic hemodynamics and involve complicated procedures [34]. Central venous pressure (CVP) is positively correlated with the amount of hemorrhage that occurs during hepatic resection [35-37]. A low CVP is obtained by administration of vasodilators, limitation of infusion, manipulation of the patient's posture (Trendelenburg position), and hypoventilation [38-40]. A low CVP level is generally referred to as lower than 5 cmH$_2$O [35, 36, 40]. In our hospital, when possible, intravenous infusion is restricted to 6 mL/kg/h in patients with chronic liver disease and the tidal volume is reduced to 5 to 8 mL/kg for hypoventilation during hepatic parenchymal transection to maintain a low CVP with a minimum urine output of at least 0.5 mL/kg/h. After completion of the transection, patients are given an infusion of crystalloids and/or colloids to render them euvolemic.

4. Surgical Procedures

4.1. From Skin Incision to Mobilization of the Liver

Previously, a bilateral subcostal incision with upward midline extension to the xiphoid, known also as a Mercedes incision, was common for hepatic resection; now, however, a J-shaped right upper quadrant incision is used in most patients, which eliminates the need for a left upper quadrant incision. The liver is mobilized by dividing the falciform, round, and triangular ligaments. When hemihepatectomy is performed, dissection of the hepatic arteries, portal vein branches, and hepatic veins is carried out by the extrahepatic method before dividing the liver parenchyma [41]. A cutting line is marked on the liver surface with a cautery knife. On the residual side of the cutting line, 1-0 polyglactin (Vicryl; Ethicon) stay sutures are placed along the line of the intended transection. Traction on the stay sutures is used to separate and expose the liver transection plane. Liver transection is performed from cauterizing the liver capsule using a cautery knife or Harmonic Scalpel (Ultracision, Ethicon Endo-Surgery).

4.2. Intraoperative Ultrasonography (IOUS)

IOUS is used to assess the intrahepatic anatomy of the hepatic vessels and the extent of the HCC, and to plan the parenchymal transection plane [42]. Considering that wide variations in the anatomy of the portal vein branches exist, IOUS is especially important to correctly define the segmental boundaries and to perform a segment-oriented hepatic resection. For the resection, the liver is divided to expose the main trunk of the hepatic vein or the ligating point of Glisson's triad under IOUS guidance. For example, in right hemihepatectomy, the exact position of the middle hepatic vein is noted during transection. Color doppler imaging of intraoperative ultrasonography is also used to check the hepatic blood flow during and after hepatic resection. It is reported that tailoring the resection area under IOUS guidance is associated with decrease in mortality and major morbidity [43, 44].

4.3. Intraoperative Cholangiography

Whenever necessary, intraoperative cholangiography is performed for left hemihepatectomy to identify any variant anatomy of the right lateral hepatic duct in relation to the left hepatic duct (Figure 5).

4.4. Surgical Techniques for Reduction of Intraoperative Blood Loss

Perioperative massive blood transfusion carries risks of causing infectious diseases, coagulatory disorder, or acute respiratory distress syndrome, and also promotes tumor recurrence due to its inhibitory effects on immunologic function [45, 46]. Reduction of blood loss is one of the goals in hepatic resection, and several technical developments have been introduced for this purpose, including the total inflow occlusion technique (Pringle's maneuver) [47] and hemihepatic vascular occlusion [48, 49]. These inflow occlusion techniques are applied at the beginning. They are applied in an intermittent manner, with 15 minutes of occlusion alternated with 5 minutes of reperfusion.

After the application of inflow occlusion, the hepatic vein could be a major source of hemorrhage during hepatic parenchymal transection. Outflow system control, ie, clamping the hepatic veins [50, 51], clamping the inferior vena cava (IVC) [52], or total hepatic vascular exclusion [53, 54] can reduce blood loss from the hepatic venous system during hepatic resection. In addition, blood loss is influenced by thoracotomy [39]. It would be reasonable to think that thoracotomy decreases CVP and blood loss because the compression effect of right lung inflation is lower, although animal experiments do not provide proof of this [36, 55]. We often perform thoracotomy in patients with HCCs located in the cranial part of the liver, such as segments 7 or 8, or with large tumors that require major hepatic resection.

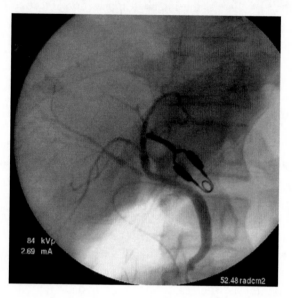

Figure 5. Intraoperative cholangiography. The clip provides information about the cutting line of the left hepatic duct. The surgeon should take account of the fact that the right lateral hepatic duct joins the left hepatic duct.

4.4.1. Total Inflow Occlusion (Pringle's Maneuver) [47]

This technique stops blood flow through the hepatic artery and portal vein by clamping the hepatoduodenal ligament using forceps with a sponge to clamp gently and avoid injury or using tape and a tourniquet.

4.4.2. Hemihepatic Vascular Occlusion [48, 49]

This technique clamps the hepatic artery and portal vein of the resected area, which can avoid portal congestion.

4.4.3. Clamping Hepatic Veins [50, 51]

This technique provides outflow control by clamping the major hepatic veins without caval occlusion, which is used in connection with inflow clamping.

4.4.4. Clamping the IVC Below the Liver [52]

This technique is used for decrease in CVP in the case of high CVP despite anesthetic management. During IVC clamping below the liver, blood pressure decreases because of central hypovolemia. The time limit for clamping is up to 15 minutes.

4.4.5. Total Hepatic Vascular Exclusion [53, 54]

This technique is used when HCC has invaded into the hepatic vein and IVC, so that it is necessary to open the vein. It involves clamping the portal pedicle and the infrahepatic and suprahepatic IVC.

4.5. Liver Hanging Maneuver

The liver hanging maneuver was first devised by Lai et al., [56] and was later modified by Belghiti et al., [57]. The original method was employed mostly for right hemihepatectomy with an anterior approach for huge liver tumors. It is a technique to transect the liver parenchyma by lifting it with a tape passed between the anterior surface of the IVC and the liver parenchyma. The tape assists in guiding the direction of the parenchymal transection and facilitates better hemorrhage control during transection of the deeper parenchyma.

A hanging tape is passed through an avascular thin route on the midline of the anterior surface of the infrahepatic portion of the IVC without any mobilization of the right liver. The space between the right hepatic vein (RHV) and the middle hepatic vein (MHV) is first dissected 2 cm downward. The dissection of the caudal portion starts with a long Kelly clamp posterior to the caudate lobe, proceeding cranially with great care along the middle plane of the IVC. The clamp appears between the RHV and MHV after 4 to 6 cm of blind dissection. The blind retrohepatic dissection along this plane is potentially hazardous. The use of ultrasonography to identify and visualize the tip of the clamp during retrohepatic dissection may overcome the pitfalls of blind passage of the clamp and minimize hemorrhage due to inadvertent injury to the IVC and short hepatic veins [58]. In addition, a safer technique for blind retrohepatic dissection using a surgical probe instead of a Kelly clamp was reported [59]. The liver hanging maneuver can be applied to left hemihepatectomy, right posterior sectionectomy, and central bisegmentectomy as a modified method [60].

The conventional approach to right hemihepatectomy requires liver mobilization. In contrast, the anterior approach using the liver hanging maneuver does not require lifting of the liver. A retrospective study of patients with large HCC has demonstrated that the anterior approach can reduce postoperative recurrence and achieve an improvement of disease-free survival [61].

4.6. Two-Surgeon Technique for Liver Parenchymal Transection [62-64]

We adopt the 2-surgeon technique to optimize parenchymal transection. The two-surgeon technique allows 2 surgeons to simultaneously participate in the parenchymal transection. The primary surgeon dissected the hepatic parenchyma from the patient's right side using an ultrasonic dissector [65-67]. The secondary surgeon operated using the monopolar soft-coagulation (SOFT COAG) system [68] from the patient's left side (Figure 6). The liver parenchyma was dissected, and the intraparenchymal vascular anatomy was defined using the ultrasonic dissector so that a decision on the hemostatic technique could be made based on the vessel size. The SOFT COAG can coagulate blood vessels ≤2 mm, but vessels thicker than 2 mm were ligated with 4-0 silk ties and/or titanium clips and cut sharply. The few larger vessels were ultrasonically dissected and controlled with 4-0/3-0 silk ties and 4-0 absorbable monofilament transfixing sutures, and sharply cut.

In addition to maximizing the efficiency of liver transection, the two-surgeon technique also creates an ideal environment for training residents and fellows in hepatic surgery. While retaining control of the dissection, the attending surgeon can help the trainee to correctly delineate the vascular and biliary anatomy within the transection plane.

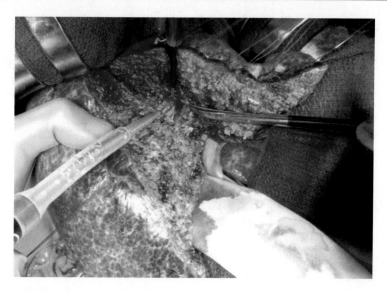

Figure 6. Two-surgeon technique. The primary surgeon holds the resected liver with the left hand (green glove) and operates using CUSA. The secondary surgeon uses SOFT COAG and scissors mainly for hemostasis and cutting coagulated vessels.

4.7. Techniques for Liver Parenchymal Transection

Various techniques of liver parenchymal transection have been used so far. These include the clamp-crush technique, ultrasonic dissector [65-67], ultrasonically activated scalpel [69], a vessel sealing system (LigaSure, Valleylab) (70), the SOFT COAG system [68], and water-cooled high-frequency monopolar electrocautery (Dissecting Sealer, TissueLink) [71]. The clamp-crush technique does not require any special instruments and is generally considered the standard form of liver parenchymal transection in Japan. As a result of many randomized clinical trials comparing different methods of parenchymal dissection, no technique offered any benefit in decreasing the morbidity or transfusion requirement [72]. Above all, the important thing in transection procedures is to stop any bleeding before proceeding. We introduce the technique of hepatic parenchymal transection using an ultrasonic dissector and SOFT COAG, aside from bipolar cautery with a saline irrigation system, which we used before SOFT COAG.

4.7.1. Ultrasonic Dissector (Cavitron Ultrasonic Surgical Aspirator System [CUSA]; Valleylab, Boulder, CO, USA) (Figure 7upper) [65-67]

The ultrasonic dissector (CUSA) has contributed to safe hepatectomy by making it easy to identify the vessels during parenchymal transection. The amplitude is set at 70% for a normal liver and at up to 100% for a cirrhotic liver, depending on the amount of fibrous tissue encountered. The rate of saline irrigation is set to 3 mL/min, whereas the suction pressure is set to 70%. The tip of the dissector is applied to the liver transection plane at a tilt and moved in a direction horizontal to the plane with minimal amplitude of movement. The exposed tiny tubular structures are cauterized by the assistant (the secondary surgeon) while the surgeon continues to apply the ultrasonic dissector without interruption. Bleeding from the major branches of the blood vessels encountered during transection is controlled temporarily with a pair of forceps by the assistant while the surgeon continues to clear the parenchyma around the blood vessel and sutures or ligates the vessel for hemostasis. Parenchymal transection with the ultrasonic dissector is not entirely bloodless. Bleeding will occur when the power output is set excessively high so that larger blood vessels are divided. Excessive bleeding from the transected area can also occur when the surgeon is anxious to proceed quickly by applying the tip of the ultrasonic dissector over a wide amplitude. This tends to occur in a trainee's early experience. Slow and cautious movement of the tip and an appropriate power output are needed.

4.7.2. SOFT COAG system (VIO 300D; ERBE Elektromedizin, Tubingen, Germany) (Figure 7middle) [68]

Conventional electrosurgical coagulation systems produce sparks and can cause carbonization and adhesions to the electrode during coagulation, which result in incomplete hemostasis. However, the SOFT COAF system automatically regulates the output voltage to below 200 V, causing the generation of Joule heat alone, which prevents development of sparks and carbonization of the tissue and reduces adhesion of the electrode to the tissue, thus resulting in greater coagulation intensities than with conventional electrosurgical coagulation systems. The VIO 300D system is set to the SOFT COAG mode at the effect of 5 and 50 W. A disk-shaped electrode is employed. SOFT COAG is particularly used for hemostasis of the hepatic vein. SOFT COAG can be safely used in areas near the major hepatic vein without damaging the venous wall, eg, in the case of pinhole bleeding of the hepatic vein and in cases where hemostasis is difficult to achieve with suturing, such as in deep bleeding due to damage resulting from the hepatic veins being pulled out. The assistant (the secondary surgeon) presses the disk-shaped electrode against the bleeding point accurately and temporarily stops the bleeding, applying heat to the point and slowly pulling it away. We have to give considerable attention to overcauterization using SOFT COAG, which results in deeper coagulation intensities than the conventional cautery knife. Therefore, coagulation for a prolonged time at one place could cause accidental damage to the Glisson sheath especially around the hilum of the liver. (Figure 8).

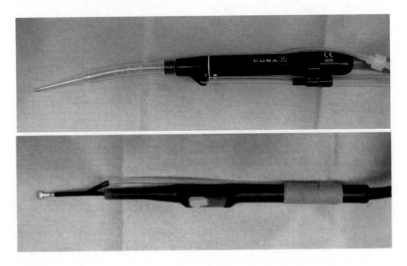

Figure 7. (Continued).

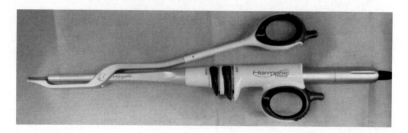

Figure 7. Surgical instruments for liver parenchymal transaction. We use (upper) an ultrasonic dissector (CUSA), (middle) a monopolar soft-coagulation system (SOFT COAG), and (lower) an ultrasonically activated scalpel (Harmonic Scalpel; Harmonic Focus Long) for liver parenchymal transaction.

4.7.3. Ultrasonically Activated Scalpel (Harmonic Scalpel; HS, Johnson and Johnson Medical, Ethicon) (Figure 7lower) [73]

The ultrasonically activated scalpel is a surgical instrument for coagulation and cutting that uses ultrasonic vibration. For liver parenchymal transaction, we use the handpiece of a coagulation shear (Harmonic Focus Long). The HS enables successful resection to be performed regardless of the condition of the liver, even when chronic hepatitis or cirrhosis exists. The HS is applied to the superficial portion of the transaction plane, excluding the root of the hepatic vein and the area near the porta hepatis. Application of the HS becomes increasingly difficult on approaching the deeper portion of the transaction plane, since it is difficult to control bleeding using the HS alone. When the deep areas of the liver are divided, there is a risk of massive bleeding if the walls of the large vessels are cut. Moreover, the HS is not appropriate for delicate procedures, such as anatomic hepatic resection, when the hepatic veins are exposed on the resected surface. Thus, division of the deep layer appears to require other techniques, such as CUSA and SOFT COAG.

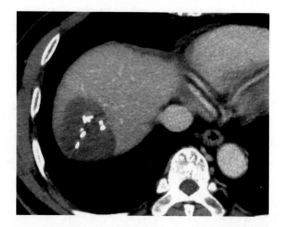

Figure 8. Damage due to SOFT COAG. This is a contrast-enhanced CT image after wedge hepatic resection of segments 7/8. The damaged area of the liver parenchyma is shown as a low-concentrated area in the remnant liver. The surgical clips indicate the transaction plane. The damage due to SOFT COAG extends 2 cm deep from the plane.

4.7.4. Bipolar Cautery with a Saline Irrigation System (B. Braun Aesculap Japan) (Figure 9) [66]

This bipolar cautery has a tiny water outlet at the tip. The water is heated between the tips, and the boiled water induces hemostasis of the tissue. The saline irrigation system prevents the tissue from sticking. Bleeding from the surface of the dissected liver parenchyma is stopped by clotting the blood with the bipolar cautery. The tissue of the small branches of Glisson sheath or small tributaries of the hepatic vein are coagulated by the bipolar cautery. Because the water droplets prevent adhesion of debris to the cautery blades, they are smoothly removed from the coagulated vessels without tearing the fragile tissue. The coagulated vessels are then easily cut by scissors. After cutting, coagulation at both ends of the vessel is preferable for obtaining complete hemostasis. This technique is valid for cord-like structures less than 1 to 2 mm in diameter. Complete hemostasis of the smaller vessels provides a dry surgical field.

The bipolar cautery is also effective for stopping oozing from cut surfaces. The tips are pressed against the oozing point, keeping the distance between the tips about 2 to 3 mm apart, and rubbing the wall while slowly pulling them away. This technique produces coagulation of the surface and is useful for obtaining complete hemostasis of the cut surfaces after hepatic resection. Thus, there are several knacks for using this instrument thoughtfully, and this method depends on the operator's skill and experience. In addition, it must be handled carefully so not to remove the coating that resists tissue sticking and controls conduction between the tips.

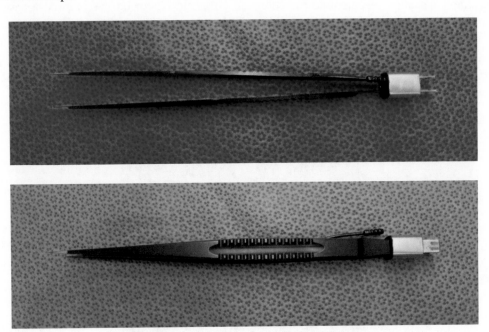

Figure 9. Bipolar cautery with a saline irrigation system. This bipolar cautery has a tiny water outlet at the tip. The water is heated up between the tips and the boiled water induces hemostasis of the tissue.

4.8. Anatomic Hepatic Resection

Hepatic resections are divided into anatomic resection and nonanatomic resection (wedge resection or resection that extends across Couinaud segmental planes). Anatomic resection was defined as resection of HCC together with the related portal vein branches and the corresponding hepatic territory. Makuuchi et al., proposed that the resected specimen should include at least the sectional or segmental portal vein associated with the HCC, because tumor dissemination from the main HCC is usually through the portal vein branches [42]. The theoretical advantage of anatomic over nonanatomic resection has been demonstrated in 2 large series in which anatomic resection was found to be an independent factor for both overall and disease-free survival [74, 75]. Anatomic resection to remove minute tumor satellites has decreased the recurrence and improved survival.

Anatomic resection procedures are classified as hemihepatectomy (right hemihepatectomy is defined as resection of Couinaud segments 5-8, and left hemihepatectomy is defined as resection of segments 2-4), sectionectomy (resection of 2 Couinaud segments), or segmentectomy (resection of 1 Couinaud segment). The principal goal of anatomic resection is an appearance of landmark vessels on the cut surface. Landmarks are defined as hepatic veins demarcating the anatomic borders of the liver segments (eg, the middle hepatic vein in hemihepatectomy [Figure 10] or the right hepatic vein in the resection of the right paramedian sector [Figure 11]).

In the EASL-EORTC clinical practice guidelines, anatomic resections are recommended. The implementation of anatomic resections according to Couinaud has ensured a surgical approach based on sound oncologic principles, although the resections are associated with a modest decrease in early recurrence [76]. Retrospective studies linking anatomic resections and better outcome should be interpreted with caution, owing to the propensity of performing wider resections in patients with well-preserved liver function. Another caution should be exercised because the surgical effort is aimed at preservation of adequate hepatic reserve through tailoring of the procedures to individual patients and tumor characteristics.

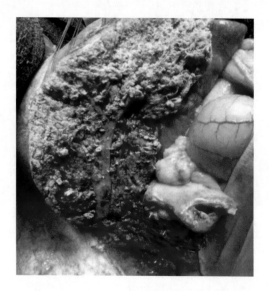

Figure 10. Anatomic hepatic resection (1). The cut surface after right hemihepatectomy. You can see the middle hepatic vein on the cut surface and the stump of the pedicle to the right liver.

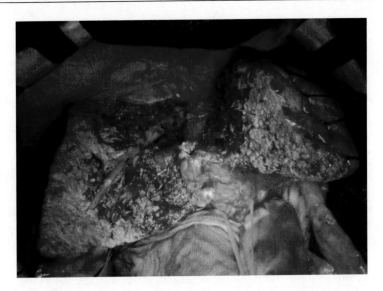

Figure 11. Anatomic hepatic resection (2). The cut surface after resection of the right paramedian sector. You can see the right hepatic vein on the cut surface, the inferior vena cava, and the stump of the pedicle to the right paramedian sector.

4.9. Bile Leakage Test

Bile leakage remains a common cause of major complication after hepatic resection. A meta-analysis indicated that a bile leakage test proved to be useful for preventing postoperative bile leakage and did not increase the incidence of complication [77]. After cholecystectomy and hepatic resection, a catheter is inserted through the cystic duct into the common bile duct and the distal common bile duct is occluded. The bile leakage test is performed using slow air injection via the catheter into the biliary tree, and a clinical judgment is then made as to whether a bile leak is present on the transected surface of the liver.

4.10. Drainage Tube

A closed silicon drain is inserted into the subphrenic or subhepatic space close to the cut surface of the liver before the closure of the abdominal wound. The drain is brought through a separate stab wound on the anterior abdominal wall and connected to a closed system without suction pressure. The abdominal drain is removed on postoperative day 4, unless there is excessive leakage of ascites or bile.

4.11. Laparoscopic Hepatectomy

Laparoscopic hepatectomy was first reported in 1993 and was initially adopted for nonanatomic liver wedge resection for peripheral benign tumors. During the past couple of decades it has been performed around the world and has been established as a safe and feasible option even for HCC. Some advantages compared to open hepatectomy have been recognized from meta-analysis, including reduction in intraoperative blood loss, less operative morbidity, and shorter length of hospitalization, especially for cirrhotic patients [78]. In addition, no significant difference was observed between laparoscopic hepatectomy and open hepatectomy for the long-term outcome of overall survival and recurrence-free survival.

5. Immediate Postoperative Management

Patients are generally administered Cefazolin as prophylactic antibiotic therapy. It is administered within 30 minutes before the skin incision, and another dose is administered 3 hours later. Additional doses are given every 3 hours thereafter during operations of longer than 3 hours' duration, and 3 days after surgery. Oral intake is started the day after the surgery. The drainage tube is removed approximately 4 days after the surgery if no abnormality is observed. The total bilirubin level of the drainage fluid is measured after the surgery, and bile leakage is diagnosed when the level exceeds 5.0 mg/dL and continues for more than 7 days [79].

6. Surgical Outcome

6.1. Perioperative Mortality and Morbidity

Technical improvements in liver surgery during the last 2 decades have decreased perioperative mortality from 15% in the 1980s to 3% to 5% in the majority of referral units. However, the risks of postoperative liver failure and fatal outcome have remained important concerns. According to the NCCN guidelines, partial hepatectomy for selected patients with HCC can be performed with low operative morbidity and mortality (in the range of ≤5%). The EASL-EORTC clinical practice guidelines describe perioperative mortality of hepatic resection in cirrhotic patients as expected to be 2% to 3%.

In Japan, after initiation of the National Clinical Database from 2011, approximately 1.2 million surgical cases from more than 3500 Japanese hospitals were collected through a Web-based data entry system. Using the database, 15,673 patients who underwent hepatic resection of 2 or more segments other than left lateral sectoriectomy were analyzed. The 30-day postoperative and in-hospital mortality rates were 1.9% and 3.8% (297 and 596 patients), respectively [80]. On the other hand, the mortality from and morbidity of hepatectomy for HCC were investigated in a large sample, using a nationwide Japanese database (the Diagnosis Procedure Combination database) [81]. For 2007 to 2008, 5270 patients who underwent hepatectomy were analyzed. The in-hospital mortality rate was 2.6% and postoperative morbidity rate was 14.5%. Increased mortality following hepatectomy was significantly associated with older age, extended lobectomy (vs. partial hepatectomy), lower hospital volume, and renal comorbidity.

6.2. Survival

HCC status defined by the number and size and by the liver functional status shows different outcomes after hepatic resection. Results of large retrospective studies have shown 5-year survival rates of more than 50% for patients undergoing hepatic resection for HCC [31, 82, 83]. Some studies suggest that hepatic resection can achieve a 5-year survival rate of approximately 70% for selected patients with preserved liver function and early stage HCC [82, 84].

The Japanese Nationwide Survey has shown that the 5-year survival rate for hepatic resection in 17,531 patients with solitary HCC was 60.2%, compared with 48.0% for 2 nodules and 30.6% for 3 or more nodules [85]. In this study, liver functional reserve was also a key factor for survival after hepatic resection in HCC, with 5-year survival rates for liver damage class A, B, and C of 59.0%, 45.3%, and 35.0%, respectively. However, it is important to point out that the HCC tumor recurrence rate at 5 years after hepatic resection has been reported to exceed 70% [82, 86]. The pattern of recurrence influences the subsequent therapy and outcome. In the case of recurrence, the patient will be reassessed according to his or her characteristics, and retreated accordingly.

Conclusion

Hepatic resection, which has been performed since early times, remains a main pillar of HCC treatment after other treatments such as radiofrequency ablation (RFA) and liver transplantation were introduced into the treatment strategy. Various techniques of hepatic resection have yielded a major progress during the last 2 decades, and it would appear that hepatic resection is technically nearly completed. Early-stage HCC is better suited for hepatic resection, whereas a more precise distribution of roles among hepatic resection, RFA, and liver transplantation will be clarified in the near future. In countries where liver transplantation is much less common, the role of hepatic resection for HCC is more important. In these countries, hepatic resection will be sometimes performed for patients with less favorable liver function. Therefore, it is necessary for surgeons to improve their skills to avoid postoperative hepatic insufficiency and mortality.

References

[1]   Benson AB 3rd, Abrams TA, Ben-Josef E, et al., NCCN clinical practice guidelines in oncology: hepatobiliary cancers. *J. Natl. Compr. Canc. Netw*. 2009; 7: 350-91.

[2]   European association for the study of the liver, European organisation for research and treatment of cancer. EASL-EORTC clinical practice guidelines: management of hepatocellular carcinoma. *J. Hepatol*. 2012; 56: 908-43. Erratum in: *J. Hepatol*. 2012; 56: 1430.

[3]   Makuuchi M, Kokudo N, Arii S, Futagawa S, Kaneko S, Kawasaki S, et al., Development of evidence-based clinical guidelines for the diagnosis and treatment of hepatocellular carcinoma in Japan. *Hepatol. Res*. 2008; 38 (1): 37–51.

[4]   Ishizawa T, Hasegawa K, Aoki T, Takahashi M, Inoue Y, Sano K, et al., Neither multiple tumors nor portal hypertension are surgical contraindications for hepatocellular carcinoma. *Gastroenterology* 2008;134:1908–1916.

[5]   Wei AC, Tung-Ping Poon R, Fan ST, Wong J. Risk factors for perioperative morbidity and mortality after extended hepatectomy for hepatocellular carcinoma. *Br. J. Surg.* 2003;90:33–41.

[6]   Eagle KA, Brundage BH, Chaitman BR, Ewy GA, Fleisher LA, Hertzer NR, et al., Guidelines for perioperative cardiovascular evaluation for noncardiac surgery. Report of the American College of Cardiology/American Heart Association Task Force on Practice Guidelines. Committee on Perioperative Cardiovascular Evaluation for Noncardiac Surgery. *Circulation.* 1996 Mar 15;93(6):1278-317.

[7]   Arii S, Yamaoka Y, Futagawa S, Inoue K, Kobayashi K, Kojiro M, et al., Results of surgical and nonsurgical treatment for small-sized hepatocellular carcinomas: a retrospective and nationwide survey in Japan. The Liver Cancer Study Group of Japan. *Hepatology* 2000;32:1224–9.

[8]   Hasegawa K, Kokudo N, Makuuchi M, Izumi N, Ichida T, Kudo M, et al., Comparison of resection and ablation for hepatocellular carcinoma: a cohort study based on a Japanese nationwide survey. *J. Hepatol.* 2013 Apr;58(4):724-9. Epub 2012 Nov 21.

[9]   Pugh RN, Murray-Lyon IM, Dawson JL, Pietroni MC, Williams R. Transection of the oesophagus for bleeding oesophageal varices. *Br. J. Surg.* 1973; 60: 646–9.

[10]   Ribero D, Curley SA, Imamura H, Madoff DC, Nagorney DM, Ng KK, et al., Selection for resection of hepatocellular carcinoma and surgical strategy: indications for resection, evaluation of liver function, portal vein embolization, and resection. *Ann. Surg. Oncol.* 2008 Apr;15(4):986-92. Epub 2008 Jan 31.

[11]   Fan ST, Lo CM, Liu CL, Lam CM, Yuen WK, Yeung C, et al., Hepatectomy for hepatocellular carcinoma: toward zero hospital deaths. *Ann. Surg.* 1999;229:322–330.

[12]   Wu CC, Cheng SB, Ho WM, Chen JT, Liu TJ, P'eng FK. Liver resection for hepatocellular carcinoma in patients with cirrhosis. *Br. J. Surg.* 2005;92:348–355.

[13]   Makuuchi M, Kosuge T, Takayama T, Yamazaki S, Kakazu T, Miyagawa S, et al., Surgery for small liver cancers. *Semin. Surg. Oncol.* 1993;9:298–304.

[14]   Imamura H, Sano K, Sugawara Y, Kokudo N, Makuuchi M. Assessment of hepatic reserve for indication of hepatic resection: decision tree incorporating indocyanine green test. *J. Hepatobiliary Pancreat Surg.* 2005;12:16–22.

[15]   Lee SG, Hwang S. How I do it: assessment of hepatic functional reserve for indication of hepatic resection. *J. Hepatobiliary Pancreat Surg.* 2005;12:38–43.

[16]   Lau H, Man K, Fan ST, Yu WC, Lo CM, Wong J. Evaluation of preoperative hepatic function in patients with hepatocellular carcinoma undergoing hepatectomy. *Br. J. Surg.* 1997; 84: 1255–9.

[17]   Liver Cancer Study Group of Japan. General Rules for the Clinical and Pathological Study of Primary Liver Cancer, Second English Edition. Tokyo: Kanehara & Co.,2003.

[18]   Farges O, Malassagne B, Flejou JF, Balzan S, Sauvanet A, Belghiti J. Risk of major liver resection in patients with underlying chronic liver disease: a reappraisal. *Ann. Surg..* 1999 Feb;229(2):210-5.

[19]   Okamoto E, Kyo A, Yamanaka N, Tanaka N, Kuwata K. Prediction of the safe limits of hepatectomy by combined volumetric and functional measurements in patients with impaired hepatic function. *Surgery.* 1984 May;95(5):586-92.

[20] Yamanaka N, Okamoto E, Kuwata K, Tanaka N. A multiple regression equation for prediction of posthepatectomy liver failure. *Ann. Surg..* 1984 Nov;200(5):658-63.

[21] Takasaki T. Development of a method of estimating postoperative hepatic functions upon hepatectomy before the operation. *Jpn J. Surg.* 1978 79:1526.

[22] Imamura H, Seyama Y, Kokudo N, Maema A, Sugawara Y, Sano K, et al., One thousand fifty-six hepatectomies without mortality in 8 years. *Arch. Surg.* 2003;138(11):1198-206.

[23] Kubota K, Makuuchi M, Kusaka K, Kobayashi T, Miki K, Hasegawa K, et al., Measurement of liver volume and hepatic functional reserve as a guide to decision-making in resectional surgery for hepatic tumors. *Hepatology.* 1997 Nov;26(5):1176-81.

[24] Mise Y, Tani K, Aoki T, Sakamoto Y, Hasegawa K, Sugawara Y, et al., Virtual liver resection: computer-assisted operation planning using a three-dimensional liver representation. *J. Hepatobiliary Pancreat. Sci.* 2013 Feb;20(2):157-64.

[25] Abulkhir A, Limongelli P, Healey AJ, Damrah O, Tait P, Jackson J, et al., Preoperative portal vein embolization for major liver resection: a meta-analysis. *Ann. Surg.* 2008 Jan;247(1):49-57.

[26] Imamura H, Shimada R, Kubota M, Matsuyama Y, Nakayama A, Miyagawa S, et al., Preoperative portal vein embolization: an audit of 84 patients. *Hepatology.* 1999 Apr;29(4):1099-105.

[27] Makuuchi M, Thai BL, Takayasu K, Takayama T, Kosuge T, Gunvén P, et al., Preoperative portal embolization to increase safety of major hepatectomy for hilar bile duct carcinoma: a preliminary report. *Surgery.* 1990 May;107(5):521-7.

[28] Madoff DC, Abdalla EK, Vauthey JN. Portal vein embolization in preparation for major hepatic resection: evolution of a new standard of care. *J. Vasc. Interv. Radiol.* 2005;16:779-90.

[29] Vauthey JN, Madoff DC, Abdalla EK. Preoperative portal vein embolization-a Western perspective. In: Blumgart LH, editor. Surgery of the liver, biliary tract and pancreas. Vol. 2. 4th ed. Philadelphia: Saunders; 2006. p. 1461-71.

[30] Abdalla EK, Barnett CC, Doherty D, Curley SA, Vauthey JN. Extended hepatectomy in patients with hepatobiliary malignancies with and without preoperative portal vein embolization. *Arch. Surg.* 2002;137:675-80.

[31] Chok KS, Ng KK, Poon RT, Lo CM, Fan ST. Impact of postoperative complications on long-term outcome of curative resection for hepatocellular carcinoma. *Br. J. Surg..* 2009 Jan;96(1):81-7.

[32] Taketomi A, Kitagawa D, Itoh S, Harimoto N, Yamashita Y, Gion T, et al., Trends in morbidity and mortality after hepatic resection for hepatocellular carcinoma: an institute's experience with 625 patients. *J. Am. Coll. Surg.* 2007 Apr;204(4):580-7.

[33] Sitzmann JV, Greene PS. Perioperative predictors of morbidity following hepatic resection for neoplasm. A multivariate analysis of a single surgeon experience with 105 patients. *Ann. Surg.* 1994 Jan;219(1):13-7.

[34] Belghiti J, Noun R, Zante E, Ballet T, Sauvanet A. Portal triad clamping or hepatic vascular exclusion for major liver resection. A controlled study. *Ann. Surg.* 1996 Aug;224(2):155-61.

[35] Jones RM, Moulton CE, Hardy KJ. Central venous pressure and its effect on blood loss during liver resection. *Br. J. Surg.* 1998 Aug;85(8):1058-60.

[36] Johnson M, Mannar R, Wu AV. Correlation between blood loss and inferior vena caval pressure during liver resection. *Br. J. Surg.* 1998 Feb;85(2):188-90.

[37] Smyrniotis V, Kostopanagiotou G, Theodoraki K, Tsantoulas D, Contis JC. The role of central venous pressure and type of vascular control in blood loss during major liver resections. *Am. J. Surg.* 2004 Mar;187(3):398-402.

[38] Wang WD, Liang LJ, Huang XQ, Yin XY. Low central venous pressure reduces blood loss in hepatectomy. *World J Gastroenterol.* 2006;12(6):935–9.

[39] Hasegawa K, Takayama T, Orii R, Sano K, Sugawara Y, Imamura H, et al., Effect of hypoventilation on bleeding during hepatic resection: a randomized controlled trial. *Arch. Surg.* 2002;137(3):311–5.

[40] Melendez JA, Arslan V, Fischer ME, Wuest D, Jarnagin WR, Fong Y, et al., Perioperative outcomes of major hepatic resections under low central venous pressure anesthesia: blood loss, blood transfusion, and the risk of postoperative renal dysfunction. *J. Am. Coll. Surg.* 1998 Dec;187(6):620-5.

[41] Makuuchi M, Yamamoto J, Takayama T, Kosuge T, Gunvén P, Yamazaki S, et al., Extrahepatic division of the right hepatic vein in hepatectomy. *Hepatogastroenterology.* 1991 Apr;38(2):176-9.

[42] Makuuchi M, Hasegawa H, Yamazaki S. Ultrasonically guided subsegmentectomy. *Surg. Gynecol. Obstet.* 1985 Oct;161(4):346-50.

[43] Torzilli G, Montorsi M, Donadon M, Palmisano A, Del Fabbro D, Gambetti A, et al., "Radical but conservative" is the main goal for ultrasonography-guided liver resection: prospective validation of this approach. *J. Am. Coll. Surg.* 2005 Oct;201(4):517-28.

[44] Torzilli G, Montorsi M, Del Fabbro D, Palmisano A, Donadon M, Makuuchi M. Ultrasonographically guided surgical approach to liver tumours involving the hepatic veins close to the caval confluence. *Br. J. Surg.* 2006 Oct;93(10):1238-46.

[45] Yamamoto J, Kosuge T, Takayama T, Shimada K, Yamasaki S, Ozaki H, et al., Perioperative blood transfusion promotes recurrence of hepatocellular carcinoma after hepatectomy. *Surgery.* 1994 Mar;115(3):303-9.

[46] Li CH, Chau GY, Lui WY, Tsay SH, King KL, Hsia CY, et al., Risk factors associated with intra-operative major blood loss in patients with hepatocellular carcinoma who underwent hepatic resection. *J. Chin. Med. Assoc.* 2003 Nov;66(11):669-75.

[47] Pringle JH. Notes on the Arrest of Hepatic Hemorrhage Due to Trauma. *Ann. Surg..* 1908 Oct;48(4):541-9.

[48] Makuuchi M, Mori T, Gunven P, Yamazaki S, Hasegawa H. Safety of hemihepatic vascular occlusion during resection of the liver. *Surg. Gynecol. Obstet.* 1987;164:155–8.

[49] Malassagne B, Cherqui D, Alon R, Brunetti F, Humeres R, Fagniez PL. Safety of selective vascular clamping for major hepatectomies. *J. Am. Coll. Surg.* 1998 Nov;187(5):482-6.

[50] Nagasue N, Yukaya H, Ogawa Y, Hirose S, Okita M. Segmental and subsegmental resections of the cirrhotic liver under hepatic inflow and outflow occlusion. *Br. J. Surg.* 1985 Jul;72(7):565-8.

[51] Cherqui D, Malassagne B, Colau PI, Brunetti F, Rotman N, Fagniez PL. Hepatic vascular exclusion with preservation of the caval flow for liver resections. *Ann. Surg.* 1999 Jul;230(1):24-30.

[52] Otsubo T, Takasaki K, Yamamoto M, Katsuragawa H, Katagiri S, Yoshitoshi K, et al., Bleeding during hepatectomy can be reduced by clamping the inferior vena cava below the liver. *Surgery*. 2004 Jan;135(1):67-73.

[53] Bismuth H, Castaing D, Garden OJ. Major hepatic resection under total vascular exclusion. *Ann. Surg*. 1989 Jul;210(1):13-9.

[54] Huguet C, Nordlinger B, Galopin JJ, Bloch P, Gallot D. Normothermic hepatic vascular exclusion for extensive hepatectomy. *Surg Gynecol Obstet*. 1978 Nov;147(5):689-93.

[55] CunninghAm. J.D, Fong Y, Shriver C, Melendez J, Marx WL, Blumgart LH. One hundred consecutive hepatic resections. Blood loss, transfusion, and operative technique. *Arch. Surg*. 1994 Oct;129(10):1050-6.

[56] Lai EC, Fan ST, Lo CM, Chu KM, Liu CL. Anterior approach for difficult major right hepatectomy. *World J. Surg*. 1996 Mar-Apr;20(3):314-7; discussion 318.

[57] Belghiti J, Guevara OA, Noun R, Saldinger PF, Kianmanesh R. Liver hanging maneuver: a safe approach to right hepatectomy without liver mobilization. *J. Am. Coll. Surg*. 2001 Jul;193(1):109-11.

[58] Kokudo N, Imamura H, Sano K, Zhang K, Hasegawa K, Sugawara Y, et al., Ultrasonically assisted retrohepatic dissection for a liver hanging maneuver. *Ann. Surg*. 2005 Nov;242(5):651-4.

[59] Takatsuki M, Eguchi S, Hidaka M, Tajima Y, Kanematsu T. A secure taping technique for a liver hanging maneuver using a surgical probe. *Surg. Today*. 2008;38(12):1155-6. Epub 2008 Nov 28.

[60] Kim SH, Park SJ, Lee SA, Lee WJ, Park JW, Hong EK, et al., Various liver resections using hanging maneuver by three glisson's pedicles and three hepatic veins. *Ann. Surg*. 2007 Feb;245(2):201-5.

[61] Wu TJ, Wang F, Lin YS, Chan KM, Yu MC, Lee WC. Right hepatectomy by the anterior method with liver hanging versus conventional approach for large hepatocellular carcinomas. *Br. J. Surg*. 2010 Jul;97(7):1070-8.

[62] Aloia TA, Zorzi D, Abdalla EK, Vauthey JN. Two-surgeon technique for hepatic parenchymal transection of the noncirrhotic liver using saline-linked cautery and ultrasonic dissection. *Ann. Surg*. 2005 Aug;242(2):172-7.

[63] Palavecino M, Kishi Y, Chun YS, Brown DL, Gottumukkala VN, Lichtiger B, et al., Two-surgeon technique of parenchymal transection contributes to reduced transfusion rate in patients undergoing major hepatectomy: analysis of 1,557 consecutive liver resections. *Surgery*. 2010 Jan;147(1):40-8.

[64] Takatsuki M, Eguchi S, Yamanouchi K, Tokai H, Hidaka M, Soyama A, et al., Two-surgeon technique using saline-linked electric cautery and ultrasonic surgical aspirator in living donor hepatectomy: its safety and efficacy. *Am. J. Surg*. 2009 Feb;197(2):e25-7.

[65] Takayama T, Makuuchi M, Kubota K, Harihara Y, Hui AM, Sano K, et al., Randomized comparison of ultrasonic vs clamp transection of the liver. *Arch. Surg*. 2001;136(8):922–8.

[66] Yamamoto Y, Ikai I, Kume M, Sakai Y, Yamauchi A, Shinohara H, et al., New simple technique for hepatic parenchymal resection using a Cavitron Ultrasonic Surgical Aspirator and bipolar cautery equipped with a channel for water dripping. *World J. Surg*. 1999 Oct;23(10):1032-7.

[67] Fan ST, Lai EC, Lo CM, Chu KM, Liu CL, Wong J. Hepatectomy with an ultrasonic dissector for hepatocellular carcinoma. *Br. J. Surg.* 1996 Jan;83(1):117-20.

[68] Itoh S, Fukuzawa K, Shitomi Y, Okamoto M, Kinoshita T, Taketomi A, et al., Impact of the VIO system in hepatic resection for patients with hepatocellular carcinoma. *Surg. Today.* 2012 Dec;42(12):1176-82.

[69] Sugo H, Mikami Y, Matsumoto F, Tsumura H, Watanabe Y, Kojima K, et al., Hepatic resection using the harmonic scalpel. *Surg Today.* 2000;30:959–62.

[70] Romano F, Franciosi C, Caprotti R, Uggeri F, Uggeri F. Hepatic surgery using the LigaSure vessel sealing system. *World J. Surg.* 2005;29:110–2.

[71] Arita J, Hasegawa K, Kokudo N, Sano K, Sugawara Y, Makuuchi M. Randomized clinical trial of the effect of a saline-linked radiofrequency coagulator on blood loss during hepatic resection. *Br. J. Surg.* 2005;92(8):954–9.

[72] Gurusamy KS, Pamecha V, Sharma D, Davidson BR. Techniques for liver parenchymal transection in liver resection. *Cochrane Database Syst. Rev.* 2009 Jan 21;(1):CD006880.

[73] Sugo H, Mikami Y, Matsumoto F, Tsumura H, Watanabe Y, Kojima K, et al., Hepatic resection using the harmonic scalpel. *Surg. Today.* 2000;30(10):959-62.

[74] Hasegawa K, Kokudo N, Imamura H, Matsuyama Y, Aoki T, Minagawa M, et al., Prognostic impact of anatomic resection for hepatocellular carcinoma. *Ann. Surg.* 2005 Aug;242(2):252-9.

[75] Regimbeau JM, Kianmanesh R, Farges O, Dondero F, Sauvanet A, Belghiti J. Extent of liver resection influences the outcome in patients with cirrhosis and small hepatocellular carcinoma. *Surgery.* 2002 Mar;131(3):311-7.

[76] Arii S, Tanaka S, Mitsunori Y, Nakamura N, Kudo A, Noguchi N, et al., Surgical strategies for hepatocellular carcinoma with special reference to anatomical hepatic resection and intraoperative contrast-enhanced ultrasonography. *Oncology* 2010;78:125–130.

[77] Wang HQ, Yang J, Yang JY, Yan LN. Bile leakage test in liver resection: A systematic review and meta-analysis. *World J. Gastroenterol.* 2013 Dec 7;19(45):8420-6.

[78] Yin Z, Fan X, Ye H, Yin D, Wang J. Short- and long-term outcomes after laparoscopic and open hepatectomy for hepatocellular carcinoma: a global systematic review and meta-analysis. *Ann. Surg. Oncol.* 2013 Apr;20(4):1203-15. Epub 2012 Oct 26.

[79] Midorikawa Y, Kubota K, Takayama T, Toyoda H, Ijichi M, Torzilli G, et al., A comparative study of postoperative complications after hepatectomy in patients with and without chronic liver disease. *Surgery.* 1999;126:484–91.

[80] Kenjo A, Miyata H, Gotoh M, Kitagawa Y, Shimada M, Baba H, et al., Risk Stratification of 7,732 Hepatectomy Cases in 2011 from the National Clinical Database for Japan. *J. Am. Coll. Surg.*, in press

[81] Sato M, Tateishi R, Yasunaga H, Horiguchi H, Yoshida H, Matsuda S, et al., Mortality and morbidity of hepatectomy, radiofrequency ablation, and embolization for hepatocellular carcinoma: a national survey of 54,145 patients. *J. Gastroenterol.* 2012; 47: 1125-33

[82] Llovet JM, Fuster J, Bruix J. Intention-to-treat analysis of surgical treatment for early hepatocellular carcinoma: resection versus transplantation. *Hepatology.* 1999 Dec;30(6):1434-40.

[83] Kianmanesh R, Regimbeau JM, Belghiti J. Selective approach to major hepatic resection for hepatocellular carcinoma in chronic liver disease. *Surg. Oncol. Clin. N. Am.* 2003 Jan;12(1):51-63.

[84] Poon RT, Fan ST, Lo CM, Liu CL, Wong J. Long-term survival and pattern of recurrence after resection of small hepatocellular carcinoma in patients with preserved liver function: implications for a strategy of salvage transplantation. *Ann. Surg.* 2002 Mar;235(3):373-82.

[85] Ikai I, Kudo M, Arii S, Omata M, Kojiro M, Sakamoto M, et al., Report of the 18th follow-up survey of primary liver cancer in Japan. *Hepatol. Res.* 2010 Nov;40(11):1043-59.

[86] Bruix J, Sherman M. Management of hepatocellular carcinoma. *Hepatology.* 2005 Nov;42(5):1208-36.

In: Therapy for Hepatocellular Carcinoma
Editor: Nobuhiro Ohkohchi

ISBN: 978-1-63117-929-7
© 2014 Nova Science Publishers, Inc.

Chapter 5

Transplantation for Hepatocellular Carcinoma

Naoki Kawagishi[*], *M.D.*
Division of Transplantation, Reconstruction, and Endoscopic Surgery,
Tohoku University Hospital, Japan

Abstract

Liver transplantation (LT) is universally accepted as the final rescue therapy for end-stage liver disease. Although there are a lot of primary diseases for the indication of LT, hepatocellular carcinoma (HCC) is one of the major indications of LT. In this chapter, LT is described on the basis of two different backgrounds i.e. Japan and western countries, and this contrast represents the living donor and the deceased donor transplantation. Milan criteria has been the gold standard criteria for HCC, but expanding the criteria has been proposed by some authors in light of favorable results noted in single center studies with variable durations of follow-up. The question still remains whether resection and LT should be considered as alternative, complimentary, or sequential in an intention-to-treat strategy. Immunosuppressants and chemotherapies on LT still remain controversial. The future direction of determining optimal LT for an individual patient requires consideration of numerous factors including liver damage, tumor stage, biomarkers, imaging techniques, and geographical transplant availability.

1. Introduction

Fifty years have passed since the first liver transplantation (LT) was performed. In the early days of LT, the main primary disease for which it was performed was hepatocellular carcinoma (HCC). The 10th liver transplant recipient in the world, a 19 month-old girl with HCC was the first to achieve extended survival [1]. (Table 1) Although tumor recurrence developed 3 months after the transplantation, she survived 400 days before dying of

---

[*] Tel.: +81-22-717-7214; Fax: +81-22-717-7217; e-mail : kawan@med.tohoku.ac.jp.

disseminated metastatic disease. In the 1970s and 1980s, novel immunosuppressants such as cyclosporine and tacrolimus enhanced organ transplantations including liver transplantation. Many end-stage liver disease patients were helped by liver transplantation, and this kind of rescue therapy spread all over developed countries. As regards HCC, after the establishment of the "Milan criteria (MC)", the indication for LT in HCC became clear. However 20 years since the publication of the MC, the indication of LC for HCC has become controversial. First of all, in terms of the first treatment for HCC, hepatic resection, ablation, and/or IVR (interventional radiology) were performed according to the condition of the liver functions. If these treatments are a contraindication, or if liver function is classified as Child-Pugh C, or the tumor recurs many times and will become untreatable in the near future, the patient becomes a candidate for LT. In Japan, the main donor source is living donors, so the background of LT is different from that in western counties. In the future, discussions about expanding the indication for and the pretreatment of HCC for achieving better long-term outcome will be necessary. In this chapter, I will discuss LT as the final treatment for HCC.

Table 1. Milestones of liver transplantation

Year	Description
1963	First human LT at the University of Colorado
1967	First successful human LT
1979	Cyclosporine introduced for kidney and liver
1987	University of Wisconsin solution for improved preservation
1988	First LDLT in Brazil
1989	Tacrolimus for organ transplantation
	First successful LDLT in Australia
	First LDLT in Japan
1992	Introduction of the modified piggyback technique
1994	First report of right lobe graft for LDLT
2002	First report of full laparoscopic donor procedure

2. Background of LT for HCC in Western Countries

LT in Japan is based on the experiences of deceased donor LT in Western countries. Here, I will introduce the historical aspects, and outline of LT for HCC in Western countries.

Thomas E. Starzl pioneered LT in 1963 for a patient with biliary atresia in Denver. Thereafter, the following 3 of 7 recipients in the 1960's had HCC [2, 3, 4, 5]. In July 1967, the 10th liver transplant recipient in the world survived for 400 days, and this case was regarded as the first successful case of LT. The recipient's primary disease was HCC. But many efforts of LT for primary liver malignancies have generally met with failure [6], and the initial enthusiasm for transplantation in patients with hepatobiliary cancer soon faded in the face of early recurrences and short-term survival. Thus, in 1989, LT for HCC was temporarily suspended in the United States [2]. In Europe, the 3-year survival of liver transplant recipients for HCC was at most 50% during the same period [7]. In the 1990s, the advent of more accurate diagnostic techniques and identification of a number of prognostic factors associated with poor outcome had provided a better understanding of the problems inherent in the application of LT for HCC. This means that restricted and proper indications of LT for HCC led to the lower recurrence and better prognosis. In 1996, Mazzaferro et al. reported in The New England Journal of Medicine that they had performed LT for a patient who had HCC within the criteria for eligibility for transplantation, i.e., the presence of a tumor 5 cm or less in diameter in patients with single hepatocellular carcinomas and of no more than 3 tumor nodules, each 3 cm or less in diameter, in patients with multiple tumors [8]. After 4 years, the actuarial survival rate was 75% and the rate of recurrence-free survival was 83%. The overall and recurrence-free survival rates at 4 years among the 35 patients (73% of the total) who met the predetermined criteria for the selection of small HCC at the pathological review of small hepatocellular carcinomas and at the pathological review of the explanted liver were 85% and 92%, respectively, whereas the rates in the 13 patients (27%) whose tumors exceeded these limits were 50% and 59%, respectively (P = 0.01 for overall survival; P = 0.002 for recurrence-free survival) [8]. The findings of Mazzaferro et al.'s report were also supported by findings from other institutions indicating that this indication was feasible for LT for HCC [9]. The MC spread worldwide as the gold standard indication that leads to the conclusion that liver transplantation is an effective treatment for small, unresectable hepatocellular carcinomas in patients with cirrhosis (Table 2). In 2002, the MELD (Model for End-Stage Liver Disease) score was introduced in the United States [10]. The MELD score was selected as the basis for the new allocation policy because of its high degree of accuracy for predicting death in patients having a variety of liver disease etiologies across a broad spectrum of liver disease severity. The MELD score consisted of total bilirubin, serum creatinine, and the International Normalized Ratio (INR). Except for the most urgent patients, all patients would be ranked continuously under the new policy according to their MELD score. Waiting time is used only to prioritize patients with identical MELD scores. Patients who were not well served by the MELD score could be prioritized through a regionalized peer review system. This new allocation policy of the United Network of Organ Sharing (UNOS) based on the model for MELD gave candidates with stage T1 or stage T2 HCC a priority MELD score beyond their degree of hepatic decompensation. This new allocation policy led to an increased incidence rate of deceased donor LT in HCC candidates. Furthermore, the 5-month dropout rate decreased significantly. In addition, the 5-month survival while waiting increased in the post-MELD period. Thus, the new MELD-based allocation policy benefited HCC candidates [11]. In 2006, the new criteria, the UCSF (University of California San Francisco) criteria, were introduced in the United States. Owing to these selection criteria, the retrospective analysis of the United Network for Organ Sharing found a significant improvement in survival over time for HCC patients undergoing LT, with a 5-year survival of 61.1% contrasting with the previously observed 5-year survival rate of 25.3% in 1987. However, some investigators suggested that the MC might be too restrictive. Indeed, the proportion of HCC patients not fulfilling the MC that could be cured by LT probably ranges from 27% to 49% [12]. The retrospective analysis of 70 consecutive patients with cirrhosis and HCC who underwent LT over a 12-year period at the UCSF prompted Yao et al. [13] to propose an expansion of the selection criteria for HCC, according to post-LT tumor characteristics. In this study, the 5-year survival rate of 60 patients with 1 lesion =<6.5 cm or 3 lesions, the largest lesion =<4.5 cm with a total tumor diameter =<8 cm on the explanted livers (UCSF criteria) was 75.2%. When transposed to the pre-LT tumor evaluation of 39 patients with non-incidental HCC meeting the UCSF criteria, the 5-year survival rate was 84%. Yao et al. concluded that these new criteria did not significantly compromise the excellent post-LT outcomes achieved by the MC. It was therefore tempting to extend the MC for patient selection for cadaveric donation [14] or for the living donor LT [15]. Another institution in the United States also reported that patients meeting the MC had similar 5-year post-transplant survival to patients meeting the UCSF criteria by preoperative imaging (79% vs. 64%; P = 0.061) and explant pathology (86% vs. 71%; P = 0.057) [16]. And the follow-up study from UCSF reported that the UCSF criteria better predict acceptable post-transplant outcome than do the MC [17]. In Europe, the results of the patients with HCC over MC showed encouraging outcomes [18]. But some other centers investigated and found that the 5-year survival was arithmetically lower in UCSF+ Milan- patients than in Milan+ patients but this difference was not significant (P = 0.10) [19]. Based on the pathological features of the explanted liver, the 5-year survival was 70.4 +/- 3.4%, 63.6 +/- 7.8%, and 34.1 +/- 3.1%, in Milan+ patients (n = 184), UCSF+ Milan- patients (n = 39), and UCSF- Milan- patients (n = 238), respectively (P < 0.001). However, the 5-year survival did not differ between the Milan+ and UCSF+ Milan- patients (P = 0.33). These results show that when applied to the pre-LT evaluation, the UCSF criteria were associated with a 5-year survival below 50%. Their applicability of the UCSF criteria was therefore limited, despite similar survival rates to those for the MC, when the explanted liver was taken into account. So there are some arguments about which criteria are best for LT for HCC, but we have to decide the criteria in accordance with the present LT and HCC clinical situations. In the last 10 years, diagnostic imaging techniques have made remarkable progress in the hepatobiliary pancreatic field. This means that indications for LT for HCC should become flexible to be in line with the progress in imaging techniques and the findings of new biomarkers.

Table 2. Overview of the criteria of LT for HCC

Institution	Year	n	Criteria	OS (within)	OS (beyond)
Milan	1996	48	One lesion = ≤ 5cm, or 2 to 3 lesions = ≤ 3cm	85 (4y)	50 (4y)
UCSF	2001	70	One nodule = ≤ 6.5cm, or = ≤ 3nodules= ≤ 4.5cm, Total tumor diameter = ≤ 8cm	75 (5y)	<30 (5y)
UCLA	2007	467	UCSF	81 (5y)	32 (5y)
Tokyo	2007	78	5 nodules = ≤ 5cm	94 (3y)	50 (3y)
Metroticket	2009	1556	Nodule size (cm) +number = ≤ 7	71 (5y)	48 (5y)
ASAN	2010	206	One nodule = ≤ 5cm, = ≤ 6 nodules, no gross vascular invasion	76 (5y)	19 (5y)
Kyoto	2013	198	= ≤ 10 nodules, all = ≤ 5cm, PIVKA-II = ≤ 400mAU/mL	82 (5y)	42 (5y)

3. Background of LT for HCC in Japan

In Japan, living donor liver transplantation (LDLT) was performed for a patient with biliary atresia who received the transplant from his father in 1989. The fourth living donor liver transplant recipient in the world, he was the pioneer of LT in Japan. From this case, the number of LDLT increased rapidly in Japan from 10 cases in 1990 to 30 cases in 1991 (Figure 1).

At first, in Japan, most of the recipients were under 18 years old, although the number of adult recipients increased gradually [20, 21]. Since the first report of adult cases with right lobe grafts, many centers in Japan began to introduce adult recipients [22]. The number of adult cases increased, and short-term survival was secured even for adult LDLT, the indication spread to HCC patients in Japan (Figure 2). Particularly from the 2000s, LDLTs were performed for approximately 100 cases of HCC annually. Even for LDLT, if the recipient's HCC were evaluated as with the MC, the patient would be predicted to have good survival.

The donor in LDLT was a family member or blood relative. Thus, the social situation was completely different from that for deceased donors, which should be distributed in an equitable manner. Namely, it was thought that it was justified if LDLT were performed for patients whose HCC was over the MC. Actually, until 2003, the number of LDLT recipients who had HCC over the MC was around 56% of all the HCC of LDLT recipients in Japan [23]. As mentioned above, LDLT for patients with HCC was accepted year by year, but the fact that social health insurance did not cover LDLT for HCC remained a big issue in Japan. In July 2004, the government permitted the inclusion of LDLT for HCC in the Japanese social insurance system if the HCC was within the MC. This doubled the number of LDLT for HCC. There were some troubles with the definition of the MC in terms of the downstaging, preoperative treatment, and histopathological findings of the explanted native liver at local insurance branches, because the government declaration did not provide precise definitions of these. But in Japan primary HCC was treated with resection, IVR, or RFA at first. Then if the liver function was decompensated, the patient was introduced to LT. From such a process, in June 2007, the criteria for social insurance indication in Japan was improved as follows: (1) maximal diameter of the tumor was calculated within 1 month before LT; (2) HCC was defined as a tumor that had low attenuation foci on plain CT, high attenuation foci in the arterial phase of enhanced CT, and low attenuation foci in the portal phase of enhanced CT. If the contrast medium was not permitted, MRI was the substitute examination; (3) concerning the treatment history, if the tumor was treated more than 3 months before the transplantation, it was not counted as the number if the tumor did not recur within 1 month before transplantation. To summarize in brief, it was changed as the above. In other words, we did not have to count the tumor, which did not recur in imaging more than 3 months after treatment in Japan.

Deceased donor liver transplantation in Japan was included in the social insurance system from 2006, while HCC was included from the beginning. To be listed as a deceased donor liver transplant candidate of HCC, the tumor should be within MC. The inspection for entry was conducted in the same manner as the LDLT insurance system. However, during the listed deceased donor candidate, image examinations should be performed every 3 or 4 months even if the tumor remained within the MC. If the HCC enlarged beyond the MC, the candidate should be withdrawn from the entry. The number of deceased donor LT for HCC in Japan was very limited at that time, just 1 case until 2006. In the future, discussions will be held about expanding the indication from the MC to others, like changing from the Milan to the UCSF criteria in the United States.

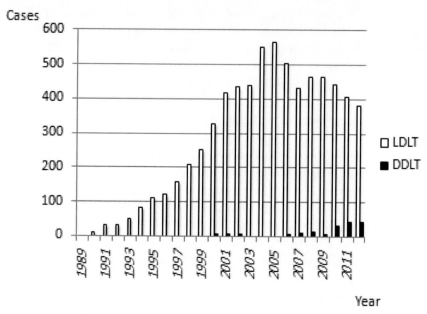

Registry of the Japanese Liver Transplantation Society 2012.

Figure 1. Liver transplantation in Japan.

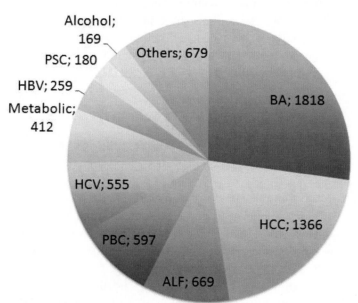

HCC is the secondary frequent primary disease for which LDLT is performed in Japan.
(Primary disease, number of cases)
BA: biliary atresia; HCC: hepatocellular carcinoma; ALF: acute liver failure; PBC: primary biliary
    cirrhosis; PSC: primary sclerosing cholangitis
(Registry of the Japanese Liver Transplantation Society 2012)

Figure 2. Primary diseases for which LDLT is performed in Japan.

4. Current Status of LT for HCC in Japan

4.1. Practical Issues

4.1.1. Living Donor Liver Transplantation

The first LDLT was performed in Brazil in December 1988 [24]. The first successful case of LDLT was the case of a Japanese parent and her child in Brisbane, Australia [25]. From the first case of LDLT in Japan in 1989, a total of more than 6000 of cases were experienced. One of the most considerable issues in LDLT is the ethical issue [26]. In 2003, the Japan Society for Transplantation renewed its ethical guidelines [27]. The major points are as follows: (1) the role of the Japan Network of Organ Transplantation was described. (2) The following ethical principles and informed consent standards should be implemented for living donors and should be confirmed by third-party personnel who have no relation or interests with the donor and/or with the recipient and who can act as an advocate of the donor. * Voluntary willingness to donate; * free from coercion; * medically and socially suitable (20 years old or older); * fully informed of the risks and benefits as a donor and; * fully informed of the risk, benefits, and alternative treatment to the recipient. (3) Living donors should be limited to relatives within the sixth degree and the third by marriage. (4) Living donation other than from those relatives should be individually approved by the Institutional Ethics Committee (IEC) and should be reviewed by the Japan Society of Transplantation (JST). (5) Donors aged between 16 and 19 years can be chosen as an exception if they are interviewed and judged to be psychosocially suitable as the donor by psychiatrists, and such transplantation should be individually approved by the IEC. Unlike living kidney donation, the living liver donation operation is much riskier and more complicated. To protect the altruistic donor and to avoid unnecessary morbidity and mortality, vigilant evaluation based on an established protocol is mandatory. A living donor should be a completely healthy person psychologically and mentally [28]. Although many patients with underlying disease have successfully undergone major hepatectomy, the same acceptance threshold could not be applied to a healthy person donating a part of the liver to another person. Even though major hepatectomy could be performed with zero perioperative mortality, concomitant morbid illness accounts for the majority of potentially fatal complications [29]. Thus, there should not be any compromise in the evaluation process and any concomitant medical illness should not be allowed for living donation.

The typical donor operational procedures of the left lateral segment are described as follows [30]: The transection line for lateral segmentectomy is along the falciform ligament, the border of segments 3 and 4. The transection line for left lobectomy without the middle hepatic vein is a few millimeters to the left of the middle hepatic vein. The transection line for a left lobectomy with the middle hepatic vein is a few millimeters to the right of the middle hepatic vein. An inverted T-shaped incision or upper middle incision is made, and the abdominal cavity is entered. Liver biopsy is performed and a pathologist is consulted. If the histology of the liver is intact, the donor operation is continued. Intraoperative ultrasound is done to confirm the hepatic veins. Hepatic arteries are isolated by using papaverine hydroxychloride to prevent arterial spasms. Intraoperative cholangiography is performed to identify the left hepatic duct and divide it. Next the portal vein is isolated and liver parenchymal transection starts without interrupting the blood supply. After division of the liver parenchyma, it will be adjusted for the procedure of the recipient's operation. The graft is observed and then the hepatic artery is divided followed by division of the left portal vein and the hepatic vein. If there is circulation deficiency of segment 4 or the Spiegel lobe after graftectomy, sometimes it is resected. Other donor graft types consist of the right lobe, left lobe, left lobe with Spiegel lobe, posterior sector, and reduced size graft of segment 2 or segment 3 [31, 32, 33, 34, 35, 36, 37, 38].

The recent interest in a minimally invasive approach to liver surgery has raised the possibility of applying these techniques to living donor operations [39, 40, 41, 42, 43]. It should be proposed that the procedure, as described, did not increase the operative risks of the procedure; instead, it decreased the potential morbidity. But we should caution that this procedure should only be considered for select donors, and that only surgical teams familiar with both living donor hepatectomy and laparoscopic liver surgery should entertain this possibility.

The Japanese Liver Transplantation Society presented its first report on donor morbidity in 2003 [44, 45]. The Society has been continuing to survey outcomes in living liver donors in Japan. The accumulated experience indicates a reduction in the incidence of donor complications, especially for right lobe resection. One donor death and 2 cases of severe after-effects related to liver donation have been reported during 18 years of living donor liver transplantation experience in Japan. The long-term outcomes of the donors, including quality of life, were investigated by some institutions [46, 47]. The donors' life was almost guaranteed regardless of the lobe the authors used as the graft.

Back-table operation is performed followed by flushing the cold preserving solution through the portal vein and hepatic artery. Flushing the solution is performed until the fluid from the hepatic vein is clear. The graft is weighed. This procedure includes graft preparation from the aspect of verification of the vascular anatomy (anomalies), potential vascular injuries, and reconstruction if needed, as well as detailed graft inspection [48]. Venoplasty is then performed to bring the venous orifice together to a common orifice. For example, despite the distance of 2 to 2.5 cm between the middle hepatic vein (MHV) and the right hepatic vein (RHV), the 2 venous openings could be brought together easily without much tension provided that the length of the extrahepatic portion of the RHV and MHV is 5 mm or more. If the MHV and RHV are not large enough for a common orifice, the liver tissue in between may be compressed and devascularized. In case segment V or VIII veins need to be reconstructed, the recipient's superficial femoral vein, native MHV, native recanalized umbilical vein, or cryopreserved veins are used for reconstruction (Figure 3) [49, 50, 51, 52]. A single biliary duct orifice in the graft is the most favorable type for duct-to-duct anastomosis. In case of 2 ductal orifices, which are close to each other, they can be joined together to form a common orifice. Ductoplasty may not be suitable for duct orifices that are more than 3 mm apart. Approximation of the 2 duct orifices in this situation may cause tension, ischemia, and subsequent stenosis of the anastomosis. Hepaticojejunostomy is then the preferred method [53]. A hepatic artery is just examined the conditions. The trimming of the arteries is done just before the anastomosis. During the back-table operation, the graft should be kept immersed in a cold preservation solution to prevent warm ischemic injury. A tip of the hepatic tissue is resected as the zero biopsy.

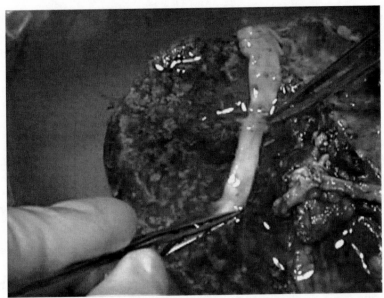

Orifices of the middle hepatic vein on the cutting surface of the right lobe are reconstructed by using the recipient's superficial femoral vein.

Figure 3. Reconstruction of the middle hepatic vein of a right lobe graft.

The recipient's operation starts with a bilateral subcostal incision with an upper midline extension to the xiphoid process also known as the Mercedes incision. The presence of a previous incision may lead to a change in the planned incision for that patient. Hilar dissection is carried out to free the right hepatic artery (RHA) at the right liver hilum, above the level of the transection of the common hepatic duct, so as to protect the blood supply to the common hepatic duct from the RHA as it crosses in front of or behind the common hepatic duct. After the division of the hepatic artery branches, the right or left side of the portal vein may be obvious. If not, dissection on both sides of the hepatoduodenal ligament is made until the portal vein is exposed. Then, dissection is kept close to the portal vein, leaving all the tissues surrounding the common hepatic duct intact. The portal vein is not divided until mobilization of the liver is completed and the liver graft is available. The common hepatic duct and the surrounding tissues are freed and transected as high as possible but not into the hilar plate, because a caudate hepatic duct may be included in the stump but missed and be the cause of bile leakage afterward. The exposed caudate hepatic veins are divided and sutured. The division of the right triangular ligament and adhesion with the right adrenal gland mobilizes the right liver. The right IVC ligament is divided. The left liver is mobilized by dividing the lesser omentum and left triangular ligament. The left caudate lobe is then lifted off from the IVC by dividing the short hepatic veins. The RHV, HHV, and LHV are then encircled. For the right graft, hepatic vein anastomosis is normally performed at the level of the right hepatic vein orifice of the recipient. For the left graft, hepatic vein anastomosis is normally performed at the level of the common trunk of the left and middle hepatic vein orifice of the recipient. After control by the vascular clamp of the portal vein, the right and left portal veins are divided. The RHV and the common trunk of the MHV and RHV are each controlled by the strong vascular clamp and divided. The venovenous bypass is rarely employed these days. The hepatic vein anastomosis is then completed with 5-0 prolene running sutures. The anastomosis of the hepatic veins has many variations between institutions [54, 55, 56]. The portal reconstruction in different LT techniques is similar, generally using an end-to-end simple portoportal anastomosis, or in a "rollover sleeve" fashion in which the edges of both donor and recipient portal veins are everted to ensure intimal approximation [57]. Arterial anastomosis varies greatly and depends on the arterial anatomy of each recipient. The goal is to perform anastomosis by using near-equal diameters of the donor and recipient arteries without rotation, surplus length, and stenosis. Before the introduction of microvascular anastomosis, the incidence of hepatic artery thrombosis had been reported to be as high as 25% [58]. After microsurgery of the hepatic artery was introduced, the incidence of the hepatic artery thrombosis was reduced to below several percent [59, 60]. The biliary anastomosis is done with interrupted or running 6–0 monofilament absorbable sutures. The technique of anastomosis is end-to-end choledocho-choledochostomy with some variations because of the diameter of the recipient or donor bile ducts. Some surgeons prefer to side cut the small bile duct when a size discrepancy exists. In the presence of a normal or small size of both the donor and the recipient bile ducts, they prefer to make an oblique cut on both sides. The purpose of the side-cut is to compensate the tissue lost during suturing, thus preventing postoperative stricture. In case of an extra large bile duct, which is seen usually in the recipient, some authors advocate to close a part of the diameter with a suture and create an anastomosis using the open part with the reduced diameter. In patients with very small common ducts or with extensive peribiliary venous collaterals, it is preferable to perform choledochojejunostomy in Roux-en-Y fashion. In recent years, microsurgical biliary reconstruction has been introduced [61, 62]. The microsurgical biliary anastomosis is performed with 6-0 Prolene sutures on a 6-0-gauge cardiovascular-point needle. The interrupted suturing technique is used for the posterior wall anastomosis first, and then the continuous suture and interrupted tie technique or combined microvascular anastomosis is used for the anterior wall. This technique is simple to use, decreases the operative time, and avoids suturing into the posterior wall as all the sutures are put into place before the knots are tied and all suture knots are tied extraluminally.

Postoperatively, patients should be transferred to the interdisciplinary intensive care unit (ICU) and maintained on ventilation support until they become normothermic and hemodynamically stable. The immunosuppressive protocol used in general is composed of steroids and tacrolimus or the combination of steroids and cyclosporine followed by mycophenolate mofetil or anti-CD25 antibody. During hospitalization, complete laboratory tests, as well as calcineurin inhibitor trough level measurements, are performed daily according to the standard protocol. Vascular patency is checked two or three times daily by duplex ultrasound during the first 7 days after LT or after an unexpected increase in the liver enzymes or deterioration of the liver function. If indicated, assessment of the arterial tree is performed either by angiography or angio-computed tomography or magnetic resonance imaging.

Complications after LT have significant impact on the early, as well as the late, postoperative course, and may range from minimal morbidities to a severe and life-threatening situation. Generally, the prognosis depends on the status of the recipient, the donor organ, and technical errors during the operation [63]. The postoperative complications can be divided into surgical and medical complications. As regards the surgical complications, the proper reconstruction of the afferent vessels is a prerequisite for successful

LTx. Poor organ inflow or outflow may result in severe postoperative complications. The nonsurgical complications include cholangitis, nonsurgical bleeding, infection, and rejection.

4.1.2. Deceased Donor Liver Transplantation

Deceased donor liver transplantation in Japan was first performed in 1964, which was not so behind that in Western countries. But heart transplantation in 1968 was very controversial in terms of the donor selection. From this heart transplantation, deceased donor organ transplantation was not performed except for kidney transplant from non-heart beating donors. But in 1997, the organ transplant law was enacted and in 1999, the first deceased donor liver transplantation was performed under the new organ transplant law [64, 65]. Although law permitted the brain dead donor, the number of deceased donors did not increase. In 2008, the "Declaration of Istanbul" recommended that countries provide transplant services for their own populations, and the Japanese government moved to change the law (Table 3) [66]. In 2009, the new organ transplant law was enacted and came into effect in July of the following year. The new law permitted brain dead donation only with the agreement of the brain-dead person's family, not based on the donor's possession of a donor card. And donors under the age of 15 were permitted. Although the Japanese transplant law was established as equal to that in Western countries, the number of deceased donors was still unsatisfactory, namely just 50 or 60 cases per year in the whole country.

Table 3. Declaration of Istanbul
(definitions of organ trafficking and transplant tourism)

Organ trafficking	The recruitment, transport, transfer, harboring, or receipt of living or deceased persons or their organs by means of the threat or use of force or other forms of coercion, of abduction, of fraud, of deception, of the abuse of power or of a position of vulnerability, or of the giving to, or the receiving by, a third party of payments or benefits to achieve the transfer of control over the potential donor, for the purpose of exploitation by the removal of organs for transplantation.
Transplant commercialism	A policy or practice in which an organ is treated as a commodity, including by being bought or sold or used for material gain.
Travel for transplantation	The movement of organs, donors, recipients, or transplant professionals across jurisdictional borders for transplantation purposes. Travel for transplantation becomes transplant tourism if it involves organ trafficking and/or transplant commercialism or if the resources (organs, professionals, and transplant centers) devoted to providing transplants to patients from outside a country undermine the country's ability to provide transplant services for its own population.

Under the above-mentioned situation, the number of deceased donor liver transplantations in Japan ranges from 40 to 50 per year, which is one tenth of the living donor liver transplantations. The practical method of deceased donor liver transplantation is described elsewhere [67, 68]; the larger graft and the bigger vessels mean it is an easier operation than LDLT.

By the assessment of the Committee of Indication for Transplantation (4 physicians, 5 surgeons, and 1 pediatrician) all candidates are reviewed on the basis of the demographic, clinical, and laboratory data including CTP score, MELD score, and disease-specific prognostic score, and each candidate is assigned clinical priority [69]. The priority of candidates is represented by a medical point system, in which points are awarded according to estimated survival: 9 points for estimated survival less than 30 days, 6 points for less than 180 days, 3 points for less than 360 days, and 1 point for over 360 days. In patients with hepatocellular carcinoma, the points were determined only by the degree of hepatic decompensation. Additional points are awarded according to ABO blood group compatibility: 1.5 points for an identical blood group and 1 point for a compatible blood group. Patients with higher total points have a higher priority for donor liver allocation. For patients with identical points, the waiting time is a liver allocation measure. Although the original CTP score used different criteria for total bilirubin levels between patients with cholestatic disease and those with other etiologies, the criteria for the CTP score in the current Japanese allocation system did not change according to the etiology of liver disease. The MELD score was calculated using the most recent version of the formula documented on the UNOS website. Liver disease etiology was not incorporated in this version of the formula. Laboratory values less than 1.0 were set to 1.0 and the maximum serum creatinine was set at 4.0 mg/dL. Serum creatinine was set at 4.0 mg/dL if the patient had received dialysis at least twice within the week prior to the serum creatinine test. The MELD score was not capped at a score of 40.

Many efforts to emphasize the deceased donor campaign have been put forward, but the number of donations in Japan is still unsatisfactory. Drastic nationwide measures are needed for the increase of deceased donor organ transplantation in this country.

4.2. Indication

In Japan, most HCC emerge on the basis of viral hepatitis. Thus, LT is the promising therapy for the patients of cirrhosis who cannot have surgical treatment. On the other hand, deceased donor LT is very limited, and the requirement for entry is restricted within the MC. And the additional conditions are as follows: (1) maximal diameter of the tumor was calculated within 1 month before LT; (2) HCC was defined the tumor that had low attenuation foci on plain CT, high attenuation foci in the arterial phase of enhanced CT, and low attenuation foci in the portal phase of enhanced CT. If contrast medium was not permitted, MRI was the substitute examination; (3) concerning the treatment history, the tumor was treated more than 3 months before transplantation, it was not counted as the number if the tumor did not recur within 1 month before transplantation.

In the 1990s, the indication of HCC for LDLT was controversial. In 1999, the Kyoto Group started the pilot study of LDLT for HCC [70]. Their exclusion criteria included only patients with extrahepatic metastasis or vascular invasion detected during preoperative evaluation. Thirty patients (54%) were in tumor, node, metastases stage IVa and 25 patients (45%) did not meet the MC at the time of LDLT. The follow-up period was 1 to 39 months (median, 11 months). The overall survival rates at 1 and 3 years were 73% and 55%, respectively, and the latter was significantly lower than that of adult right lobe LDLT without HCC (71% at 3 years). Fourteen patients died because of postoperative complications without tumor recurrence. Thirty-six patients survived without recurrence and 6 patients had recurrence. Among the 6 patients with recurrence, 4 had survived for 11 to 36 months after LDLT. In the analysis of patients who survived longer than 3 months after transplantation, 19 of 20 patients within the MC survived without recurrence. However, 15 of 20 patients beyond the criteria also survived without recurrence for 3 to 33 months (median, 12 months) and 3 of 5 patients with recurrence survived for 11 to 36 months (median, 20 months). Histopathologic grading and microscopic portal venous invasion had a significant negative impact on tumor recurrence. And they concluded that because many patients who did not meet the MC survived without tumor recurrence after transplantation, different patient selection criteria are necessary in LDLT to save those with advanced HCC. In the setting of LDLT for HCC treatment, the relationship between the recipient and donor is altruism; the graft is never shared with the third party, and over MC may be acceptable. But there should be scrupulous informed consent including the possibility with early recurrence of HCC.

In July 2004, the government permitted the inclusion of LDLT for HCC in the Japanese social insurance system if the HCC was within the MC. For decades, this restriction of social insurance led the indication of LDLT for HCC within the MC. But some institutions tried to perform transplants for patients exceeding the MC. The Kyoto Group proposed the Kyoto criteria, involving a combination of tumor number equal or less than 10, maximal diameter of each tumor equal or less than 5 cm, and serum des-gamma-carboxy prothrombin levels equal to or less than 400 mAU/mL. The group has used these criteria since January 2007 [71]. One hundred ninety-eight patients with HCC who underwent LDLT from February 1999 through December 2011 were enrolled in this study. Tumor biology was significantly less aggressive in patients within the Kyoto criteria. They concluded that the Kyoto criteria are useful expanded criteria for LDLT for HCC and could help to achieve favorable outcomes. The Tokyo group proposed the Tokyo criteria as follows: up to 5 HCC nodules with a maximum diameter of 5 cm (the 5-5 rule) [72]. A total of 78 adult patients underwent adult living donor liver transplantation between April 1996 and October 2005. The Kyushu group proposed other criteria, known as Kyushu University criteria as follows: tumor nodule equal to or less than 5 cm and des-gamma-carboxy prothrombin equal to or less than 300 mAU/mL [73].

Concerning the progress of the imaging devices and the results from the high volume center, the indication for LDLT for HCC will expand over the MC in the future. But it needs in-depth analysis and discussions.

4.3. Practical Issues about LT of HCC

The procedure of the LT was described in detail in the former section. Here, we describe the particular procedure of LT for HCC. In the case of HCC recipients, particularly for patients over the MC, laparotomy is incised normally but whether lymphnode metastasis or peritoneal dissemination is present should be checked carefully. So in LDLT, the donor's operation starts after the recipient's laparotomy. Immunosuppressants are the same as for other primary diseases. Although transarterial chemoembolization is sometimes performed before LT, anastomosis of vessels and biliary ducts are done as normal. In the early period, neoadjuvant or adjuvant chemotherapy was administered in Japan, but these days, chemotherapy during LT is considered on a case-by-case basis. If the recurrent tumor is resectable, surgical resection is strongly recommended.

Most HCC patients have viral hepatitis such as HBV or HCV. In terms of HBV, the early experience with liver transplantation for HBV-related disease was that the majority of patients developed recurrent infection in the early postoperative period [74]. However, over the last 20 years, the improvement of specific prophylactic therapy has almost settled the problem of recurrent hepatitis B. Namely, injection of high doses of HBIG (hepatitis B immunoglobulin) and nucleoside analogue administration have contributed to prolong the survival of HBs positive recipients so that at present this is equal to that of recipients with other primary diseases. On the other hand, this therapy is very expensive, which leads to poor compliance. These factors led to the development of alternative strategies of prophylactic therapy for hepatitis B. But from 2008, HBIG was approved by the social insurance system in Japan. In recent years, alternative prophylactic treatment is under investigation [75].

Recurrence of HCV infection is nearly universal and often occurs immediately after transplantation. Indeed, the prevalence of chronic HCV in HCV-positive liver transplant recipients is 70% to 90% after 1 year, and the progression of fibrosis is accelerated, which means that 8% to 44% of patients progress to allograft cirrhosis within 5 to 10 years [76]. Therefore, graft and patient survival are significantly reduced for HCV-positive recipients in comparison with HCV-negative recipients. But in recent years, direct-acting antivirals (DAA) such as protease inhibitors, polymerase, or other nonstructural protein inhibitors represent a new era in HCV-associated liver disease [77, 78]. These agents are astonishingly promising for HCV recipients.

Another important primary disease of LT for HCC is nonalcoholic steatohepatitis (NASH). NASH has the possibility of recurrence after LT, but no effective prophylaxis is available for it so far. Maintaining low body weight, good control of diabetes mellitus, this kind of clinical stability is needed after LT.

4.4. Outcome

A Japanese nationwide survey was performed in 2004, and results published in 2007 [79, 80, 81]. In 2004, it included 318 cases, and in 2007, 653 cases (Table 4, 5). The cases were followed until the end of June 2006, with a median follow-up period of 21.5 months (range, 6 - 97.8 months). The median age was 56 years (range, 21-70 years). A total of 476 patients (72.9%) were male, and 177 (27.1%) were female. HCV infection was a leading cause of liver cirrhosis, occurring in 385 recipients (59%), vs. HBV for 199 (30%). Half the patients had advanced liver failure (Child-Pugh class C), whereas 30% were Child-Pugh class B, and 10% were Child-Pugh class A. Of the 653 recipients, at the time of the last follow-up, 497 (76.1%) were alive without (n = 451) or with (n = 46) HCC recurrence; 156 (23.9%) had died of recurrent HCC (n = 46) or for other reasons (n = 110). Actuarial patient survival was 82.6% at 1 year, 72.6% at 3 years, and 68.9% at 5 years; actuarial disease-free survival (DFS) was 77.4% at 1 year, 65.1% at 3 years, and 61.5% at 5 years. By univariate analysis, pretransplantation serum levels of alpha-fetoprotein (AFP) and protein induced by vitamin K absence or antagonism factor II (PIVKA II), MELD score, and tumor characteristics of explanted livers (e.g., number and size of tumors, differentiation, and vascular invasion) were found to be important risk factors for patient survival. By multivariate analysis, AFP and PIVKA II were found to be independent risk factors for patient survival. Survival of patients who pathologically satisfied (n = 337) and exceeded (n = 316) the MC were 86.9% and 78.0% at 1 year, 82.7% and 63.6% at 3 years, and 77.6% and 60.2% at 5 years, respectively. Ninety-two recipients (14.1%) developed recurrence after LDLT. The cumulative recurrence rate was 9.2% at 1 year, 19.9% at 3 years, and 21.6% at 5 years. By univariate analysis, tumor stage, age, AFP, PIVKA II, and pathological characteristics of the tumors (e.g., number and size of tumors, distribution, vascular invasion, and differentiation) were closely associated with HCC recurrence. By multivariate analysis, AFP, PIVKA II, vascular invasion, and number, distribution, and size of tumors were found to be independent risk factors for recurrence. The recurrence rate of the patients who were within and beyond the MC were, 1.0% and 17.7% at 1 year, 4.6% and 34.2% at 3 years, and 4.6% and 37.3% at 5 years, respectively. Ninety-two recipients (14.1%) developed recurrence after LDLT. The cumulative recurrence rate was 9.2% at 1 year, 19.9% at 3 years, and 21.6% at 5 years. By univariate analysis, tumor stage, age, AFP, PIVKA II, and pathological characteristics of the tumors (e.g., number and size of tumors, distribution, vascular invasion, and differentiation) were closely associated with HCC recurrence. By multivariate analysis, AFP, PIVKA II, vascular invasion, and number, distribution, and size of tumor were found to be independent risk factors for recurrence. The recurrence rate of the patients who were within and beyond the MC were, 1.0% and 17.7% at 1year, 4.6% and 34.2% at 3 years, and 4.6% and 37.3% at 5 years, respectively. Neither pretransplantation treatments nor the type of modalities showed any influence on patient survival and recurrence rate, as compared with those of the recipients who received no treatment.

Table 4. Japanese national survey

n=653	1-year (%)	3-year (%)	5-year (%)
Patient survival	82.6	72.6	68.9
Disease-free survival	77.4	65.1	61.3
Recurrence rate	9.2	19.9	21.6

Table 5. Japanese national survey (classified by the Milan criteria)

n=653	1-year (%)	3-year (%)	5-year (%)
Patient survival			
Milan (within)	86.9	82.8	77.8
(beyond)	78.0	63.1	60.4
Disease-free survival			
Milan (within)	86.7	80.5	75.9
(beyond)	67.6	50.1	47.1

The Kyoto Group reported their data [71]. The 5-year overall survival for patients within the Kyoto criteria (n = 147; 82%) was greater than that for the 49 patients exceeding them (n = 49; 42%; p < .001). The 5-year recurrence rate for patients within the Kyoto criteria (4.4%) was less than that for patients exceeding them (51%; p < .001). Intention-to-treat analysis of the 62 patients who underwent LDLT after implementation of the Kyoto criteria showed that the 5-year overall survival rate and the recurrence rate were 82% and 7%, respectively. The Tokyo group reported their data [82]. At the University of Tokyo, patients are selected on the basis of a maximum tumor number of 5 with a maximum diameter of less than 5 cm. Between 1996 and July 2008, 336 adult patients underwent LDLT; of these, 100 (30%) had HCC (82 men and 18 women; median age, 56 years). MELD scores ranged from 2 to 34 (median 13). In the explanted specimens, the median tumor number was 2.8 and the median tumor size was 2.6 cm. During the median observation period of 45 months, 7 patients died with HCC recurrence and another 14 died without recurrence. Patient survival at 3 and 5 years was 79% and 78%, respectively, which was comparable to that of patients without HCC (n = 236; 89% and 86%, p = 0.08). The Kyushu group reported that the recurrence-free survival rates at 5 years after LDLT in the patients who met the MC (n = 55) and in those who did not (n = 54) were 95.6% and 65.7%, respectively (p = 0.0001). Of the patients who met the MC, recurrence was noted in only 1 patient (1.9%) but no risk factors, such as serum des-gamma-carboxy prothrombin levels, were evaluated [73].

5. Current Status of LT for HCC in Western Countries

After the proposal of the MC in 1996, these criteria were parsed well in LT as the treatment modality for their HCC. Worldwide adoption of the MC, as a standard improved 5-year patient survival, grew to more than 70% [83, 84]. The original group conducted a systematic review of the published literature over 15 years, revealing that patient selection according to the MC is an independent prognostic factor for outcome after liver transplantation for HCC [85]. A recent international consensus conference (involving 300 experts from 5 continents) recommended the MC as the current benchmark for the selection of HCC patients for liver transplantation and the basis for comparison with other suggested criteria [86]. This boundary has been challenged, with many suggesting that these criteria are too restrictive and the number of requirements could achieve comparable survival rates. Subsequently, slightly expanded criteria—the University of California, San Francisco (UCSF), criteria—were proposed [13]. These patients were found to have survival rates of 90% and 75%, at 1 and 5 years, respectively. This study was corroborated and even expanded at different centers, including a study at UCLA, which also demonstrated the applicability of preoperative imaging, as opposed to explant pathology, in the new expanded criteria [16]. Although patient survival was improved by adoption of the MC and/or the UCSF criteria, the high number of candidate dropouts due to the shortage of organs remained an important problem. Thus, in 2002, the United Network for Organ Sharing (UNOS) staging classification was introduced under the Model for End-Stage Liver Disease (MELD) organ allocation policy. The classification includes T0 (no tumors), T1 (single tumor equal to or less than 1.9 cm), T2 (single tumor equal to or less than 5 cm, or within 2 to 3 tumors equal to or less than 3cm), T3 (single tumor more than 5 cm, or within 2 to 3 tumors equal to or more than 3 cm), T4A (more than 4 nodules of any size), and T4B (any stage with macroscopic vascular invasion). Patients with T2 tumors receive 21 MELD points. The outcome of the recipients with UNOS tumor stage T2 or less is equivalent to that obtained with recipients within the MC.

In 2009, Mazzaferro et al. [87] made an interesting contribution to this controversy in their retrospective review of pathology after liver transplantation for HCC in 1556 patients; 1112 of these patients had tumors that did not fulfill the MC. In a subgroup of 283 patients not meeting the MC whose tumors were within the up-to-7 criteria (i.e., HCCs with a maximum score of 7, with the score being the sum of the size of the largest tumor and the total number of tumors) and were not characterized by microvascular invasion, the overall 5-year survival rate was 71.2%. Despite the inherent methodological concerns associated with retrospective pathological assessments of the tumor burden, this study provides further support for liver transplantation for patients with HCC lesions not meeting the MC because the limits for the extension of the MC were chosen to achieve a survival rate similar to that for patients with HCC meeting the MC. In addition, a 70% threshold for the 5-year survival rate was chosen, and this is similar to the rate expected for patients undergoing liver transplantation for other, noncancerous conditions. Thus, acceptable survival rates may be achieved if patients fulfill the "up to seven" criteria, which states that the sum of the number of tumor nodule (s) and the diameter of the largest tumor must not exceed 7. An algorithm, the "Metroticket Calculator," was then developed to predict survival after liver transplantation for different computations of tumor size, numbers of nodules, and the presence or absence of microvascular invasion. While this algorithm explains the biological basis behind the good survival rates in some individual patients selected for transplantation according to additional criteria, this approach has its limitations. In particular, the study in which the "up to seven" and "Metroticket Calculator" methods were suggested was a retrospective analysis of pathological data that excluded other prognostic parameters such as tumor grade.

Expanding the criteria for HCC has been proposed by some authors in light of favorable results noted in single-center studies with variable durations of follow-up. However, in most regions, candidates that exceed the MC are not given priority on the transplant waiting list in comparison with those who meet the MC. The rate of removal from the transplant waiting list due to either tumor progression or death is an important factor to consider when one is evaluating organ allocation policy and has been estimated to range from 20% to 30% [88]. A retrospective cohort of patients listed for LT with a diagnosis of HCC between January 1998 and March 2006 was identified from Organ Procurement Transplant Network data [89]. Analysis was performed from the time of listing. Adjusted Cox models were used to assess the relative effect of potential confounders on removal from the waiting list as well as survival from the time of wait listing. A total of 4482 patients with HCC were placed on the liver waiting list during the study period. Of these, 65% underwent transplantation, and 18% were removed from the list because of tumor progression or death. The overall 1- and 5-year intent-to-treat survival for all patients listed was 81% and 51%, respectively. The 1- and 5-year survival was 89% and 61% for those listed with tumors meeting the MC versus 70% and 32% for those exceeding the MC (p < 0.0001). On multivariate analysis, advanced liver failure manifested by Child-Pugh class B or C increased the risk of death, while age < 55 years, meeting the MC, and obtaining a liver transplant were associated with better survival. They concluded that the current criteria for liver transplantation of candidates with HCC lead to an acceptable 5-year survival rate while limiting the dropout rate. Another group investigated the intention-to-treat survival curve of the HCC group overlapped that of the benign group (5-year survival rates were 73% and 71%, respectively; p = NS). At the time of listing, 103 study group patients were within the MC; among these patients, 29 (28%) showed tumor progression beyond MC before OLT. Simulating the dropout of these 29 patients at the time of diagnosis of tumor progression, we compared the dropout probability of the 103 patients within MC with that of the control group. As a result, the 1- and 2-year dropout rates became 37% and 53%, respectively, in the study group, which were significantly higher than those for the controls (p < .01). They concluded that HCC patients on the waiting list showed a significantly greater dropout rate than did subjects with benign cirrhosis when overly restrictive radiologic dropout criteria were used [90].

So most of the institutions currently perform bridging strategies, which include neoadjuvant chemotherapy, transarterial chemoembolization, radiofrequency ablation, surgical resection, sorafenib, or combination therapy, in order to decrease dropout rates and prevent tumor progression [91, 92, 93]. Randomized trials will be extremely difficult to design and execute in light of the documented risk of tumor progression that understandably engenders strong reluctance on the part of most transplant physicians to withhold ablative treatment for candidates awaiting transplantation. And the second goal for the use of local ablative strategies has been to downstage HCC patients. Although down-staging can refer to reducing the tumor burden of patients who fall within the MC, the more controversial application of down-staging is to bring HCC patients who, at initial diagnosis, fall outside of the MC into criteria that they can qualify for liver transplantation. At present, there is no evidence for the superiority of ablation/resection over TACE, but some studies showed better results for the former in achieving a complete response. The response to neo-adjuvant treatments should be evaluated through the mRECIST criteria, but few studies adopted these criteria and did not properly analyze factors affecting response. Simultaneous evaluation of the impact of neo-adjuvant therapies on dropout rates, post-LT HCC recurrence, and patient survival is rarely reported. Tumor stage and volume, alpha-fetoprotein levels, response to treatments and liver function affect pre-LT outcomes. These same factors, together with vascular invasion and poor tumor differentiation, are major determinants of poor post-LT outcomes. Owing to the low number of prospective studies with well-defined entry criteria and the variability of results, the role of down-staging is still to be defined. Novel molecular markers seem promising for the estimation of prognosis and/or response to treatments. With the persistent scarcity of organ donors, neo-adjuvant treatments can help identify patients with different probabilities of cancer progression, and consequently balance the priority of HCC and non-HCC candidates through revised additional scores for HCC [94].

Resection versus LT is another big issue. The question remains whether these 2 modalities should be considered as alternative, complimentary, or sequential in an intention-to-treat (ITT) strategy (Table 6). Particularly, early HCC and Child-Pugh class A cirrhosis remains controversial in Western countries. Therefore, evidence-based guidelines need to be followed when planning a curative strategy in early HCC cirrhotic patients. A specialized, hepatobiliary center has the responsibility of providing information and following best practice guidelines based on large cohort studies in patients who underwent either resection or LT as first-line treatment. Moreover, not only overall survival (OS) but also recurrence-free survival (RFS) (which is the chief determinant of long-term survival) must to be considered when proposing the treatment strategy. A report from Stanford University presented a retrospective matched case cohort study comparing long-term survival outcomes between consecutive transplant-eligible HCC patients treated with resection versus LT using ITT and as treated models [95]. Resection patients were matched to LT patients by age, sex, and etiology of HCC in a 1:2 ratio. The study included 171 patients (57 resection and 114 LT). Resection patients had greater post treatment tumor recurrence than did the LT patients (43.9 vs. 12.9 %; p < 0.001). In the as-treated model of the pre-model for the end-stage liver disease (MELD) era, LT patients had a significantly better 5-year survival rate than did the resection patients (100 vs. 69.5 %; p = 0.04), but no difference was seen in the ITT model. In the multivariate Cox proportional hazards model, inclusive of age, sex, ethnicity, tumor stage, and MELD era (pre-MELD vs. post-MELD), treatment with resection was an independent predictor of poorer survival (HR 2.72; 95 % CI, 1.08–6.86). They concluded that transplant-eligible HCC patients who received LT had significantly better survival than did those treated with resection, suggesting that patients who can successfully remain on an LT listing and actually undergo LT have better outcomes. A French group reported that from 1990 to 2010, 198 patients with early HCC in cirrhosis underwent either resection (group R, n = 97) or LT (group T, n = 101) as the primary procedure [96]. Their policy was to prioritize Child-Pugh A patients with peripheral lesions for resection rather than for LT. Patient and tumor characteristics, and outcomes, were studied. And the results were as follows: A longer diagnosis-to-surgery interval, more Child Pugh B/C patients, and more tumor nodules (on histopathological examination) were found in group T patients. The postoperative mortality (4.1% vs. 3.0%, $P = 0.72$) and rate of major complications (19.1% vs. 24.7%, p = 0.35) were similar in groups R and T, respectively, whereas tumor recurrence was higher in group R (62% vs. 10% in group T, p < 0.0001). The 5-year OS (75% vs. 52%, p =0.0008) and RFS (72% vs. 20%, p < 0.0001) was better in group T; similarly, more patients were disease free at the last follow-up (27% vs. 62%, p < 0.0001). Resection as the surgical procedure, tumor diameter 3 cm or more on histology, and microvascular tumor invasion were poor prognostic factors for OS and RFS. Including dropout patients from the LT list in the analysis, the outcomes in group T were still better (70% and 61% vs. 51% and 36% at 5 and 10 years, p = 0.01). And they concluded that on an ITT basis, LT is associated with the best survival outcomes in patients with early HCC in cirrhosis. Resection may achieve comparable OS in patients with single HCC in cirrhosis sized smaller than 3 cm; however, the RFS still remains lower than that in patients of group T.

Table 6. Intention-to-treat analysis of survival after LT versus liver resection

		LT		LR	
Authors	Child-Pugh	n	OS (%, 5-y)	n	OS (%, 5-y)
Llovet (1999) [119]	A	37	71	77	51
Bigourdan (2003) [120]	A	17	71	20	36
Poon (2007) [121]	A,B,C	43	44	204	60
Shah (2007) [122]	A,B	140	64	121	56
Cillo (2007) [123]	A,B,C	40	63	131	31
Del Gaudio (2008) [124]	A,B,C	293	58	80	66
Baccarani (2008) [125]	A,B,C	48	72	38	27
Sapisochin (2013) [126]	A,B,C	122	49 (10-y)	95	33 (10-y)

So far, the hepatic resection and transplantation remain the cornerstone curative therapies for patients with HCC. In patients with early-stage tumors and advanced liver disease, transplantation is clearly the treatment of choice with 5-year survival rates of roughly 70%. Liver transplantation, however, is limited by organ shortage and the inherent risk of transplantation and immunosuppression. In patients without cirrhosis or in patients with cirrhosis with preserved liver function and the absence of portal hypertension and tumors beyond the MC, resection remains the treatment of choice when feasible. Although recurrence following resection is common, several recent reports have documented 5-year overall survival rates following resection for very-early- and early-stage tumors similar to that for liver transplantation. Overall survival rates beyond 5 years, however, may be significantly worse for patients undergoing resection. The essential challenge is determining which therapeutic modality is best for patients with relatively early-stage tumors who could tolerate resection. Numerous factors must be considered including tumor size, multifocality, medical comorbidity, and geographic factors that affect waitlist time and organ availability [97].

LDLT offers a timely alternative to DDLT for patients with HCC; however the indication for it and its prevalence are controversial. In terms of the ITT analysis, some groups reported that their study included 183 consecutive patients with HCC who were listed for liver transplantation over a 9-year period [98]. Tumor recurrence was the primary endpoint. At listing, patient and tumor characteristics were comparable in the 2 groups (LDLT, n=36; DDLT, n=147). Twenty-seven (18.4%) patients dropped out, all from the DDLT waiting list, mainly due to tumor progression (19/27 [70%] patients). The mean waiting time was shorter in the LDLT group (2.6 months vs. 7.9 months; p = 0.001). The recurrence rates in the two groups were similar (12.9% and 12.7%, p = 0.78), and there was a trend toward a longer time to recurrence after LDLT (38 months vs. 16 months, p = 0.06). Tumors exceeding the University of California, San Francisco (UCSF) criteria, tumor grade, and microvascular invasion were independent predictive factors for recurrence. On an ITT basis, the OS in the 2 groups was comparable. Patients beyond the Milan and UCSF criteria showed a trend toward worse outcomes with LDLT than with DDLT (p = 0.06). They concluded that the recurrence and survival outcomes after LDLT and DDLT were comparable on an ITT analysis. Shorter waiting time preventing dropouts is an additional advantage with LDLT. LDLT for HCC patients beyond the validated criteria should be proposed with caution. And another author investigated that between January 1996 and September 2009, 345 patients with HCC were identified: 287 (83%) had DDLT and 58 (17%) had LDLT [99]. The OS rates were calculated with the Kaplan-Meier method, whereas competing risks methods were used to determine the HCC recurrence rates. The LDLT and DDLT groups were similar with respect to most clinical parameters, but they had different median waiting times (3.1 vs. 5.3 months, p = 0.003) and median follow-up times (30 vs. 38.1 months, p = 0.02). The type of transplant did not affect any of the measured cancer outcomes. The OS rates at 1, 3, and 5 years were equivalent: 91.3%, 75.2%, and 75.2%, respectively, for the LDLT group and 90.5%, 79.7%, and 74.6%, respectively, for the DDLT group (p = 0.62). The 1-, 3-, and 5-year HCC recurrence rates were also similar: 8.8%, 10.7%, and 15.4%, respectively, for the LDLT group and 7.5%, 14.8%, and 17.0%, respectively, for the DDLT group (p = 0.54). A regression analysis identified microvascular invasion (but not the graft type) as a predictor of HCC recurrence. They concluded that in well-matched cohorts of LDLT and DDLT recipients, LDLT and DDLT provide similarly low recurrence rates and high survival rates for the treatment of HCC. But still some investigators report that LDLT gives poorer outcome than DDLT in HCC patients [100].

Immunosuppressive agents, particularly calcineurin inhibitors, were thought to enhance tumor progression. Some reports investigated that high CsA exposure favors tumor recurrence; therefore, CsA blood levels should be kept to the effective minimum in HCC patients [101]. A binder of mTOR has been developed as an anticancer agent, owing to its ability to inhibit cell growth, proliferation, angiogenesis, and metabolism [102, 103]. Encouraging results from a retrospective comparison of HCC patients treated with sirolimus to patients treated with calcineurin inhibitors showed a post-LT survival benefit without any differences in the incidence of major complications [104, 105].

HCC has been thought to be a chemotherapy-resistant tumor, but some studies have tried to prove the effectiveness of neoadjuvant chemotherapy [106, 107]. A number of studies showed promising preliminary results for adjuvant chemotherapy, but most of the studies came with poorer outcomes than expected. Recently, sorafenib, an inhibitor of multikinases and receptors, appears to function by blocking tumor-cell proliferation and angiogenesis and increasing the rate of apoptosis. The UCLA group reported on 8 patients who underwent liver transplant for hepatocellular carcinoma between May 2007 and April 2009, and tolerated adjuvant therapy with sorafenib were matched with patients who did not receive sorafenib according to age, sex, year of transplant, tumor burden, and presence of vascular invasion [108]. During follow-up, there were no episodes of rejection in either group. Eight patients were able to tolerate a predetermined duration of therapy. During a mean (± standard deviation [SD]) follow-up of 17.75 ± 6.26 months, 1 of 8 patients (12.5%) treated with sorafenib developed hepatocellular carcinoma recurrence. During a mean (± SD) follow-up of 31.63 months (± 22.30 months), 4 of 8 matched controls (50.0%) developed hepatocellular carcinoma recurrence. Disease-free 1-year survivals for the sorafenib and control groups were 85.7% and 57.1%, respectively. Overall, the 1-year survivals for the sorafenib and the control group were 87.5% and 62.5%. And another group reported that sorafenib was effective for recurrent HCC after LT [109]. With the demonstration of the promise of this active systemic agent in advanced HCC, it remains to be seen what role sorafenib will play after resection and after LT. Further studies are expected.

Recently, imaging techniques and devices have made remarkable progress. Advanced imaging techniques for HCC are being developed to improve recipient selection. Some authors reported that dual-contrast MRI (DC-MRI) showed significantly better diagnostic performance in transplantation candidates for the detection of HCCs, particularly small HCCs, than both multidetector row CT (MDCT) and super paramagnetic iron oxide (SPIO)-enhanced MRI (S-MRI). However, for assessing the appropriateness of a transplantation recipient based on the MC, MDCT, S-MRI, and DC-MRI showed comparable diagnostic accuracy without a statistical difference [110]. Some authors reported that PET/CT-positive status was an independent prognostic factor for disease-free survival influencing early recurrence in multivariate analysis (HR 3.945; 95% CI 1.196-13.016; p = 0.024). $^{(18)}$F-fluorodeoxyglucose positron emission tomography/computed tomography ($^{[18]}$F-FDG-PET/CT) is an independent and significant predictor of early tumor recurrence in LDLT for HCC [111]. These kinds of progression will be performed in the future.

Biomarkers have been proposed to be better than preoperative imaging in predicting post transplant HCC recurrence. AFP, DCP and other proposed biomarkers include innumerable other molecular markers using proteins ranging from those involved in cell proliferation, cell adhesion and extracellular matrix, angiogenesis, cell surface markers, and transcription factors among others. AFP is the most widely used marker. Some authors reported that poor differentiation and higher AFP levels are indicators of poor prognosis after liver transplantation [112], and others reported that the absolute serum AFP level and changes in the serum AFP level strongly predict post transplant survival independently of the tumor burden [113]. DCP is studied in Japan, but it has received minimum consideration in Western countries.

6. Other Liver Tumors

6.1. Cholangiocarcinoma

Cholangiocarcinoma arises from the bile duct epithelium, and historically, treatment options for this devastating disease have been limited. Resection is the standard of care, although many patients present with unresectable disease owing to involvement of the bilateral hilar structures, or to underlying parenchymal liver disease (primary sclerosing cholangitis). Even when resection is possible, the 5-year survival is only 20% to 40%. While initially endorsed as an indication for orthotopic LT, the experience with LT alone was disappointing owing to a high rate of tumor recurrence (53% to 84%) and thus, perihilar cholangiocarcinoma became a contraindication to LT. However, inspired by small reports of long-term survival noted in patients who received radiotherapy alone, first the University of Nebraska [114] and later the Mayo Clinic [115] developed a protocol using neoadjuvant chemoradiation followed by LT. This protocol includes selected patients with unresectable early stage (I – II) perihilar cholangiocarcinoma, who consecutively undergo external beam radiotherapy (EBRT) combined with radiosensitizing chemotherapy (ie, 5-Flouracil), brachytherapy with endoscopically placed Iridium-192 beads, maintenance chemotherapy (ie, oral capecitabine), staging surgery to rule out metastases, and finally LT. Subsequent reports consistently showed 5-year recurrence-free survival of approximately 70%. Recently the result from 12 centers were published; they collected and analyzed data from 12 large-volume transplant centers in the US that met the inclusion criteria of treating 3 or more patients with perihilar cholangiocarcinoma using neoadjuvant therapy followed by LT from 1993–2010 (n = 287 total patients) [116]. Center-specific protocols and medical charts were reviewed on-site. The patients completed external radiation (99%), brachytherapy (75%), radio sensitizing (98%), and/or maintenance chemotherapy (65%). Seventy-one patients dropped out before liver transplantation (rate of 11.5% in 3 months). Intent-to-treat survival was 68% and 53%, 2 and 5 years after therapy, respectively; post transplantation, recurrence-free survival rates were 78% and 65%, respectively. Patients outside the UNOS criteria (those with tumor mass >3 cm, transperitoneal tumor biopsy, or metastatic disease) or with a prior malignancy had significantly shorter survival times ($p < .001$). There were no differences in outcomes among patients based on differences in operative staging or brachytherapy. Although most patients came from 1 center (n = 193), the other 11 centers had similar survival times after therapy. They concluded that patients with perihilar cholangiocarcinoma who were treated with neoadjuvant therapy followed by liver transplantation at the 12 US centers had a 65% rate of recurrence-free survival after 5 years, demonstrating this therapy to be highly effective. An 11.5% dropout rate after 3.5 months of therapy indicates the appropriateness of the MELD exception. Rigorous selection is important for the continued success of this treatment.

6.2. Epithelioid Hemangioendothelioma

Hepatic epithelioid hemangioendothelioma (HEHE) is a rare malignant tumor of endothelial origin that may arise in the liver. The clinical course of HEHE is unpredictable, and reliable prognostic clinical and histopathological features are limited. Nearly 90% of patients present with bilobar and multifocal disease, and 37% present with extra hepatic involvement; thus, less than 10% of patients are candidates for resection [117]. Interestingly, the presence of an extra hepatic tumor is not a contraindication to hepatic replacement and does not correlate with survival. The data from single-institution series are limited, but compiled reviews have reported 1- and 10-year survival rates of 96% and 72%, respectively. Long-term survival is possible despite the presence of extrahepatic metastasis; therefore patients with HEHE should be considered candidates for LT.

6.3. Metastatic Colorectal Liver Tumor

LT for colorectal cancer (CRC) liver metastases is no longer considered owing to the poor outcome observed up to the 1990s. According to the European Liver Transplant Registry (ELTR), 1- and 5-year survival following Lt for CRC liver metastases performed before 1995 was 62% and 18%, respectively. However, 44% of graft loss or patient deaths were not related to tumor recurrence. Over the last 20 years, there has been dramatic progress in patient survival after LT; thus, it could be anticipated that survival after LT for CRC secondaries today would far exceed the outcome of past experience. By using new imaging techniques for proper patient selection, modern chemotherapy, and aggressive multimodal treatment against metastases, long-term survivors and even a cure could be expected in the Norway group [118]. Preliminary data from a pilot study show an overall survival rate of 94% after a median follow up of 25 months. While long-term survival after the first LT is 80% all indications confounded, 5-year survival after repeated LT is no more than 50% to 55%. If patients transplanted for CRC secondaries can reach the latter survival rate, it could be difficult to discriminate them in the liver allocation system and live donation could be an option. However, further investigations should be performed in terms of the metastatic colorectal tumor.

6.4. Others

Hepatic involvement from neuroendocrine tumors can be treated with LT when metastases are unresectable or for palliation of medically uncontrollable symptoms [117]. Five-year survival rates as high as 90% have been reported, and the Ki67 labeling index can be used to predict outcomes after LT. Hepatoblastoma is the most common primary hepatic malignancy in children. There exist subtle differences in the timing of chemotherapy between US and European centers; however, the long-term survival rate after transplantation ranges from 66% to 77%. Fibrolamellar hepatocellular carcinoma is a distinct liver malignancy best treated by surgical resection. However, there is an increasing amount of data supporting LT when resection is contraindicated. In the treatment of either primary or metastatic hepatic sarcomas, unacceptable survival and recurrence rates currently prohibit the use of LT.

Conclusion

LT for HCC is an acceptable treatment option in selected patients. Even if an individual patient who does not meet the Milan criteria might benefit from LT, the limited number of donor organs currently limits the indications for LT to patients who have the greatest likelihood of survival after surgery. LT in patients with HCC should, therefore, be restricted to those who are expected to have the same postoperative survival as that of patients with other end-stage liver diseases. In another words, if the donor source expands, the indication of LT for HCC will be changed.

References

[1]   Starzl TE. Experience in Hepatic Transplantation. Philadelphia, *WB Saunders,* 1969:350-355.
[2]   Stone MJ, Fulmer M, Klintmalm GB: Transplantation for primary hepatic malignancy. Transplantation of the liver. *Elsevier Saunders Philadelphia,* 2005: 211-231.
[3]   Starzl TE, Marchioro TL, von Kaulla KN, Hermann G, Brittain RS, Waddell WR. : Hemotransplantation of the liver in humans. *Surg Gynecol Obstet.* 1963:117(Dec):659-676.
[4]   Starzl TE, Marchioro TL, Rowlands TD Jr., Kirkpatrick CH, Wilson WE, Rifkind D, et al. Immunosuppression after experimental and clinical homotransplantation of the liver. *Ann Surg.,* 1964:160(Sep):411-439.
[5]   Demirleau, Noureddine, Vignes, Prawerman, Reziciner, Larraud, et al. Tentative d'homogreffe hepatique (Attempted hepatic homograft). *Mem Acad Chir* (Paris) ,1964: 90(Jan):117-119.
[6]   Starzl TE, Demetris AJ, Van Thiel D. Liver Transplantation. *N Engl J Med ,* 1989: 321(15,16):1014-1022, 1092-1099.
[7]   Bismuth H, Chiche L, Adam R, Castaing D, Diamond T, Dennison A. Liver resection versus transplantation for hepatocellular carcinoma in cirrhotic patients. *Ann Surg.,* 1993: 218(2):145-151.
[8]   Mazzaferro V, Regalia E, Doci R, Andreola S, Pulvirenti A, Bozzetti F, Montalto F, Ammatuna M, Morabito A, Gennari L. Liver transplantation for the treatment of small hepatocellular carcinomas in patients with cirrhosis. *N Engl J Med.* ,1996: 334(11):693-699.
[9]   Mor E, Kaspa RT, Sheiner P, Schwartz M. Treatment of hepatocellular carcinoma associated with cirrhosis in the era of liver transplantation. *Ann Intern Med.* 1998:129(8):643-653.
[10] Freeman RB Jr, Wiesner RH, Harper A, McDiarmid SV, Lake J, Edwards E, et al. The new liver *Liver Transpl.* 2002:8(9):851-8.
[11] Sharma P, Balan V, Hernandez JL, Harper AM, Edwards EB, Rodriguez-Luna H, et al. Liver transplantation *Liver Transpl.* 2004:10(1):36-41.
[12] Marsh JW, Dvorchik I. Liver organ allocation for hepatocellular carcinoma: are we sure? *Liver Transpl* 2003:9(7):693-696.

[13]   Yao FY, Ferrell L, Bass NM, Watson JJ, Bacchetti P, Venook A, et al. Liver
       transplantation for hepatocellular carcinoma: expansion of the tumor size limits does
       not adversely impact survival. *Hepatology.* 2001, 33(6):1394-1403.

[14]   Kneteman NM, Oberholzer J, Al Saghier M, Meeberg GA, Blitz M, Ma MM, et al.
       Sirolimus-based immunosuppression for liver transplantation in the presence of
       extended criteria for hepatocellular carcinoma. *Liver Transpl* 2004:10(10):1301-1311.

[15]   Broelsch CE, Frilling A, Malago M. Should we expand the criteria for liver
       transplantation for hepatocellular carcinoma—yes, of course! *J Hepatol*
       2005;43(4):569-573.

[16]   Duffy JP, Vardanian A, Benjamin E, Watson M, Farmer DG, Ghobrial RM, et al. Liver
       transplantation criteria for hepatocellular carcinoma should be expanded: a 22-year
       experience with 467 patients at UCLA. *Ann Surg.,* 2007:246(3):502-511.

[17]   Yao FY, Ferrell L, Bass NM, Bacchetti P, Ascher NL, Roberts JP. Liver
       transplantation for hepatocellular carcinoma: comparison of the proposed UCSF
       criteria with the Milan criteria and the Pittsburgh modified TNM criteria. *Liver
       Transpl.* 2002;8(9):765-74.

[18]   Herrero JI, Sangro B, Pardo F, Quiroga J, Iñarrairaegui M, Rotellar F, et al. Liver
       transplantation in patients with hepatocellular carcinoma across Milan criteria. *Liver
       Transpl.,* 2008: 14(3):272-278.

[19]   Decaens T, Roudot-Thoraval F, Hadni-Bresson S, Meyer C, Gugenheim J, Durand F,
       et al. Impact of UCSF criteria according to pre- and post-OLT tumor features: analysis
       of 479 patients listed for HCC with a short waiting time. *Liver Transpl.*
       2006;12(12):1761-9.

[20]   Hashikura Y, Makuuchi M, Kawasaki S, Matsunami H, Ikegami T, Nakazawa Y, et al.
       Successful living-related partial liver transplantation to an adult patient. *Lancet.*
       1994;343(8907):1233–1234.

[21]   Kawasaki S, Makuuchi M, Matsunami H, Hashikura Y, Ikegami T, Nakazawa Y, et al.
       Living related liver transplantation in adults. *Ann Surg.* 1998;227(2): 269–274.

[22]   Yamaoka Y, Washida M, Honda K, Tanaka K, Mori K, Shimahara Y, et al. Liver
       transplantation using a right lobe graft from a living related donor. *Transplantation.*
       1994;57(7):1127–1130.

[23]   Todo S, Furukawa H; Japanese Study Group on Organ Transplantation. Living donor
       liver transplantation for adult patients with hepatocellular carcinoma: experience in
       Japan. *Ann Surg.,* 2004;240(3):451-461.

[24]   Raia S, Nery JR, Mies S. Liver transplantation from live donors. *Lancet.*
       1989;8661(2):497.

[25]   Strong RW, Lynch SV, Ong TH, Matsunami H, Koido Y, Balderson GA. Successful
       liver transplantation from a living donor to her son. *N Engl J Med.* 1990;322(21):1505-
       7.

[26]   Singer P, Siegler M, Whitingto P, Lantos J, Emond J, Thistlethwaite R, et al. Ethics of
       Liver Transplantation with Living Donors. *N Engl J Med* 1989; 321(9):620-622

[27]   Kato S. [Ethical guidelines of the Japan Society for Transplantation]. *Nihon Rinsho.*
       2005;63(11):1899-907.

[28]   Abecassis M, Adams M, Adams P, Arnold RM, Atkins CR, Barr ML, et al. Consensus
       statement on the live organ donor. *JAMA.* 2000;284(22):2919-26.

[29] Akabayashi A, Slingsby BT, Fujita M. The first donor death after living-related liver transplantation in Japan. *Transplantation* 2004;77(4):634.

[30] Kawagishi N, Ohkohchi N, Fujimori K, Doi H, Sakurada M, Kikuchi H,et al. Safety of the donor operation in living-related liver transplantation: analysis of 22 donors. *Transplant Proc.* 1998 ;30(7):3279-80.

[31] Kokudo N, Sugawara Y, Imamura H, Sano K, Makuuchi M. Tailoring the type of donor hepatectomy for adult living donor liver transplantation. *Am J Transplant.* 2005;5(7):1694-703.

[32] Yamaoka Y, Washida M, Honda K, Tanaka K, Mori K, Shimahara Y, et al. Liver transplantation using a right lobe graft from a living related donor. *Transplantation.* 1994;57(7):1127-30.

[33] Marcos A, Fisher RA, Ham JM, Shiffman ML, Sanyal AJ, Luketic VA, et al. Right-lobe living donor liver transplantation. *Transplantation* 1999; 68(6): 798–803.

[34] Takayama T, Makuuchi M, Kubota K, Sano K, Harihara Y, Kawarasaki H. Living related transplantation of left liver plus caudate lobe. *J Am Coll Surg* 2000; 190(5): 635.

[35] Sugawara Y, Makuuchi M, Takayama T, Imamura H, Kaneko J. Right lateral sector graft in adult living-related liver transplantation. *Transplantation* 2002; 73(1): 111.

[36] Lo C-M, Fan S-T, Liu C-L, Wei WI, Lo RJ, Lai CL, et al. Adult-to-adult living donor liver transplantation using extended right lobe grafts. *Ann Surg* 1997; 226(3): 261–270.

[37] Kanazawa H, Sakamoto S, Fukuda A, Uchida H, Hamano I, Shigeta T, et al. Living-donor liver *Transplantation.* 2013;95(5):750-4.

[38] Urahashi T, Mizuta K, Sanada Y, Wakiya T, Yasuda Y, Kawarasaki H. Liver graft volumetric changes *Pediatr Transplant.* 2012;16(7):783-7.

[39] Rotellar F, Pardo F, Benito A, Martí-Cruchaga P, Zozaya G, Lopez L, et al. Totally laparoscopic right-lobe hepatectomy for adult living donor liver *Am J Transplant.* 2013;13(12):3269-73.

[40] Samstein B, Cherqui D, Rotellar F, Griesemer A, Halazun KJ, Kato T, et al. Totally laparoscopic full left hepatectomy for living donor liver *Am J Transplant.* 2013;13(9):2462-6.

[41] Yu YD, Kim KH, Jung DH, Lee SG, Kim YG, Hwang GS. Laparoscopic live donor left lateral sectionectomy is safe and feasible for pediatric living donor liver *Hepatogastroenterology.* 2012;59(120):2445-9.

[42] Eguchi S, Takatsuki M, Soyama A, Hidaka M, Tomonaga T, Muraoka I, Kanematsu T. Elective living donor liver *Surgery.* 2011;150(5):1002-5.

[43] Thenappan A, Jha RC, Fishbein T, Matsumoto C, Melancon JK, Girlanda R, et al. Liver allograft outcomes after laparoscopic-assisted and minimal access *Am J Surg.* 2011;201(4):450-5.

[44] Hashikura Y, Ichida T, Umeshita K, Kawasaki S, Mizokami M, Mochida S, et al. Donor complications associated with living donor liver transplantation in Japan. *Transplantation.* 2009;88(1):110-4.

[45] Umeshita K, Fujiwara K, Kiyosawa K, Makuuchi M, Satomi S, Sugimachi K, et al. Operative morbidity of living liver donors in Japan. *Lancet.* 2003;362(9385):687-90.

[46] Miyagi S, Kawagishi N, Fujimori K, Sekiguchi S, Fukumori T, Akamatsu Y, et al. Risks of donation and quality of donors' life after living donor liver transplantation. *Transpl Int.* 2005;18(1):47-51.

[47]   Morooka Y, Umeshita K, Taketomi A, Shirabe K, Maehara Y, Yamamoto M, et al. Reliability and validity of a new living liver *Surg Today.* 2013;43(7):732-40.

[48]   Mehrabi A, Fonouni H, Müller SA, Schmidt J. Current concepts in transplant surgery: liver transplantation today. *Langenbecks Arch Surg.* 2008;393(3):245-60.

[49]   Sato K, Sekiguchi S, Fukumori T, Kawagishi N, Akamastu Y, Enomoto Y, et al. Experience with recipient's superficial femoral vein as conduit for middle hepatic vein reconstruction in a right-lobe living donor liver transplant procedure. *Transplant Proc.* 2005;37(10):4343-6.

[50]   Tashiro H, Itamoto T, Ohdan H, Oshita A, Fudaba Y, Ishiyama K, et al. Reconstruction of the middle hepatic vein tributaries draining segments V and VIII of a right liver graft by using the recipient's own middle hepatic vein and vascular closure staples. *Surg Today.* 2008;38(3):289-91.

[51]   Soejima Y, Shimada M, Suehiro T, Yoshizumi T, Kishikawa K, Maehara Y. Reconstruction of the middle hepatic vein tributaries using the recipient's recanalized umbilical vein in right-lobe living-donor liver transplantation. *Surgery.* 2006;139(3):442-5.

[52]   Sugawara Y, Makuuchi M, Akamatsu N, Kishi Y, Niiya T, Kaneko J, et al. Refinement of venous reconstruction using cryopreserved veins in right liver grafts. *Liver Transpl.* 2004;10(4):541-7.

[53]   Akamatsu N, Sugawara Y, Hashimoto D. Biliary reconstruction *Transpl Int.* 2011;24(4):379-92.

[54]   Mori A, Kaido T, Ogura Y, Ogawa K, Hata K, Yagi S, et al. Standard hepatic vein *Liver Transpl.* 2012;18(5):602-7.

[55]   Ikegami T, Shirabe K, Yoshiya S, Soejima Y, Yoshizumi T, Uchiyama H, Toshima T, Motomura T, Maehara Y. One-step reconstruction *Surg Today.* 2013;43(7):769-76.

[56]   Sugawara Y, Makuuchi M, Imamura H, Kaneko J, Kokudo N. Outflow reconstruction *Liver Transpl.* 2003;9(3):306-9.

[57]   Imamura H, Makuuchi M, Sakamoto Y, Sugawara Y, Sano K, Nakayama A, et al. Anatomical keys and pitfalls in living donor liver *J Hepatobiliary Pancreat Surg.* 2000;7(4):380-94.

[58]   Broelsch CE, Whitington PF, Emond JC, Heffron TG, Thistlethwaite JR, Stevens L, et al. Liver transplantation in children from living related donors. Surgical techniques and results. *Ann Surg.* 1991;214(4):428-37; discussion 437-9.

[59]   Hatano E, Terajima H, Yabe S, Asonuma K, Egawa H, Kiuchi T, et al. Hepatic artery *Transplantation.* 1997;64(10):1443-6.

[60]   Sakamoto Y, Harihara Y, Nakatsuka T, Kawarasaki H, Takayama T, Kubota K, et al. Rescue of liver *Br J Surg.* 1999;86(7):886-9.

[61]   Lin TS, Concejero AM, Chen CL, Chiang YC, Wang CC, Wang SH, Liu YW, Yang CH, Yong CC, Jawan B, Cheng YF. Routine microsurgical biliary reconstruction *Liver Transpl.* 2009;15(12):1766-75.

[62]   Lin TS, Chiang YC. Combined microvascular anastomosis: experimental and clinical experience. *Ann Plast Surg.* 2000;45(3):280-3.

[63]   Eghtesad B, Kadry Z, Fung J. Technical considerations in liver transplantation: what a hepatologist needs to know (and every surgeon should practice). *Liver Transpl.* 2005;11(8):861-71.

[64] Kawasaki S, Hashikura Y, Ikegami T, Nakazawa Y, Miwa S, Kubota T, et al. First case of cadaveric liver *J Hepatobiliary Pancreat Surg.* 1999;6(4):387-90.

[65] Watts J. Japan *Lancet.* 1999;353(9155):821.

[66] Steering Committee of the Istanbul Summit. Organ trafficking *Lancet.* 2008;372(9632):5-6.

[67] Groth CG, Starzl TE. Liver transplantation Postgrad Med. 1973;53(1):202-10.

[68] Calne RY. Early days of liver *Am J Transplant.* 2008;8(9):1775-8.

[69] Genda T, Ichida T, Sakisaka S, Sata M, Tanaka E, Inui A, et al. Waiting list mortality *J Gastroenterol.* 2013 Mar 12. [Epub ahead of print]

[70] Kaihara S, Kiuchi T, Ueda M, Oike F, Fujimoto Y, Ogawa K, et al. Living-donor liver transplantation for hepatocellular carcinoma. *Transplantation.* 2003;75(3 Suppl):S37-40.

[71] Kaido T, Ogawa K, Mori A, Fujimoto Y, Ito T, Tomiyama K, et al. Usefulness of the Kyoto criteria *Surgery.* 2013;154(5):1053-60.

[72] Sugawara Y, Tamura S, Makuuchi M. Living donor liver *Dig Dis.* 2007;25(4):310-2.

[73] Shirabe K, Taketomi A, Morita K, Soejima Y, Uchiyama H, Kayashima H, et al. Comparative evaluation of expanded criteria for patients with hepatocellular carcinoma *Clin Transplant.* 2011;25(5):E491-8.

[74] Todo, S., Demetris, A.J., Van Thiel, D., Teperman, L., Fung, J.J., Starzl, T.E. Orthotopic liver transplantation for patients with hepatitis B virus-related liver disease. *Hepatology,* 1991; 13(4):619-626.

[75] Kawagishi N, Takeda I, Miyagi S, Satoh K, Akamatsu Y, Sekiguchi S, et al. Nucleoside analogue therapy following one-year course of hepatitis B immunoglobulin in preventing hepatitis B virus reactivation after living donor liver transplantation. *Tohoku J Exp Med.* 2010;222(4):275-9.

[76] Takada Y, Uemoto S. Living donor liver *Surg Today.* 2013;43(7):709-14.

[77] Coilly A, Roche B, Samuel D. Current management *Liver Int.* 2013;33 Suppl 1:56-62.

[78] Coilly A, Roche B, Dumortier J, Leroy V, Botta-Fridlund D, Radenne S, et al. Safety and efficacy of protease inhibitors *J Hepatol.* 2014;60(1):78-86.

[79] Todo S, Furukawa H; Japanese Study Group on Organ Transplantation. Living donor liver *Ann Surg.* 2004;240(3):451-9; discussion 459-61.

[80] Todo S, Furukawa H, Tada M; Japanese Liver Transplantation Study Group. Extending indication: role of living donor liver transplantation for hepatocellular carcinoma. *Liver Transpl.* 2007;13(11 Suppl 2):S48-54.

[81] Furukawa H, Shimamura T, Suzuki T, Taniguchi M, Nakanishi K, Yamashita K, Kamiyama T, Matsushita M, Todo S. Liver transplantation *J Hepatobiliary Pancreat Sci.* 2010;17(5):533-8.

[82] Sugawara Y, Kokudo N. Surgical treatment of hepatocellular carcinoma: comparison of resection and transplantation. *Oncology.* 2008;75 Suppl 1:119-23.

[83] Llovet JM, Fuster J, Bruix J. Intention-to-treat analysis of surgical treatment for early hepatocellular carcinoma: resection versus transplantation. *Hepatology.* 1999 Dec;30(6):1434-40.

[84] Jonas S, Bechstein WO, Steinmüller T, Herrmann M, Radke C, Berg T, et al. Vascular invasion and histopathologic grading *Hepatology.* 2001 May;33(5):1080-6.

[85] Mazzaferro V, Bhoori S, Sposito C, Bongini M, Langer, Miceli R,et al: Milan criteria in liver transplantation for hepatocellular carcinoma: An evidence-based analysis of 15 years of experience. *Liver Transpl* 2011;17(Suppl 2):S44–S57.

[86] Clavien PA, Lesurtel M, Bossuyt PM, Gores, Langer, Perrier A, et al: Recommendations for liver transplantation for hepatocellular carcinoma: an international consensus conference report. *Lancet Oncol* 2012;13(1):e11–e22.

[87] Mazzaferro V, Llovet JM, Miceli R, Bhoori S, Schiavo M, Mariani L, et al.; for Metroticket Investigator Study Group. Predicting survival after liver transplantation in patients with hepatocellular carcinoma beyond the Milan criteria: a retrospective, exploratory analysis. *Lancet Oncol* 2009;10(1)35-43.

[88] Bruix J, Sherman M. Management of hepatocellular carcinoma. *Hepatology* 2005;42(5):1208-1236.

[89] Pelletier SJ, Fu S, Thyagarajan V, Romero-Marrero C, Batheja MJ, Punch JD, et al. An intention-to-treat analysis of liver *Liver Transpl.* 2009;15(8):859-68.

[90] Vitale A, Boccagni P, Brolese A, Neri D, Srsen N, Zanus, et al. Progression of hepatocellular carcinoma before liver transplantation: dropout or liver transplantation? *Transplant Proc.* 2009;41(4):1264-7.

[91] Heckman JT, Devera MB, Marsh JW, Fontes P, Amesur NB, Holloway SE, et al. Bridging locoregional therapy for hepatocellular carcinoma prior to liver transplantation. *Ann Surg Oncol* 2008;15(11):3169-3177.

[92] Belghiti J, Carr BI, Greig PD, Lencioni R, Poon RT. Treatment before liver transplantation for HCC. *Ann Surg Oncol* 2008; 15(4):993-1000.

[93] Pompili M, Francica G, Rapaccini GL. Bridge treatments of hepatocellular carcinoma in cirrhotic patients submitted to liver transplantation. *Dig Dis Sci* 2008;53(10):2830-2831.

[94] Cescon M, Cucchetti A, Ravaioli M, Pinna AD. Hepatocellular carcinoma locoregional therapies for patients in the waiting list. Impact on transplantability and recurrence rate. *J Hepatol.* 2013;58(3):609-18.

[95] Robert W, James W, Antonia V, Aijaz A, Clark B, Amy G, et al. Primary Surgical Resection Versus Liver Transplantation for Transplant-Eligible Hepatocellular Carcinoma Patients. *Dig Dis Sci.* 2013 Nov 27. [Epub ahead of print]

[96] Adam R, Bhangui P, Vibert E, Azoulay D, Pelletier G, Duclos-Vallée JC, et al. Resection or transplantation for early hepatocellular carcinoma in a cirrhotic liver: does size define the best oncological strategy? *Ann Surg.* 2012;256(6):883-91.

[97] Earl TM, Chapman WC. Hepatocellular Carcinoma: resection *Semin Liver Dis.* 2013;33(3):282-92.

[98] Bhangui P, Vibert E, Majno P, Salloum C, Andreani P, Zocrato J, et al. Intention-to-treat analysis of liver transplantation for hepatocellular carcinoma: living versus deceased donor transplantation. *Hepatology.* 2011;53(5):1570-9.

[99] Sandhu L, Sandroussi C, Guba M, Selzner M, Ghanekar A, Cattral MS, et al. Living donor liver *Liver Transpl.* 2012;18(3):315-22.

[100] Park MS, Lee KW, Suh SW, You T, Choi Y, Kim H, et al. Living-donor liver transplantation associated with higher incidence of hepatocellular carcinoma recurrence than deceased-donor liver transplantation. *Transplantation.* 2014;97(1):71-7.

[101] Vivarelli M, Cucchetti A, Piscaglia F, La Barba G, Bolondi L, Cavallari A, Pinna AD. Analysis of risk *Liver Transpl.* 2005;11(5):497-503.

[102] Guba M, von Breitenbuch P, Steinbauer M, Koehl G, Flegel S, Hornung M, et al. Rapamycin inhibits primary and metastatic tumor growth by antiangiogenesis: involvement of vascular endothelial growth factor. *Nat Med.* 2002;8(2):128-35.

[103] Yuan R, Kay A, Berg WJ, Lebwohl D. Targeting tumorigenesis: development and use of mTOR inhibitors in cancer therapy. *J Hematol Oncol.* 2009;2:45.

[104] Zimmerman MA, Trotter JF, Wachs M, Bak T, Campsen J, Skibba A, et al. Sirolimus-based immunosuppression *Liver Transpl.* 2008;14(5):633-8.

[105] Toso C, Merani S, Bigam DL, Shapiro AM, Kneteman NM. Sirolimus-based immunosuppression is associated with increased survival after liver transplantation for hepatocellular carcinoma. *Hepatology.* 2010;51(4):1237-43.

[106] Seehofer D, Nebrig M, Denecke T, Kroencke T, Weichert W, Stockmann M, et al. Impact of neoadjuvant transarterial chemoembolization on tumor recurrence and patient survival after liver transplantation for hepatocellular carcinoma: a retrospective analysis. *Clin Transplant.* 2012;26(5):764-74.

[107] Pokorny H, Gnant M, Rasoul-Rockenschaub S, Gollackner B, Steiner B, Steger G, et al. Does additional doxorubicin chemotherapy improve outcome in patients with hepatocellular carcinoma treated by liver transplantation? *Am J Transplant.* 2005;5(4 Pt 1):788-94.

[108] Saab S, McTigue M, Finn RS, Busuttil RW. Sorafenib as adjuvant therapy for high-risk hepatocellular carcinoma in liver transplant recipients: feasibility and efficacy. *Exp Clin Transplant.* 2010;8(4):307-13.

[109] Pfeiffenberger J, Koschny R, Hoffmann K, Mehrabi A, Schmitz A, Radeleff B, Stremmel W, Schemmer P, Ganten TM. Sorafenib treatment is save and may affect survival of recurrent hepatocellular carcinoma after liver transplantation. *Langenbecks Arch Surg.* 2013;398(8):1123-8.

[110] Lee DH, Kim SH, Lee JM, Park HS, Lee JY, Yi NJ,et al. Diagnostic performance of multidetector row computed tomography, superparamagnetic iron oxide-enhanced magnetic resonance imaging, and dual-contrast magnetic resonance imaging in predicting the appropriateness of a transplant recipient based on Milan criteria: correlation with histopathological findings. *Invest Radiol.* 2009;44(6):311-21.

[111] Lee SD, Kim SH, Kim YK, Kim C, Kim SK, Han SS, et al. (18)F-FDG-PET/CT predicts early tumor recurrence in living donor liver transplantation for hepatocellular carcinoma. *Transpl Int.* 2013 Jan;26(1):50-60.

[112] Yaprak O, Akyildiz M, Dayangac M, Demirbas BT, Guler N, Dogusoy GB, et al. AFP level and histologic differentiation predict the survival of patients with liver transplantation for hepatocellular carcinoma. *Hepatobiliary Pancreat Dis Int.* 2012 Jun;11(3):256-61.

[113] Berry K, Ioannou GN. Serum alpha-fetoprotein level independently predicts posttransplant survival in patients with hepatocellular carcinoma. *Liver Transpl.* 2013 Jun;19(6):634-45.

[114] Sudan, DeRoover A, Chinnakotla S, Fox, Shaw B Jr, McCashland T, et al. Radiochemotherapy and transplantation allow long-term survival for nonresectable hilar cholangiocarcinoma. *Am J Transplant.* 2002 Sep;2(8):774-9.

[115] De Vreede I, Steers JL, Burch PA, Rosen CB, Gunderson LL, Haddock MG, et al. Prolonged disease-free survival after orthotopic liver transplantation plus adjuvant chemoirradiation for cholangiocarcinoma. *Liver Transpl.* 2000 May;6(3):309-16.

[116] Darwish Murad S, Kim WR, Harnois DM, Douglas DD, Burton J, Kulik LM, et al. Efficacy of neoadjuvant chemoradiation, followed by liver transplantation, for perihilar cholangiocarcinoma at 12 US centers. *Gastroenterology.* 2012 Jul;143(1):88-98.

[117] Grossman EJ, Millis JM. Liver transplantation for non-hepatocellular carcinoma malignancy: Indications, limitations, and analysis of the current literature. *Liver Transpl.* 2010 Aug;16(8):930-42.

[118] Foss A, Adam R, Dueland S. Liver transplantation for colorectal liver metastases: revisiting the concept. *Transpl Int.* 2010 Jul;23(7):679-85.

[119] Llovet JM, Fuster J, Bruix J. Intention-to-treat analysis of surgical treatment *Hepatology.* 1999;30(6):1434-40.

[120] Bigourdan JM, Jaeck D, Meyer N, Meyer C, Oussoultzoglou E, Bachellier P, et al. Small hepatocellular carcinoma in Child A cirrhotic patients: hepatic resection versus transplantation. *Liver Transpl.* 2003;9(5):513-20.

[121] Poon RT, Fan ST, Lo CM, Liu CL, Wong J. Difference in tumor *Ann Surg.* 2007;245(1):51-8.

[122] Shah SA, Cleary SP, Tan JC, Wei AC, Gallinger S, Grant DR, et al. An analysis of resection *Ann Surg Oncol.* 2007;14(9):2608-14.

[123] Cillo U, Vitale A, Brolese A, Zanus G, Neri D, Valmasoni M, et al. Partial hepatectomy as first-line treatment *J Surg Oncol.* 2007;95(3):213-20.

[124] Del Gaudio M, Ercolani G, Ravaioli M, Cescon M, Lauro A, Vivarelli M, et al. Liver transplantation *Am J Transplant.* 2008;8(6):1177-85.

[125] Baccarani U, Isola M, Adani GL, Benzoni E, Avellini C, Lorenzin D, et al. Superiority of transplantation *Transpl Int.* 2008;21(3):247-54.

[126] Sapisochin G, Castells L, Dopazo C, Bilbao I, Minguez B, Lázaro JL, et al. Single HCC *Ann Surg Oncol.* 2013;20(4):1194-202.

In: Therapy for Hepatocellular Carcinoma
Editor: Nobuhiro Ohkohchi

ISBN: 978-1-63117-929-7
© 2014 Nova Science Publishers, Inc.

Chapter 6

Transcatheter Arterial Chemoembolization

*Shiro Miyayama**

Department of Diagnostic Radiology, Fukuiken Saiseikai Hospital,
Wadanaka-cho, Fukui, Japan

Abstract

Transcatheter arterial chemoembolization (TACE) is an effective therapeutic option for inoperable hepatocellular carcinoma (HCC) and has been performed worldwide mainly for intermediate-stage HCC patients with Child-Pugh A/B class. With recent advances in catheter-guidewire technologies, angiographic units, and chemoembolic agents, the techniques and outcomes of TACE have rapidly progressed. Several different types of chemoembolic agents are used in TACE. In Asia, TACE with Lipiodol and gelatin sponge particles is mainly performed, while, in Western countries, TACE with drug-eluting microspheres is a standard procedure and radioembolization is another option. There is a wide variety of TACE techniques; however, superselective TACE is a standard technique worldwide for localized tumors. Cone-beam computed tomography, as well as TACE-guidance software, helps to improve the technical success of TACE. The combination of antiangiogenics and TACE is also expected as a promising method. On the other hand, TACE induces several complications; therefore, physicians should also be well aware of such complications.

1. Introduction

Since the first procedure performed by Yamada et al. in 1977 [1], transcatheter arterial chemoembolization (TACE) for inoperable hepatocellular carcinoma (HCC) has developed

* Corresponding author: Shiro Miyayama, M.D. Department of Diagnostic Radiology, Fukuiken Saiseikai Hospital, 7-1, Funabashi, Wadanaka-cho, Fukui 918-8503, Japan, Tel: +81-776-23-1111, Fax: +81-776-28-8519, Email: s-miyayama@fukui.saiseikai.or.jp.

mainly in Japan (Table 1). In 2002, two randomized controlled trials (RCT) demonstrated that TACE showed a survival benefit compared with best supportive care [2, 3] (Table 2). Two meta-analyses also demonstrated the clinical usefulness of TACE in prolonging HCC patients' survival [4, 5]. Now, TACE is one of the most effective therapeutic options for inoperable HCC and is performed worldwide. According to a nationwide registered survey conducted between 2004 and 2005 by the Liver Cancer Study Group of Japan [6], 17986 new cases of HCC were registered during the period. Among these cases, hepatectomy was performed in 31.7% of the patients, percutaneous ablation in 30.6%, and TACE in 31.7% as the initial therapy. TACE and the intrahepatic arterial injection of a mixture of Lipiodol (Lipiodol Ultrafluide; Andre Guerbet, Aulnay-sous-Bois, France) and the anticancer drug alone also served as treatment for intrahepatic recurrent tumors in 58.3% of patients who developed after previous treatments. Moreover, TACE is performed as pre-radiofrequency (RF) ablation treatment [7, 8]. Therefore, TACE is the most commonly performed therapeutic option for HCC in Japan and it directly contributes to prolonging the life span of patients.

Table 1. Development of cTACE in Japan

Author	Year of publication	Topics in TACE	Overall survival (%)			
			1-yr	2-yr	3-yr	4-yr
Yamada, et al.	1983	TACE using anticancer agents + GS	44%			
Nakakuma et al.	1983	Lipiodol accumulation in HCC				
Ohishi et al.	1985	Establishment of cTACE				
Nakamura et al.	1988	Lipiodol in the portal vein after TACE				
Uchida et al.	1990	Segmental TACE	91%	67%	67%	
Matsui et al.	1993	Subsegmental TACE	100%	92%	78%	67%*
Takayasu et al.	2001	Unified DSA and CT system	93%	77%	77%**	
Miyayama et al.	2007	Ultraselective TACE				
Irie et al.	2013	B-TACE				

* Maximum tumor diameter ≤4 cm, ** maximum tumor diameter ≤5 cm.

Table 2. Randomized controlled trials proven the survival benefit of TACE

Study	Year of publication	No. of patients	Overall survival (%)		
			1-yr	2-yr	P
Lo et al.	2002				
TACE (cisplatin, Lipiodol, gelfoam)		40	57	31	.002
Best supportive care		39	32	11	
Llovet et al.	2002				
TACE (doxorubicin, Lipiodol, gelfoam)		40	82	63	.009*
TAE (gelfoam)		37	75	50	
Best supportive care		35	63	27	

* TACE vs. best supportive care (TAE vs. best supportive care = N.S.; TACE vs. TAE = N.S.).

The concepts and techniques of TACE still differ among countries, as do the etiology of HCC and patients' baseline background. In Asia, TACE is performed on demand on the basis of imaging findings. On the other hand, TACE is repeated 6- to 8-week intervals in Western countries. This suggests that TACE is considered a locoregional therapy in Asia, but a chemotherapy in Western countries. The most commonly used embolic agents also differ between the two regions. These differences among countries and/or regions make direct comparison of each outcome difficult.

2. Rationale for TACE

Moderately to poorly differentiated HCC tissue is supplied only by arterial blood [1, 9]. On the other hand, the normal liver parenchyma is supplied by both arterial and portal blood. For these reasons, embolization of the hepatic artery can theoretically be expected to result in selective ischemic necrosis of the tumor tissues. This is a principal rationale for TACE.

However, HCC frequently recurs after TACE, and this is the reason why TACE is classified as a palliative treatment for HCC (Figure 1). One important cause of tumor tissue surviving after TACE is thought to be the portal venous supply to tumors appearing when the hepatic artery is embolized. Ekelund et al. [10] investigated the blood supply in rats with experimental liver tumors after arterial embolization with gelatin sponge powder or ethanol. They found that the portal venous blood supply to tumors clearly increased after arterial embolization. Goseki et al. [11] immunohistochemically demonstrated that HCC treated with TACE was supplied by the portal blood by using 5 bromo-2'-deoxyuridine (BrdU) intraoperatively injected into the portal vein immediately before hepatectomy. Furthermore, some of the capsular and/or extracapsular invasion of tumor cells is supplied by both the hepatic artery and the portal vein [12]. Well-differentiated tumor portions fed by both the artery and the portal vein are also present in early-stage HCC, mainly at the periphery of the tumor. In addition, HCC frequently develops microsatellite metastases around the tumor, even in a small tumor [13] (Figure 2). These microsatellite lesions are also supplied by both the hepatic artery and the portal vein. These tumor tissues supplied by both the hepatic artery and the portal vein can survive after embolization of the hepatic artery alone, and reversed portal blood through tumor drainage and the surrounding hepatic sinusoids may exaggerate the tumor survival [10]. The surviving tumor enlarges and receives arterial blood from the recanalized embolized artery, other adjacent arteries, or extrahepatic collaterals. If the arterial branches are severely damaged and extrahepatic collaterals cannot develop, the tumor may be fed by portal blood [14, 15] (Figure 3). Ideally, embolization of both the artery and the portal vein is necessary to completely necrotize the tumor [16, 17]; however, because of the invasiveness and technical complexity of these methods, their methods have largely been abandoned. To improve the local control effects of TACE, several new techniques have been developed in Japan [12, 18-23].

3. Devices, Equipment, Drugs, and Embolic Agents Used in TACE

3.1. Catheters and Guidewires

Initially, TACE was performed at the lobar or proper hepatic artery using a 6-F angiographic catheter [1]. In the 1980s, a coaxial catheter technique using a 3-F microcatheter was developed, and since then, the TACE procedure has made rapid progress. Uchida et al. [20] reported the usefulness of TACE at the segmental artery of the hepatic artery (segmental TACE) in 1990 and Matsui et al. [21] reported the excellent therapeutic effects of TACE at the subsegmental artery of the hepatic artery (subsegmental TACE) in 1993. In 2007, we reported TACE techniques at the most distal level of the subsubsegmental artery of the hepatic artery (ultraselective TACE) using a 2-F tip microcatheter [18].

Now, several microcatheters with a tip <2-F are commercially available in Japan. In addition, a triaxial catheter technique has been used for vessels that are difficult to select even by a coaxial catheter technique [22]. Moreover, several types of 1.8- or 3.3-F tip microballoon catheters that can pass through a 4- or 5-F angiographic catheter have been developed for the use of balloon-occluded TACE (B-TACE) or balloon-assisted TACE [19, 23]. With the advancement of microcatheter-guidewire technologies, it is possible to perform pin-point embolization to a highly limited tumor-bearing area. As a result, TACE has become more effective and less invasive [24].

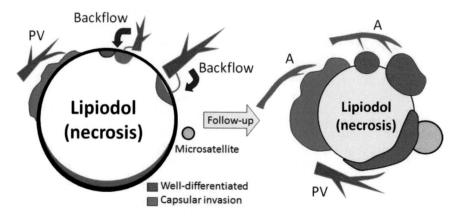

Figure 1. Schematic presentation of the mechanism of tumor recurrence (survival) after TACE. The tumor portions fed by both the arterial and the portal blood may survive after arterial blockage and the reversed portal blood flow through the drainage and surrounding sinusoids may also promote tumor survival. The surviving tumor enlarges and receives arterial blood from the recanalized embolized artery, other adjacent arteries, or extrahepatic collaterals. If the arterial branches are severely damaged and extrahepatic collaterals cannot develop, the tumor may be fed by the portal blood.

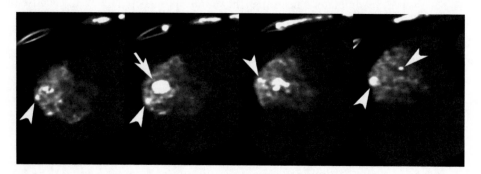

Figure 2. Microsatellite lesions around a small tumor. Unenhanced CT obtained 1 week after ultraselective TACE shows that dense Lipiodol accumulation in the microsattelite lesions (arrowheads) around a 14-mm-diameter tumor (arrow).

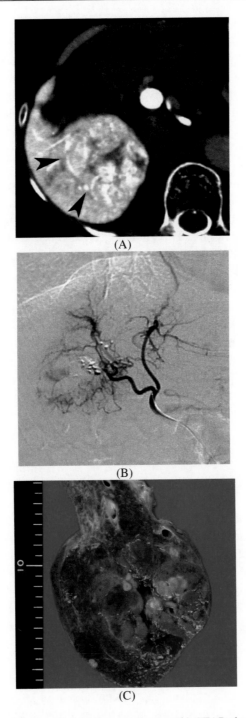

(A)

(B)

(C)

Figure 3. Recurrent HCC mainly supplied by the portal vein. (A) CTAP obtained during the 9th TACE shows a 6-cm-diameter tumor mainly supplied by the portal blood in the right hepatic lobe (arrowheads). Small areas with decreased portal blood are also seen in the tumor. (B) Proper hepatic arteriogram shows attenuation of the right hepatic artery by previous TACE and small tumor stains corresponding to the areas with decreased portal blood on CTAP. (C) The autopsy specimen shows moderately-differentiated HCC.

3.2. Intraprocedural CT

Computed tomography (CT) observation during intraarterial contrast material injection is useful for precise imaging diagnosis and for decision making regarding the treatment strategy for HCC. CT during arterial portography (CTAP) is the most reliable imaging modality for the diagnosis of malignant hepatic lesions, and it provides useful information concerning not only the number of HCC lesions but also the malignancy grades of hepatocyte nodules originating in the cirrhotic liver. CTAP can clearly depict a moderately to poorly differentiated HCC lesion, which is a good candidate for TACE, as a hypoattenuating nodule because of a lack of intratumoral portal blood [9]. In contrast, such a tumor shows hypervascularity on CT during hepatic arteriography (CTHA) [9, 25]. Additionally, corona enhancement around the tumor is seen on the late phase CTHA which represents venous drainage through the hypervascular HCC nodule [25], and is one of the most reliable findings to distinguish between HCCs and arterioportal shunts [26]. Corona enhancement is also important to determine the safety margin for treatment [27, 28]. These imaging techniques can depict small foci of HCC that cannot be demonstrated on digital subtraction angiography (DSA). In addition, CT during selective arteriography of the extrahepatic collateral pathway can depict whether the selected vessel is feeding the tumor. CT obtained immediately after TACE also helps to confirm the completeness of TACE. However, performing CT during the TACE procedure is complicated and time consuming because it is necessary to transfer the patient from the angiography room to the CT room. A unified CT and DSA system can resolve this problem [29], but it is relatively expensive and is not widely distributed.

3.3. Cone-Beam CT Technology

Cone-beam CT (CBCT) technology is an alternative method of obtaining CT images using an angiographic C-arm system equipped with a large flat-panel detector that rotates around the patient. Several CBCT techniques can be performed during the TACE procedure: during arterial portography (CBCTAP), during hepatic arteriography (CBCTHA), and after Lipiodol injection (LipCBCT) [27, 28, 30-33]. All three techniques correspond to CTAP, CTHA, and Lipiodol-CT obtained by a conventional CT scanner. Corona enhancement can also be depicted with high frequency on the 2nd-phase CBCTHA images [27]. Even an angiographically occult small tumor can be detected and completely treated under CBCT guidance [32] (Figure 4). An advantage of CBCT is reduction of the irradiation dose compared with conventional CT [30]. In addition, TACE guidance software using CBCT data helps not only to improve the technical success of TACE but also to reduce the physicians' labor [33, 34] (Figure 4). On the other hand, CBCT has some disadvantages [31]. CBCT images have several noises, in particular at the central portion of the field of view (FOV). In addition, CBCT images are low contrast, and motion artifacts mainly caused by inadequate breath-holding deteriorates the image quality. Artifacts from the catheter, contrast material in the vessels, or densely accumulated Lipiodol are also seen. The FOV of CBCT is also too small to observe the entire liver. Therefore, CBCT examination should not be used for the preoperative workup for HCC patients.

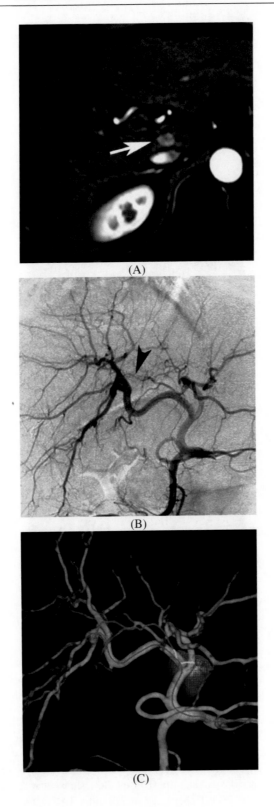

(A)

(B)

(C)

Figure 4. (Continued).

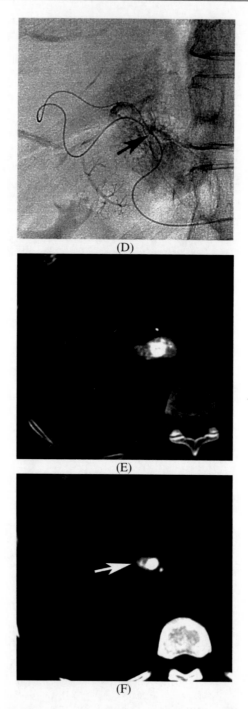

Figure 4. Ultraselective TACE for angiographically occult HCC under CBCT guidance. (A) Arterial phase gadoxetic acid-enhanced MR image shows a tumor 1.5 cm in diameter in the caudate lobe (S1) (arrow). (B) Common hepatic arteriogram shows no tumor stains. (C) AFD software can clearly identify the tumor feeder. (D) The caudate artery (A1) was selected (arrowhead on A) and TACE was performed. The arrow indicates the catheter tip. (E) LipCBCT shows that the tumor is completely embolized with a safety margin. (F) CT obtained 3 months after TACE shows that Lipiodol is densely accumulated not only in the tumor but also in the surrounding liver parenchyma (arrow).

3.4. Anticancer Agents

Several anticancer agents are usually used in TACE, although RCT and meta-analysis have provided no evidence that TACE is more effective than transcatheter arterial embolization (TAE) (bland TAE) [3-5].

3.4.1. Doxorubicin

Doxorubicin (Adriamycin; Kyowa Hakko Kirin, Tokyo, Japan) is an anticancer agent produced by *Streptomyces peucetius*, classified as an anthracycline antibiotic. It forms a complex with DNA by intercalation of its planar rings between nucleotide base pairs, with consequent inhibition of DNA, RNA, and protein synthesis. The side effects include bone marrow suppression, alopecia, and cardiotoxicity [35]. Development of another type of cancer (acute myelogeneous leukemia) and a certain blood disorder (myelodysplastic syndrome) have been reported [36].

3.4.2. Epirubicin

Epirubicin hydrochloride (Pharmorubicin; Pfizer, Tokyo, Japan) is a cell-permeable anthracycline antitumor antibiotic. It is a stereoisomer (4'-epi-isomer) of doxorubicin that exhibits reduced cardiotoxicity [37]. Epirubicin also inhibits nucleic acid and protein synthesis.

3.4.3. Mitomycin

Mitomycin (Mitomycin C; Kyowa Hakko Kirin) is an anticancer antibiotic produced by *Streptomyces caespitosus*. It is a DNA crosslinking and damaging agent that inhibits DNA synthesis and induces apoptosis in a variety of cells [38]. The most serious adverse effect of mitomycin is bone marrow suppression, and gastrointestinal disturbance, alopecia, and skin reactions commonly occur.

3.4.4. Cisplatin

Cisplatin is a platinum-containing chemotherapeutic agent. The main mode of action resembles that of an alkylating agent with production of crosslinks between the two strands of DNA in the double helix so that DNA cannot be replicated and the cells cannot divide [39]. In Japan, a fine-powder formulation of cisplatin (DDP-H; IA-call, Nippon Kayaku, Tokyo, Japan) is commercially available. Cisplatin requires pre-and post-hydration because of renal toxicity and has severe side effects including thrombocytopenia, hepatic failure, renal failure, and hypersensitivity reactions. The incidence of hypersensitivity reactions increases when the number of the treatment cycles using cisplatin is increased [40].

3.4.5. Carboplatin

Carboplatin (Nippon Kayaku) belongs to the group of platinum-based antineoplastic agents, like cisplatin, and interacts with DNA to interfere with DNA repair. The great benefit of carboplatin is its reduced side effects, particularly the elimination of nephrotoxic effects [41]. Nausea and vomiting are less severe as compared with cisplatin and more easily controlled.

3.4.6. Miriplatin

Miriplatin hydrate (Miripla; Dainippon Sumitomo, Osaka, Japan) is an anticancer agent for treatment of HCC by intrahepatic arterial injection suspended in Lipiodol. It is commercially available in Japan and China. Miriplatin is a lipophilic platinum complex, and 1,2-diaminocyclohexane platinum(II) dichloride, the active platinum compound that binds to the nuclear DNA of tumor cells causing cytotoxicity, is gradually released from miriplatin/Lipiodol accumulated in the tumor. Therefore, miriplatin can theoretically reduce the adverse effects of platinum and does not require additional hydration. In an experimental study reported by Kishimoto et al. [42], however, only 5.9% of the platinum that was initially contained in miriplatin/Lipiodol was released into saline after 28-days' incubation. In addition, the high viscosity of miriplatin/Lipiodol may stall the flow of the tumor-feeding branch and lead to incomplete TACE. Warming of miriplatin/Lipiodol can reduce its viscosity and can improve the penetration of miriplatin/Lipiodol into the tumor sinusoids [43]. It is also reported that damage to the arteries by miriplatin is weaker than that by other anticancer agents. However, the local control effect of miriplatin is also weaker than that of other anticancer agents [44-46]. The slow release of active platinum and less arterial damage are thought to be the reasons for the high frequency of tumor recurrence after TACE with miriplatin.

3.4.7. Other Anticancer Agents

Mitoxantrone (Novantron; Takeda, Osaka, Japan) and oxaliplatin (Elplat; Yakuruto, Tokyo, Japan) are infrequently used in TACE [47]. SMANCS, a reaction product of a copolymer of styrene-maleic acid conjugated to neocarzinostatin, had been used in TACE in Japan since 1982 [48]; however, production of SMANCS ceased in 2013.

3.5. Embolic Agents

3.5.1. Lipiodol

Lipiodol is a poppyseed oil used as radiopaque contrast material in lymphangiography, hysterosalpingography, and sialography. Nakakuma et al. [49] first reported long-term selective retention of Lipiodol in HCC tissues after intraarteial injection during surgical hepatic artery ligation. Thereafter, Ohishi et al. [50] established the efficacy of Lipiodol in TACE for HCC not only for the embolic material but also for usefulness for evaluation of post-TACE changes in the tumor and diagnosis of small daughter nodules. Until now, Lipiodol has been widely used in TACE, and in 2013 in Japan, it was approved for National Health Insurance reimbursement for TACE.

Lipiodol plays an important role in TACE (Figure 5). Lipiodol is a semi-fluid embolic agent and can block the tumor sinusoids. It can also flow into the surrounding portal venules and hepatic sinusoids through the peribiliary plexus and the drainage route from hypervascular HCC [18, 51, 52]. This can evoke strong ischemic effects not only on the tumor but also on the normal liver parenchyma. In Japan, customarily, the total amount of Lipiodol should not exceed 10 mL in a single TACE session to avoid severe complications [20]. On the other hand, a larger amount of Lipiodol is usually used in Western countries because it is considered as a drug carrier rather than as an embolic agent [53].

One to three anticancer agents are mixed with Lipiodol as a suspension or an emulsion to aim drug-eluting effect; however, these agents are lost from Lipiodol in a very short period (<4 hours) except for miriplatin, which is a lipophilic anticancer agent [42], unlike drug-eluting beads [54]. Two types of a Lipiodol emulsion can be prepared: water in an oil emulsion (WOE) and oil in a water emulsion (OWE). Both WOE and OWE are plastic fluids and WOE has a high yield stress compared with OWE [55]. This yield stress conveys the potential to occlude a thin tube at a low pressure gradient as a solid-like embolic agent. Moreover, the oily droplet size of WOE is larger than that of OWE. Therefore, WOE has stronger embolic effects than OWE. We usually use a WOE mixed 2-10 mL of Lipiodol with contrast material one-third the quantity of Lipiodol that dissolves 10-30 mg of epirubicin and 2-6 mg of mitomycin C.

Lipiodol is retained and concentrated in necrotic tumor tissues over a long period [56], and it helps to detect tumor recurrence on CT when a defect of Lipiodol accumulation in the tumor is found. Lipiodol is usually cleared from the liver parenchyma by Kupffer cells [57]; however, it is also retained over a long period in the hepatic parenchymal necrosis induced by TACE [18] (Figures 4, 6). Beam-hardening artifacts from dense Lipiodol accumulation deteriorate the image quality of CT, whereas Lipiodol does not influence the quality of the magnetic resonance (MR) image [58] (Figure 7).

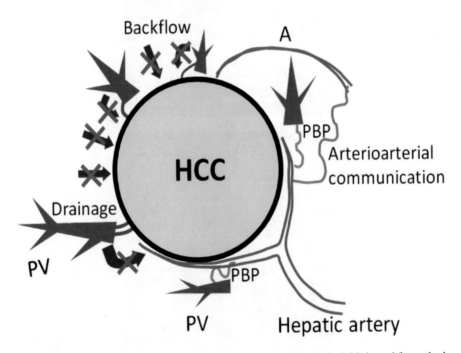

Figure 5. Schematic presentation of the role of Lipiodol in cTACE. Lipiodol injected from the hepatic artery flows into the portal vein through the peribiliary vascular plexus and tumor drainage and can block the reversed portal blood supply to the tumor from the surrounding portal venules and sinusoids. Lipiodol also passes through the arterioarterial communications. As a result, blockage of both the arterial and the portal blood flow can be achieved.

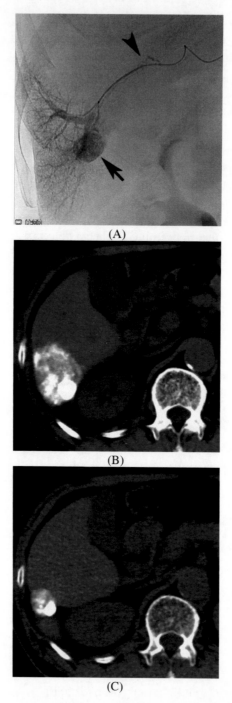

(A)

(B)

(C)

Figure 6. Visualization of the portal vein and lymphatic vessels during ultraselective TACE.
(A) During TACE of a small HCC (arrow), the portal veins are markedly opacified with Lipiodol. The hepatic lymphatic vessel is also demonstrated (arrowhead). (B) Unenhanced CT obtained 1 week after TACE shows dense Lipiodol accumulation in the tumor and surrounding liver parenchyma.
(C) Unenhanced CT obtained 6 months after TACE shows atrophy of the liver parenchyma with Lipiodol retention.

In some European and Asian countries excluding Japan, ^{131}I-labeled Lipiodol (1850-2400 MBq) administered by intraarterial injection 8 to 12 weeks after HCC resection is attempted as an adjuvant treatment. ^{131}I-Lipiodol emits γ-radiation with a mean penetration of 4 mm, potentially delivering a sufficient dose of radiation to the remnant liver and eradicating microscopic lesions. In a prospective study by Boucher et al. [59], the disease-free survival curves statistically differed between the ^{131}I-Lipiodol adjuvant therapy (n = 38) and control (n = 38) groups ($P < .03$) (2 -, 3-, and 5-year disease-free survival in the ^{131}I-Lipiodol group vs. the control group; 76.9%, 62.6%, and 41.7%, respectively, vs. 47.4%, 34.4%, and 27.1%, respectively). However, the overall survival curves did not significantly differ between the two groups ($P = .09$).

3.5.2. Gelatin Sponge

Gelatin sponge (GS) is the most commonly used embolic agent in Asia, especially for TACE. Previously in Japan, a GS sheet (Gelfoam: Pfizer, Tokyo, Japan; Spongel: Astellas, Tokyo, Japan) was cut with scissors (cutting method) or crushed by pumping using a three-way stopcock valve and two 2.5-mL syringes (pumping method) into approximately 0.5-1-mm cubes and used as an embolic agent. Now, a 1- or 2-mm-diameter ready-made spherical GS particle (Gelpart; Nippon Kayaku) is commercially available. In addition, these ready-made particles or handmade particles prepared by the cutting method can be crushed into approximately 0.2- to 0.5-mm particles by the pumping method and these are used for superselective TACE [18, 19].

GS is widely recognized as a temporary occlusive agent because it is resolvable. GS is composed of bovine or porcine collagen [60]; therefore, these materials may cause many antibody-mediated reactions. In an experimental study by Sato and Yamada [61], acute inflammatory reactions developed around the GS particles immediately after intravascular injection, followed by granulomatous arteritis with massive infiltration of mononuclear and giant cells within 20 days. Proliferation of fibroblasts into thrombi occurred after 1 week, and then, the GS was surrounded by a proliferated intima after 2 weeks. Thereafter, the GS was gradually resorbed and the occluded lumen became recanalized. However, attenuation of the embolized vessels occurs owing to arteritis and intimal proliferation and permanent vascular occlusion may develop when a dense packing of GS is performed [60].

The manually prepared GS particles have jagged edges and the particle size is not uniform; therefore, occluding points of the targeted vessels cannot be expected. The size of a ready-made particle is also too large to embolize the tumor vessels. It may occlude the proximal vessels before reaching the tumor vessels; therefore, the performance of GS particles as an embolic agent is inferior to that of microspheres [62].

3.5.3. Polyvinyl Alcohol

Polyvinyl alcohol (PVA) particles (Cook, Bloomington, IN, USA; Boston Scientific, Natick, MA, USA) are made from a PVA sheet. The particles are filtered with sieves and are available in sizes ranging from 100 to 1000 μm [63]. Because PVA particles have an irregular nature and vary in size, they tend to aggregate, occluding vessels more proximally than might be expected on the basis of the calibrated size. Catheter occlusion can also develop; therefore, dilution of particles, proper suspension, and slow infusion are required [64].

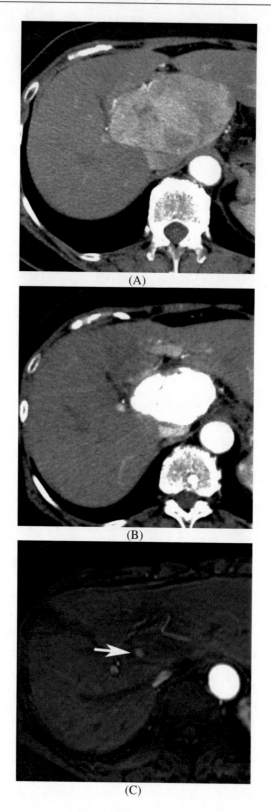

Figure 7. (Continued).

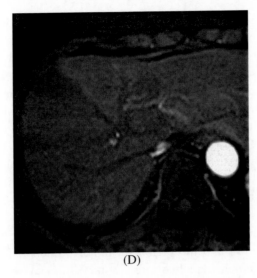

(D)

Figure 7. Efficacy of MR imaging after cTACE. **(A)** Arterial-phase CT shows a large tumor 10.2 cm in diameter in S1. Serum levels of alpha-fetoprotein (AFP) and protein induced in vitamin K absence II (PIVKA-II) were 15775 mg/mL and 7556 AU/mL, respectively. Two stepwise TACE sessions including TACE of the right IPA were performed (not shown). **(B)** Arterial-phase CT obtained 5 months after the 1st TACE shows that the tumor is reduced in size with dense Lipiodol accumulation. No viable tumors can be detected. **(C)** However, arterial-phase gadoxetic acid-enhanced MR image obtained 6 months after the 1st TACE shows a small viable portion in the tumor (arrow). Additional TACE was performed 1 year after the 1st TACE (not shown). **(D)** Arterial-phase gadoxetic acid-enhanced MR image obtained 1 year and 3 months after the 1st TACE shows the disappearance of the viable tumor. The serum levels of AFP and PIVKA-II were normalized (7 mg/mL and 14 AU/mL, respectively).

PVA particles provide permanent occlusion of the embolized vessels and the results are an inflammatory reaction and focal angionecrosis, with vessel fibrosis developing over time [64]. As a result, extrahepatic collateral pathways may markedly develop [65]. PVA particles are mainly used in Western countries; others than in China, they are not used for TACE in Asia.

3.5.4. Microspheres (Beads)

Various kinds of microspheres are commercially available in Western countries and some part of Asia. Several microspheres became available in 2014 in Japan. Microspheres are permanent embolic agents made from an acrylic polymer matrix or from PVA hydrogel [54, 62, 66-70]. Unlike GS and PVA particles, microspheres are smooth and spherical in shape, and fragmentation is not observed. The particles are precisely calibrated in sizes ranging from 40 to 1300 μm and can embolize vessels with diameters almost equal to the particle size. Some microspheres can also be loaded with anticancer agents. DC Bead (Biocompatibles UK, Farnham, UK) is a bead with negatively charged functional groups that allows the loading of several positively charged anticancer drugs, such as doxorubicin, epirubicin, and irinotecan. Forty-three percent of loaded anticancer agents are eluted at 28 days, and 89% at 90 days [54]. Drug release is sustained to allow long-term local release within the tumor and minimize the systemic levels of the drug. Hepasphere (Biosphere, Rockland, MA, USA) is a nonbiodegradable, spherical, dry particle, which swells within several minutes of absorbing the nonionic contrast material by up to approximately 4 times its original dry size [62]. This microsphere is elastic compared with DC Bead, and it deforms and conforms to the vessel lumen. During the absorbing of contrast material, water-soluble chemotherapeutic agents can be loaded by its reservoir effect, as well as the loading of positively charged anticancer agents. Hepashere releases anticancer agents earlier than DC bead [66]. Maeda et al. [67] reported that cisplatin loaded into Hepasphere was released within 24 hours. Embozene-TANDEM (CeloNova BioSciences, Newnan, GA, USA) is another drug-eluting bead, and it can be loaded with positively charged anticancer agents. This bead can release anticancer agents more slowly than DC Bead [68].

Experimental studies show that smaller-sized microspheres induce more necrosis of the hepatic parenchyma. In addition, smaller-sized drug-eluting beads induce more necrosis of the hepatic parenchyma than the same-sized bland beads or larger-sized drug-eluting beads [69]. As mentioned above, one of the important technical problems of TACE only with a particulate embolus in HCC is the suspected reversal of flow from the surrounding hepatic sinusoids and portal venules into the peripheral tumor portion following TACE [10]. For tumor tissues, smaller particles are likely to occlude in distal vessels, resulting in more localized chemotherapeutic delivery and good imaging response [70], although the risk of unexpected complications may increase.

3.5.5. Ethanol

TAE with a mixture of Lipiodol and ethanol (TEA) has been shown to be an effective treatment for inoperable HCC [71, 72]. In a randomized controlled study performed by Yu et al. [72], Lipiodol retention in the tumor was greater in the TEA group than in the TACE group ($89.5 \pm 10.7\%$ vs. $47.5 \pm 21.2\%$; $P < .0001$). The tumor progression rate at 1 year was higher in the TACE group (5/30 vs. 0/30; $P = .0261$). One- and 2-year overall survival rates were higher in the TEA group (93.3% and 80.0%, respectively, vs. 73.3% and 43.3%, respectively; $P = .0053$). However, TEA has not been widely recognized or performed in Japan, because the local tumor control of TEA reported in a study from Japan was almost equal to that of subsegmental TACE [21].

3.5.6. Yttrium-90 Microsphere

Radioembolization with yttrium-90 (Y90) microspheres, a pure beta-emitter with a 64.1-hour physical half-life, injected through the hepatic artery for HCC has been developed [73]. This treatment is not an embolotherapy but rather a form of brachytherapy, and the target dose to the liver will be 100 to 120 Gy. Two Y90-microsphere devices are commercially available, but not in Japan: TheraSphere (MDS Nordion, Ottawa, Canada) is 20 to 30 μm in diameter and made of glass with a minimally embolic device and higher specific activity, and SIR-Spheres (Sirtex Medical, Sydney, Australia) is 20 to 60 μm in diameter (95% of particles are 30-35 μm) and made of resin with moderately embolic and lower specific activity. Radioembolization with Y90-microspheres has potential risks of pneumonitis and treatment-induced liver dysfunction such as bilirubin elevation. In addition, the size of the microsphere is extremely small compared with other embolic agents; therefore, checking for the hepatopulmonary shunt and prophylactic embolization of arteries supplying the extrahepatic organs, such as the stomach, duodenum, pancreas, and gallbladder, are required before treatment [74]. One to two weeks prior to radioembolization, a simulation of the actual treatment is also required using technetium-99m labeled macroaggregated albumin (^{99m}Tc-MAA) particles that are roughly the size of the microspheres to detect extrahepatic shunting to the lung or the gastrointestinal tract. Additional prophylactic embolization or dose reduction is recommended in cases of unfavorable ^{99m}Tc-MAA scintigraphy.

3.5.7. Other Embolic Agents

Autologous blood clot is used as an embolic agent, especially for HCC patients with advanced cirrhosis. Since autologous blood clot is a temporary occlusive agent that resolves within 2 to 3 hours and does not damage the hepatic artery, it can be used in patients with Child-Pugh C class [75]. In particular, TACE with autologous blood clot (short occlusion time-TACE: S-TACE) is effective for tumors ≤5 cm [76].

Degradable starch microsphere (DSM), an embolic agent 40 to 45 μm in diameter made from potato starch, induces transient occlusion of the arteriolar capillary bed. Since DSM is degraded by serum amylase, the duration of occlusion in the hepatic arteries by DSM is limited to 80 minutes. Thus, DSM seldom injures the hepatic artery. DSM is usually used with anticancer drugs, sometimes with Lipiodol, and this treatment is mainly indicated for advanced cases [77].

TAE with N-butyl-2-cyanoacrylate (NBCA, Histoacryl Blue; B. Baum, Melsungen, Germany) has also been reported [78]. NBCA is a permanent embolic agent and polymerizes instantaneously on contact with blood or epithelium. The polymerization time can be controlled by changing the dilution ratio mixed with Lipiodol, and the ratios between 1:3 and 1:10 are used according to the desired occlusion level. However, hypoxia induced by complete arterial occlusion may stimulate vascular endothelial growth factor (VEGF) production by the tumor, leading to additional blood supply from the extrahepatic collateral pathways that cannot be embolized because of the small caliber and feeding to other organs [78]. As a result, re-intervention becomes difficult. Therefore, NBCA is inappropriate for TAE of HCC except in cases of uncontrollable tumor bleeding.

4. Indication and TACE Strategy

4.1. Indication

TACE is indicated for inoperable hypervascular HCC in patients with Eastern Cooperative Oncology Group (ECOG) performance status (PS) 0 to 2. On the basis of the Barcelona Clinic Liver Cancer (BCLC) staging system, TACE is recommended for intermediate-stage HCC (stage B): 2 or 3 tumors >3 cm or more than 3 lesions in patients with Child-Pugh A or B class [79]. According to the consensus meeting of the 45th annual meeting of the Japan Society of Hepatology, HCC with tumor thrombus in the second or third portal branch or HCC within the Milan criteria (single tumor ≤5 cm or multiple but less than 3 tumors ≤3 cm each) in patients aged ≤65 years with Child-Pugh C class is indicated for TACE, in addition to BCLC-B HCC [80]. TACE is also indicated for smaller tumors when curative treatment, such as hepatectomy or RF ablation, is contraindicated owing to severe associated disease and/or aging, as well as to the tumor location (Figure 4). Furthermore, TAE/TACE is indicated for hemostasis of spontaneously ruptured HCCs (Figure 8) [81, 82].

4.2. Contraindication

Main portal vein occlusion, hyperbilirubinemia >3.0 mg/dL, refractory massive ascites or pleural effusion, uncontrollable hepatic encephalopathy, and poor performance status (ECOG PS ≥3) are contraindicated for TACE. The presence of bile duct dilatation or a history of endoscopic papillotomy or bilioenteric anastomosis is also contraindicated for TACE because of the high risk of liver abscess formation after TACE [83]. TACE is usually contraindicated for patients who have extrahepatic disease as well as intrahepatic tumors; however, it is indicated for patients whose intrahepatic tumors are thought to become the main cause of death (liver-dominant disease).

4.3. Consensus of the TACE Strategy

Intermediate-stage HCC includes various tumor conditions. It is important to change the technique and magnitude of TACE in individual cases, although there is no consensus on how to change the TACE techniques according to the tumor spread. For localized small or intermediate-sized tumors (for example, ≤6 cm and less than 5 lesions), curative TACE should be performed as selectively as possible to achieve good tumor control and to reduce adverse effects. For large but localized tumors (for example, >6 cm and less than 3 lesions), curative TACE should also be performed. In such conditions, stepwise TACE sessions with intervals of at least 3 weeks are recommended to avoid severe complications [84] (Figures 7, 9). Bland TAE is another option for elderly patients. For bilobar multiple lesions, mild embolization of the entire liver is required. In such conditions, the two hepatic lobes should be treated in separate treatment sessions 2 to 8 weeks apart to reduce adverse effects. For far advanced (large and bilobar) tumors, palliative TACE/TAE for mass reduction or prevention of tumor rupture should be performed.

5. TACE Technique

The procedure is usually performed via the femoral artery. After local anesthesia, the femoral artery is punctured and catheterized. After performing diagnostic arteriography and CT examination including possible extrahepatic collaterals, TACE is performed. Now, in Japan, almost all TACE procedures are performed using a 1.7- to 2.4-F tip microcatheter through a 3- to 5-F angiographic catheter under CT or CBCT guidance as well as DSA.

Before injection of chemoembolic agents, 0.5 mL of 2% lidocaine (Terumo, Tokyo, Japan) is usually injected through the catheter to prevent pain and vasospasm [21]. In addition, opioid analgesics are widely used for control of TACE/TAE-related pain during or after the procedure [85].

The endpoint of TACE is occlusion of the tumor feeders and disappearance of target tumor stains on DSA. Confirmation of the embolized areas using CT or CBCT is also useful for determination of the endpoint [28].

TACE techniques are wide-ranging. The types of embolic agents and catheter positioning strongly influence the therapeutic or adverse effects of TACE. Therefore, TACE techniques are usually classified according to these factors.

5.1. Classification of TACE According to Embolic Agent

5.1.1. Conventional TACE

In Asia, a mixture of Lipiodol and anticancer drugs and GS particles have been mainly used as embolic agents. This technique is called "conventional TACE (cTACE)." A nationwide survey by the TACE Study Group of Japan showed that >90% of TACE treatments for HCCs included Lipiodol [86]. Regarding the dose of Lipiodol used for a single TACE session, the average dose (mL) is roughly equal to the sum of the target tumor diameters (cm) [20, 86], but it should not exceed 10 mL. For localized tumors, a mixture of Lipiodol and anticancer drugs is slowly injected through a microcatheter introduced into the tumor-feeding branch until abundant visualization of the surrounding portal vein and/or marked retardation of the arterial flow is seen. Subsequently, 0.2- to 0.5-mm GS particles are injected until complete blockage of the arterial flow is achieved. Although the size of the GS particles is too large to occlude the tumor vasculatures, Lipiodol can make up for this weak point of GS particles as an embolic agent. HCC nodules frequently have multiple feeding branches. For such tumors, the main feeding branch should be embolized last because the dense retention of Lipiodol and contrast material in the tumor and liver parenchyma just after TACE makes it difficult to confirm the residual tumor on DSA [18], or even on CBCT [28]. In addition, the most proximal feeder should be embolized last to avoid the inadvertent occlusion of another feeder by overflowed embolic agents. In cases of multiple HCC nodules (less than 5), selective/superselective TACE is performed for each nodule. For multiple tumors (6 or more), TACE is performed at the more proximal level using a mixture of Lipiodol and 1-mm GS particles.

Although a definitive statement regarding treatment with or without chemotherapy cannot be made without an adequately powered prospective trial [3], 1 to 3 anticancer agents mixed with Lipiodol are usually used in TACE. Doxorubicin is the most popular anticancer agent used in TACE worldwide. In Japan, epirubicin is the most common anticancer agent (74%) followed by doxorubicin, mitomycin C, cisplatin, and others [87]. Miriplatin is another anticancer drug that is composed of a lipophilic platinum complex [42]. Although TACE has a long history in Japan, the most effective and least toxic regime for TACE has not yet been established.

Consensus is also lacking about the most suitable dosage of anticancer drugs for TACE. Lu et al. [88] randomized 34 patients who elected to undergo preoperative superselective TACE with low-dose (2 mg of mitomycin C, 10 mg of epirubicin, and 100 mg of carboplatin) (n = 16) and high-dose (10 mg of mitomycin C, 40 mg of epirubicin, and 300 mg of carboplatin) regimens. They found that there were no significant differences in early tumor response ($P > .05$), necrosis rates (mean ± standard deviation, 88.4 ± 11.1% vs. 87.1 ± 12.5%, $P > .05$), and apoptosis index (11.0 ± 4.0% vs. 10.7 ± 3.9%, $P > .05$) between the low-dose and high-dose TACE groups. Their results suggest that superselective TACE with low-dose anticancer drugs is feasible and effective and, arguably, could be advocated. Until now, however, further studies have not been performed to determine the more effective regime and optimal dosages.

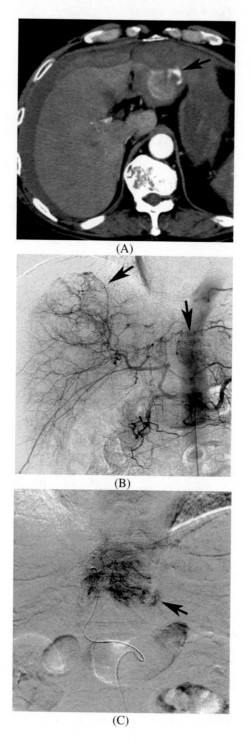

(A)

(B)

(C)

Figure 8. (Continued).

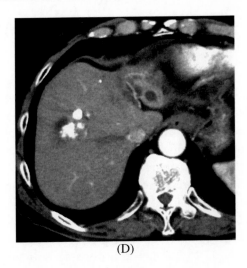

(D)

Figure 8. TAE for ruptured HCC. (A) Arterial-phase CT shows massive peritoneal bleeding and extravasation of contrast material from HCC 4 cm in diameter in the left lateral segment (arrow). Another tumor 5.5 cm in diameter is also seen in the right hepatic lobe (not shown). (B) Emergency angiography shows two tumor stains (arrows). (C) Selective arteriogram of the lateral inferior subsegmental artery of the left hepatic artery shows a tumor stain and extravasation of contrast material (arrow). Bland TAE with GS was performed. Three weeks later, the tumor in the right hepatic lobe was treated with cTACE (not shown). Thereafter, two additional TACE sessions were performed for the recurrent and newly developed tumors. (D) Arterial-phase CT obtained 3 years and 6 months after the 1st TAE shows good control of both tumors. No other viable tumors are depicted.

5.1.2. TACE Using Drug-Eluting Beads

In Western countries, TACE using doxorubicin loaded drug-eluting beads (DEBDOX) has become a standard technique for the treatment of intermediate-stage HCC. DEBDOX is a novel drug delivery embolization system that has been designed to deliver a higher and more sustained release of the drug directly into the tumor and a low release of the drug into the systemic circulation with calibrated tumor vessel obstruction. However, the survival benefit of DEBDOX in comparison with cTACE has not been proven by RCTs [53, 89].

The technical recommendations represent the consensus of a panel of experts and are aimed at defining standards for an appropriate and consistent use of DEBDOX [90]. For disease within the Milan criteria, each single treatment should include a planned dose of up to 75 mg doxorubicin loaded into one vial of DC Bead. For disease beyond the Milan criteria, each single treatment should include a planned dose of up to 150 mg of doxorubicin loaded into two vials of DC Bead. In bilolar or very large tumors, the two hepatic lobes can be treated in separate TACE sessions. Use of 100 to 300 μm beads is recommended for a standard procedure. In small tumors, smaller particles are ideal for precise embolization; however, in cases with significant arterioportal or arteriovenous shunting, embolization of the shunt using GS particles or metallic coils should be performed before microsphere administration. One milliliter of DEBDOX is diluted with at least 5 to 10 mL of contrast material and should be slowly injected through the catheter at 1 mL of DEBDOX suspension/min without reflux. Superselective catheterization is preferable, but wedging of the catheter should be avoided. The embolization endpoint is near stasis of the tumor-feeding artery (i.e., the contrast column should clear within 2–5 heartbeats), not complete occlusion of the tumor feeders. The safety of DEBDOX-TACE through the extrahepatic collaterals has not been established.

5.1.3. Bland TAE

The rationale for bland TAE is not only to create tumor regression by terminal vessel blockage with small particles alone, but also to minimize post-embolization syndrome, which is often seen after cTACE [91]. However, the survival benefit of bland TAE is still unclear. TAE using GS particles was not significant compared with conservative management on RCT and meta-analysis [3-5]. This unfavorable result might have been caused by the large particle size of the GS. Now, this procedure is mainly performed for hemostasis of spontaneously ruptured HCC [81], because Lipiodol and anticancer drugs may severely damage the liver in patients in the shock state. Small-sized microspheres can provide occlusion of the distal intratumoral vessels and achieve massive tumor necrosis. Osuga et al. [62] reported that TAE using Hepashere particles of 53 to 212 μm in a dry state was safe and effective for large HCCs and postprocedural pain was definitely mild compared with cTACE. Bonomo et al. [92] also reported good local tumor control using 40- and 100-μm Embozene microspheres. However, the risk of fatal respiratory complications caused by passing through the arteriovenous shunt may increase when smaller particles are used [92-94].

A recent prospective randomized study by Malagari et al. [95] demonstrated that TACE using doxorubicin-eluting beads presents a better local response, fewer recurrences, and a longer time to progression (TTP) than bland TAE with same-sized microspheres ($P = .008$). This results show that the addition of an anticancer agent(s) in transarterial HCC embolization is based on the assumption that chemotherapeutics augment the antitumoral action of ischemia, counteracting the stimulation of neoangiogenesis resulting from hypoxia due to embolization. However, no significant benefit to survival of doxorubicin-eluting bead TACE was found, partly because of a short follow-up.

5.2. Classification of TACE by Catheter Positioning

5.2.1. Selective/Superselective TACE

Selective TACE is generally defined as TACE that is performed at the segmental artery of the hepatic artery, and superselective TACE as TACE at the distal portion of the subsegmental artery of the hepatic artery. Among these, TACE at the subsegmental artery is called subsegmental TACE [21], and it is a standard technique worldwide for small HCCs. If cTACE is performed at the more distal level of the subsubsegmental artery, it is called ultraselective TACE. The efficacy of selective/superselective cTACE for localized HCC has been established. When Lipiodol is injected at the distal level of the hepatic artery, some Lipiodol flows into the portal veins and can block the portal blood flow [18, 51]. This leads not only to massive necrosis of the tumor but also to atrophy of the surrounding liver parenchyma ("medical segmentectomy" effect [21]). Additionally, the superselective technique can also reduce the liver damage. In a report by Matsui et al. [21], complete necrosis could be achieved in approximately 70% of tumors ≤4 cm in diameter by a single subsegmental TACE session and no severe complications developed. Golfieri et al. [96] also reported that complete necrosis and necrosis ≥90% were more frequently (approximately 2 times) observed after selective/superselective TACE compared with nonselective TACE ($P =$ .013 and $P = .008$, respectively).

5.2.2. Nonselective TACE

Nonselective TACE is defined as TACE that is performed at the lobar or proper hepatic artery, and it is indicated for multiple unilobar or bilobar tumors. However, there are no definite criteria about the upper limit of the number and diameter of tumors that can be treated with selective/superselective TACE. Even in nonselective TACE, the tip of a catheter should be placed distal to the orifice of the cystic artery. In addition, injection of embolic agents into other arteries supplying the extrahepatic organs should be avoided. In bilobar tumors, the two hepatic lobes can be treated in separate treatment sessions with intervals of at least 2 to 8 weeks. A large tumor located on the liver surface or near the hepatic hilum should be preferentially treated to prevent tumor rupture or portal venous invasion. If the tumor distribution can be localized after nonselective TACE, subsequent TACE should be performed on demand in a superselective fashion (Figure 10).

5.2.3. TACE through the Extrahepatic Collateral Pathways

HCC is frequently supplied by the extrahepatic collateral vessels [65, 97-107]. An extrahepatic collateral pathway mainly develops after interruption of the hepatic artery by surgical ligation, arterial injury induced by repeated TACE, or placement of a catheter for hepatic arterial infusion. Adhesion between the liver and other organs exaggerates the degree of the extrahepatic collaterals. An extrahepatic blood supply to HCC also develops according to the anatomical location and size of the HCC although the hepatic artery is intact [99] (Figure 11). In particular, extrahepatic collateral supplies develop early at the bare area of the liver [100]. Extrahepatic collateral supplies can inhibit the effectiveness of TACE; therefore, these should be adequately searched and embolized for transcatheter management of HCC to be effective.

In our previous analysis [98], TACE through the extrahepatic collaterals was attempted in 386 (16.6%) of 2329 procedures (Table 3). The incidences of the collateral source to HCC were 83% from the right inferior phrenic artery (IPA) (Figure 9), 24% from the cystic artery (Figure 11), 13% from the omental artery, 12% from the right renal capsular artery and left IPA (Figure 8), 8% from the right internal artery (IMA) and right intercostal arteries (Figure 12), and 7% from the right inferior adrenal artery. The right middle adrenal artery, right or left gastric arteries, middle or right colic artery (Figure 13), 3 and 9 o'clock artery, and left IMA were also infrequent extrahepatic collateral pathways that were found in <4% of procedures. The incidence of development of each collateral pathway may depend on the size of the area that is attached to the liver in addition to the tumor location and size. Previous extrahepatic collateral TACE also exaggerates the development of another extrahepatic collateral supply [100]. Therefore, the incidence may easily change according to the patient and tumor background. In addition, atherosclerotic change or previous catheter manipulation frequently causes stenosis or occlusion of the orifice of the IPA. In such conditions, the IPA is reconstructed mainly through the retroperitoneal branches arising from the dorsal pancreatic artery, adrenal arteries, left gastric artery, and patent contralateral IPA [101]. Each anastomosis branch may make the network, and some may simultaneously opacify the IPA. The less tortuous access route should be selected to complete TACE.

Table 3. Extrahepatic collateral pathways observed in 2329 TACE procedures of 719 patients

Artery	No. of procedures	No. of patients	Technical Success rates (%)
Right inferior phrenic	285	145	96
Cystic	60	43	70
Omental	34	23	74
Left inferior phrenic	30	22	93
Right renal capsular	28	21	100
Right intercostal	22	14	53
Right inferior adrenal	19	13	100
Right internal mammary	16	15	100
Left gastric	8	7	63
Right middle adrenal	7	7	100
Right gastric	7	5	71
Right or middle colic	6	5	67
3 and 9 o'clock	4	4	75
Right lumbar	3	3	100
Left internal mammary	1	1	100

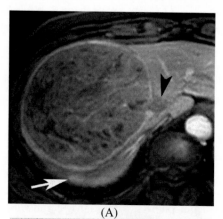

(A)

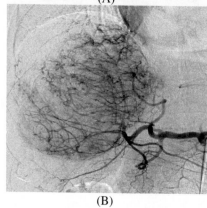

(B)

Figure 9. (Continued).

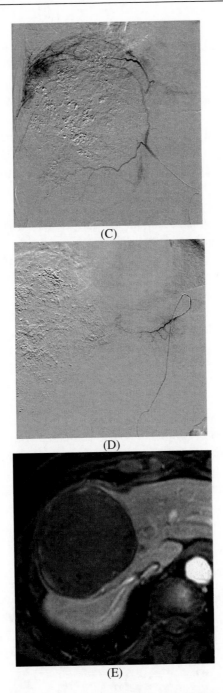

Figure 9. Stepwise TACE for large HCC. (**A**) Arterial-phase gadoxetic acid-enhanced MR image shows a tumor 13.5 cm in diameter with intrahepatic metastasis (arrow) and hepatic vein tumor thrombus (arrowhead). Serum levels of AFP and PIVKA-II were 8 mg/dL and 6405 AU/mL, respectively. (**B**) Celiac arteriogram shows a large tumor stain. (**C, D**) The right IPA and the anteromedial limb of the left IPA also supply the tumor. Three stepwise TACE sessions were performed (not shown). (**E**) Arterial-phase gadoxetic acid-enhanced MR image shows complete tumor remission. Serum levels of tumor markers were normalized after TACE (3 mg/dL and 22 AU/mL, respectively).

There is a close relationship between the tumor location and suspicious extrahepatic collaterals [98]. Tumors located on the posterior surface of the right lobe and near the diaphragm are likely to be fed by the right IPA. The right intercostal and lumbar arteries also supply them, especially when the right IPA is attenuated by repeated TACE. Blood supply from the right IMA is also seen when the tumor is located beneath the diaphragm or at the anterior chest wall. Tumors located near the right renal fossa are fed by the right renal capsular, middle adrenal, and inferior adrenal arteries. Tumors located on the anterior surface of the right hepatic lobe or on the lower edge of the left hepatic lobe are fed by the omental or colic artery. Tumors in the lateral segment of the left hepatic lobe are fed by the right or left gastric artery in addition to by the left IPA. The cystic artery mainly feeds tumors located near the gallbladder fossa, but it infrequently supplies tumors in the right lobe or medial subsegment of the liver at a distance from the gallbladder fossa when the hepatic artery is attenuated [102]. In addition, a small hepatic branch frequently arises from the cystic artery [108]. Tumors arising in the caudate lobe tend to be fed by the right IPA, right renal capsular artery, and gastric artery. In particular, recurrent tumors in the Spiegel lobe are frequently fed by the proximal branch of the right IPA [103].

TACE can be performed only when the tumor-feeding branch arising from these extrahepatic collaterals is selected. In our previous analysis, the feeding branch arising from the right intercostal artery is the most difficult type of branch to catheterize [98]. With advances in catheter-guidewire technology, it has become possible to introduce a microcatheter into almost all such small feeders [84] (Figure 12). For TACE through the cystic, colic, or gastric artery, the microcatheter should be deeply advanced until the stain in the gallbladder or alimentary tract wall has disappeared (Figures 11, 13). Infused dosage of chemoembolic agents should be properly reduced compared with TACE of the hepatic artery, and complete blockage of the tumor feeders should be avoided. Furthermore, an emulsion of Lipiodol and anticancer drugs should not be injected into the skin-supplying branch derived from the IMA and intercostal artery because it may cause skin necrosis [98, 104]. These extrahepatic collaterals usually anastomose each other; therefore, careful observation is needed during the injection of the embolic agents to avoid unexpected procedure-related complications [105].

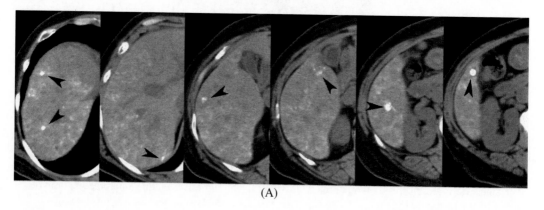

(A)

Figure 10. (Continued).

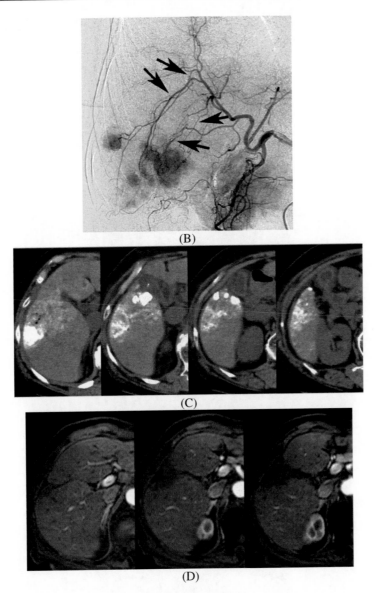

(B)

(C)

(D)

Figure 10. Changes in TACE techniques according to the tumor distribution. (**A**) Unenhanced CT obtained 1 week after nonselective TACE of the right hepatic lobe shows seven small tumors (arrowheads). Three tumors are also in the left hepatic lobe, and nonselective TACE was performed 1 month later (not shown). (**B**) Several tumors in the right hepatic lobe recurred 1 year and 6 months after the 1st TACE, and superselective TACE was performed through four branches, including through a branch of the cystic artery (arrows). (**C**) CT obtained 1 week after the 3rd TACE shows dense Lipiodol accumulation in the tumors. Thereafter, six additional TACE procedures were performed for recurrent or newly developed tumors (not shown). (**D**) Arterial-phase gadoxetic acid-enhanced MR image obtained 8 years and 10 months after the initial TACE shows the atrophy of the embolized area. No viable tumors are depicted.

We believe that TACE through extrahepatic collateral pathways contributes to prolonging the life span of patients; however, the evidence to support its usefulness is insufficient. The importance of extrahepatic collateral TACE may increase in long-term survivors who have undergone multiple TACE sessions, as well as in patients with large HCC [84]. Indeed, the incidence of blood supply from minor extrahepatic collaterals, such as the left IMA and right lumbar artery, has recently been increasing [106, 107].

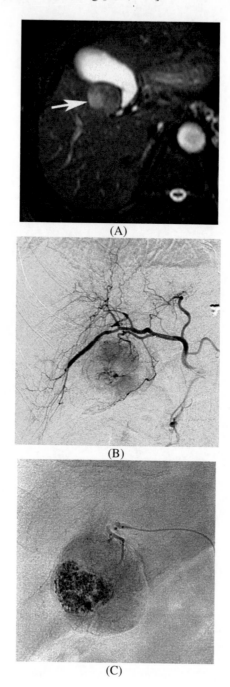

(A)

(B)

(C)

Figure 11. (Continued).

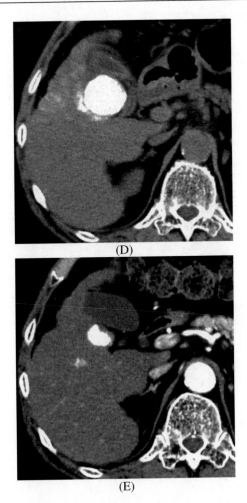

(D)

(E)

Figure 11. HCC initially supplied by the cystic artery. (**A**) T2-weighted MR image shows a tumor 3.6 cm in diameter near the gallbladder (arrow). (**B**) Right hepatic arteriogram shows a tumor stain supplied by the cystic artery. (**C**) The feeding branch was selected and embolized. A branch of the anterior inferior subsegmental artery of the right hepatic artery (A5) was also embolized (not shown). (**D**) Unenhanced CT obtained 1 week after TACE shows dense Lipiodol accumulation in the tumor. (**E**) Arterial-phase CT obtained 8 years after TACE shows that the tumor is reduced in size without recurrence.

6. Technical Variations in cTACE

Several technical variations in cTACE have been developed to enhance the local control effect. These techniques are performed under nonphysiological blood circulation and can make good use of the characteristics of Lipiodol as "a semi-fluid embolic agent." Therefore, these techniques should not be applied to microsphere TAE/TACE.

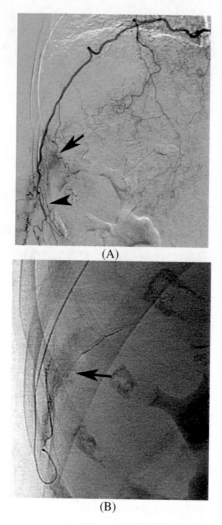

(A)

(B)

Figure 12. Recurrent HCC supplied by the right intercostal artery. (A) Arteriogram of the right 10th intercostal artery shows a tumor stain (arrow) supplied by a small branch (arrowhead). (B) TACE was performed after selective catheterization. The arrow indicates the tumor.

6.1. TACE under Balloon Occlusion of the Hepatic Vein

In an experimental study by Kanazawa et al. [109], arteriogram during hepatic vein occlusion demonstrated a greater number of peripheral arterial branches in the occluded area than in the non-occluded areas. Prolonged hepatogram showing hepatofugal opacification of the portal branches was also observed in the occluded area. They speculated that temporary segmental hepatic vein occlusion might improve the therapeutic effects of hepatic arterial infusion.

Higashihara and Okazaki [12] developed TACE under balloon occlusion of the hepatic vein (Figure 14). When the hepatic vein is occluded, the portal veins act as the drainage of the arterial blood because of the pressure gradient between the artery and portal vein. Therefore, chemoembolic agents injected from the hepatic artery can also flow into the portal vein through the transsinusoidal and arterioportal communications. As a result, simultaneous embolization of both the hepatic artery and the portal vein can be achieved and the therapeutic effects of TACE may improve. They treated 83 patients with 98 HCC lesions (mean diameter, 3.3 cm) with TACE under balloon occlusion of the hepatic vein and the 3-, 5- and 8-year survival rates of 76 of the patients were 83.4%, 64.6%, and 54.2%, respectively. Their results were almost equal or superior to those for patients treated by hepatectomy. However, their technique is not widely distributed because the procedure was complicated and some tumors located in the boundary between subsegments had multiple different subsegmental feeding arteries and multiple draining veins.

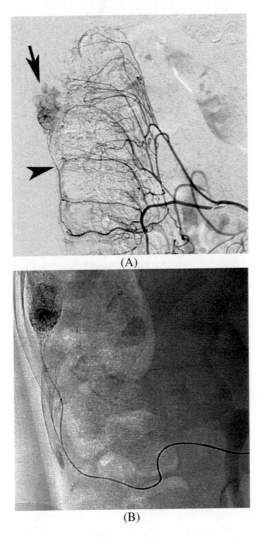

(A)

(B)

Figure 13. Recurrent HCC supplied by the right colic artery. **(A)** Arteriogram of the right colic artery shows a tumor stain (arrow) supplied by a small branch (arrowhead). **(B)** After selective catheterization into the tumor-feeding branch, TACE was performed without complications.

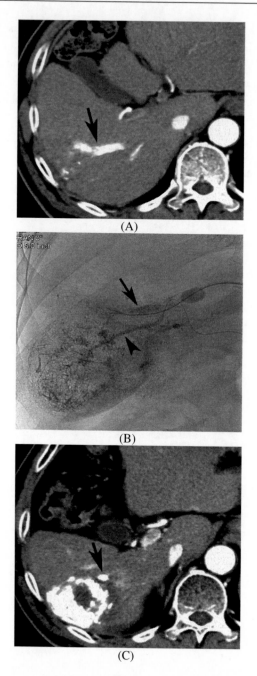

Figure 14. TACE under balloon occlusion of the hepatic vein. **(A)** Arterial-phase CT shows an enhanced tumor in the right hepatic vein accompanied by an arteriovenous shunt (arrow). **(B)** The posterior segmental artery of the right hepatic artery was embolized under right hepatic vein occlusion. TACE of a branch of A5 was also performed under right hepatic vein occlusion (not shown). The arrow indicates Lipiodol accumulation in the right hepatic vein tumor thrombus and the arrowhead indicates the microcatheter tip. **(C)** Arterial-phase CT obtained 10 months after TACE shows Lipiodol accumulation in the tumor thrombus without recurrence (arrow).

6.2. Ultraselective TACE

Ultraselective TACE is defined as TACE that is performed at the most distal level of the subsubsegmental artery of the hepatic artery [18]; however, this term does not merely mean "TACE performed at the most distal level of the hepatic artery." In ultraselective TACE, embolic agents distally flow away not only by the physiological blood flow but also by the injection force because a microcatheter in the small vessel can block the backflow of embolic agents by its mass effect. This condition enables passive embolic agent injection; therefore, the dose of Lipiodol reaching into the portal veins increases and blockage of both the arterial and the portal blood flow can be achieved, and it may cause infarction of the nontumorous liver parenchyma (Figures 4, 6, 15). When the flow of the tumor-feeding branch is unexpectedly stopped before adequate portal vein visualization is achieved, 0.5 μg of prostaglandin E1 (Liple; Mitsubishi Pharma, Osaka, Japan) or 2% lidocaine is administered through the catheter to increase arterial flow. In addition, the microcatheter is advanced more distally to achieve a "semi-wedged condition," if possible. Now, we routinely use an angled 1.7-F tip microcatheter (ASAHI Veloute; Asahi Intecc, Seto, Japan) for TACE, and selective catheterization into the distal subsubsegmental artery is possible in 98.5% of small tumors [33].

We focused on the relationship between tumor recurrence and portal vein visualization during TACE (Figure 16). Portal vein visualization was divided into 3 grades on the spot radiograph: grade 0, no visualization; grade 1, visualization adjacent to the tumor; and grade 2, visualization of the whole or extending embolized area [18, 110]. The therapeutic effects for grade 2 were excellent, and the 5-year local recurrence rate was 19%. That of the grade 1 group was 42%; however, local recurrence was frequently seen in the grade 0 group, including several cases showing incomplete embolization. The local recurrence rates of tumors with markedly visualized portal veins during TACE were significantly lower than those of tumors with slight or no portal vein visualization ($P = .015$ and $P < .0001$, respectively) [110]. Although we aimed at grade 2 visualization in almost all tumors during the procedure, 47% of tumors were classed as grade 2, 42% as grade 1, and 11% as grade 0. Our results suggest that the grade of portal vein visualization is not intentionally controlled in some tumors, and this is a significant limitation of our method. Overflow of embolic materials into the portal vein may also partly depend on the underlying arterioportal communication, tumor vascularity, and arterial blood flow of individual patients [18]. However, we speculate that catheter positioning is the most important factor to influence portal vein visualization because the incidence of grade 2 visualization has increased after introduction of a 1.7-F tip microcatheter in ultraselective TACE.

In addition to inflow into the portal vein, Lipiodol also passes through the anastomosis between the hepatic arterial branches (Figure 17), sometimes in the extrahepatic collaterals [105, 111]. For these reasons, injection of Lipiodol with slight force at a distal portion of the hepatic artery can enhance the therapeutic effect of TACE. Histologically, peritumoral massive parenchymal necrosis is found in the surgically resected tumor with marked portal vein visualization by Lipiodol during ultraselective TACE (Figure 15) [112]. Additionally, hypovascular tumor portions of early-stage HCC also frequently become necrotic following ultraselective TACE [113]. Ultraselective TACE can treat not only the tumor but also the tumor drainage area by overflowed Lipiodol, where HCC cells spread mainly via the portal system and form intrahepatic satellite lesions [13, 114] (Figure 2). Therefore, this technique may contribute to the prevention of tumor spread via the portal system or control preexisting microsatellite lesions, and may reduce the incidence of locoregional tumor recurrence.

Lipiodol accumulation in the hepatic lymphatic system is also demonstrated during ultraselective TACE without clinical significance (Figure 6) [115].

6.3. Balloon-Occluded TACE

Balloon-occluded TACE (B-TACE) was first reported by Irie et al. [19] (Figure 18). They found that inflow of Lipiodol increased in the tumor but decreased in the liver parenchyma when TACE was performed under selective occlusion of a tumor-feeding branch using a microballoon catheter. They measured the balloon-occluded arterial stump pressure (BOASP) and limited inflow of Lipiodol occurred when BOASP ≤ 64 mmHg was obtained. The decreased pressure gradient between the artery and portal vein and the high viscosity of Lipiodol emulsion may be reasons for the limited inflow of Lipiodol into the liver parenchyma. The concepts of ultraselective TACE and B-TACE are similar because both procedures aim at nonphysiological embolization. However, ultraselective TACE aims at injection of Lipiodol emulsion into the tumor and surrounding liver parenchyma through both the artery and the portal vein; conversely, B-TACE aims at selective Lipiodol accumulation in the tumor from the artery alone. Therefore, Lipiodol is slowly injected and injection is intentionally stopped before portal vein opacification in B-TACE. We speculate that the portal veins may also be markedly visualized during B-TACE when a large amount of Lipiodol is forcefully injected; however, it may deteriorate the liver function because the embolized area of B-TACE is usually large compared with that of ultraselective TACE.

The local control effects and overall survival rates of B-TACE have not yet been reported. B-TACE is likely to attenuate the arteries more strongly than conventional cTACE; therefore, the use of miriplatin is recommended because its damage to the arteries is weaker than that of other anticancer drugs [116]. On the other hand, disappearance of tumor staining on DSA obtained under balloon occlusion is also seen in some tumors. Therefore, the efficacy and indications of B-TACE have still not been established.

7. Periprocedural Management

7.1. Pre-Procedural Management

The diagnosis of HCC and indication of TACE should be decided on the basis of dynamic CT and/or MR imaging findings. Laboratory data, including serum tumor markers, are examined in all patients before TACE. Sonography is also performed to check for the presence of ascites, if necessary. A wide spectrum antibiotic is prophylactically administered immediately before the TACE procedure. Pre-hydration is also required when cisplatin is used.

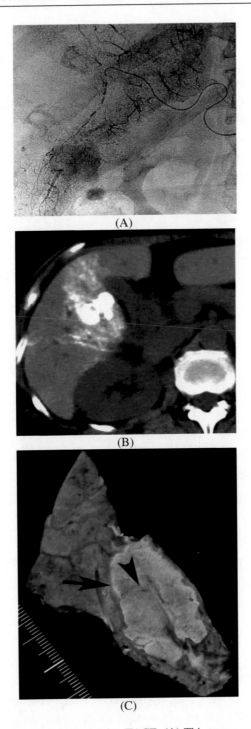

(A)

(B)

(C)

Figure 15. Peritumoral necrosis after ultraselective TACE. (**A**) This tumor was supplied by two feeding arteries (not shown). First, the tumor-feeding branch of the posterior inferior subsegmental artery of the right hepatic artery (A6) was embolized (not shown). Second, the tumor-feeding branch of A5 was embolized. The portal veins appeared to be markedly extending the embolized area during TACE. (**B**) Unenhanced CT obtained 1 week after TACE shows dense Lipiodol accumulation in the tumor. (**C**) The surgical specimen shows not only complete necrosis (arrowhead) but also peritumoral necrosis surrounding the tumor (arrow). (Reprinted, with permission, from reference 112.).

7.2. Post-Procedural Management

After TACE with cisplatin, post-hydration is necessary. Laboratory data are examined in all patients 2 to 3 days after TACE, 1 week after TACE, and every 1 to 3 months after TACE. Blood culture and continuous administration of an antibiotic are recommended if infectious complications are clinically suspected. Sonography or CT should also be performed to check for any complications, if necessary. The serum levels of liver enzymes are elevated 1 to 3 days after TACE; however, these usually return to baseline levels within 1 to 2 weeks. In subsegmental and ultraselective TACE for small tumors, no substantial changes in liver function are observed. Post-embolization syndrome should be adequately managed conservatively.

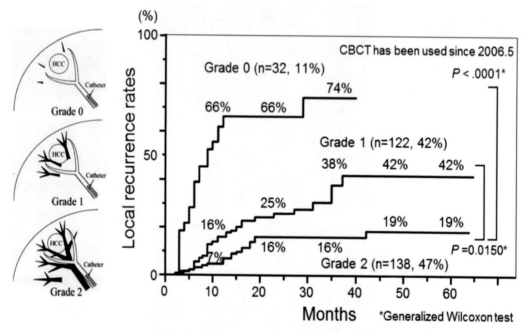

Figure 16. Relationship between the grades of portal vein visualization and local tumor recurrence (Reprinted, with permission, from references 18 and 110.).

7.3. Evaluation of Therapeutic Response

CT or CBCT should be performed at the end of TACE or within 1 week to check for embolized area. In cTACE, Lipiodol is highly radiopaque and its distribution can clearly indicate the embolized area. However, distinction between contrast material and Lipiodol is impossible on CT or CBCT images obtained immediately after TACE. It is also frequently impossible to distinguish whether Lipiodol is distributed through the artery or the portal vein if ultraselective TACE is performed [117]. Therefore, there is a possibility that the embolized areas may be overestimated on CT or CBCT obtained at the end of TACE.

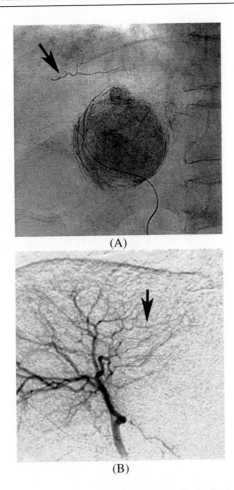

(A)

(B)

Figure 17. Passage of Lipiodol through arterioarterial anastomosis during ultraselective TACE.
(A) During TACE of a small branch of the medial subsegmental artery, another artery is retrogradely opacified with Lipiodol (arrow). **(B)** The artery is a branch of the anterior superior subsegmental artery of the right hepatic artery (arrow).

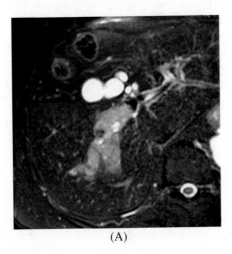

(A)

Figure 18. (Continued).

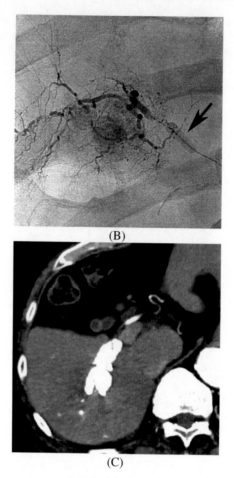

(B)

(C)

Figure 18. B-TACE for HCC invading the right portal vein. **(A)** T2-weighted MR image shows a tumor in the right portal vein. Serum levels of AFP and PIVKA-II were 3018 mg/dL and 774 AU/mL, respectively. **(B)** B-TACE was performed at the posterior segmental artery of the right hepatic artery. The arrow indicates the balloon. Subsequently, A1 was also embolized (not shown). **(C)** Arterial phase CT obtained 1 month after B-TACE shows good tumor control. Serum levels of AFP and PIVKA-II were normalized 4 months after B-TACE (7 mg/dL and 19 AU/mL, respectively).

Table 4. Liver damage classification proposed by the Liver Cancer Study group of Japan

Item	Grade of liver		
	A	B	C
Ascites	None	Controllable	Uncontrollable
Serum bilirubin level (mg/dL)	<2.0	2.0-3.0	>3.0
Serum albumin level (g/dL)	>3.5	3.0-3.5	<3.0
ICG15 (%)	<15	15-40	>40
Prothrombin activity (%)	>80	50-80	<50

2 or more items scoring the same grade occurred in the 2 grades, the higher grade is adopted as the degree of liver damage. ICG15 (%) = indocyanine green retention rate at 15 minutes.

Table 5. TNM stage of HCC proposed by the Liver Cancer Study Group of Japan

T1	Filling 3 factors
T2	Filling 2 factors
T3	Filling 1 factors
T4	Filling 0 factors
Stages	
I	T1 N0 M0
II	T2 N0 M0
III	T3 N0 M0
IV-A	T4 N0 M0 or any T N1 M0
IV-B	Any T N0-1 M1

T factor; 1, Single; 2, <2 cm; 3, no vascular invasion.

In DEB-TACE and bland TAE, evaluation of the embolized areas is frequently difficult on unenhanced CT or CBCT. Dual-phase CBCT examination performed at the end of TACE; i.e., the 1st-phase CBCT without contrast material injection and 2nd-phase CBCT with contrast material injection, can depict the embolized areas as unenhanced regions [118]. Evaluation of the embolized areas is important to check for technical errors, such as missing a small hepatic or extrahepatic tumor feeder.

Dynamic CT or MR imaging 1 to 2 months after embolization should be performed to evaluate the early response of tumors as well as evaluation of serum tumor markers. The modified Response Evaluation Criteria in Solid Tumors (mRECIST) should be used for response classification [119]. In tumors with dense Lipiodol accumulation, it is sometimes difficult to detect peritumoral recurrence because of the beam-hardening artifacts from Lipiodol. MR imaging is mandatory for precise evaluation of tumor response [58] (Figure 7). Thereafter, CT and MR imaging as well as blood tests should be performed every 2 to 3 months. Ideally, CT and MR imaging should be performed in turn. When residual or recurrent tumors are demonstrated on the follow-up images, TACE should be repeated if possible.

8. Outcomes

8.1. Outcomes of cTACE/TAE

8.1.1. Efficacy Results from Multicenter Prospective Cohort Studies

TACE shows higher survival rates in patients with fewer tumor numbers, smaller tumor size, and better liver function [87, 120]. According to the nationwide registered survey conducted between 1994 and 2001 by the Liver Cancer Study Group of Japan [120], TACE was performed in 8510 patients as an initial therapy. For the overall survival of this cohort, the median and 1-, 3-, 5-, and 7-year survival rates were 34 months, 82%, 47%, 26%, and 16%, respectively. With regard to the degree of liver damage classification (Table 4), the 5-year survival rates of grades A, B, and C were 33%, 21%, and 8%, respectively, with statistical significance ($P < .0001$).

According to the TNM staging system (Table 5), the 5-year survival rates in stages I, II, III, and IV-A were 47%, 32%, 20%, and 10%, respectively, with significant differences among them ($P < .0001$). With regard to the survival rates classified by the combination of degree of liver damage and the TNM staging system, the 5-year survival rates of grade A in stages I, II, III, and IV-A were 52%, 39%, 27%, and 10%, respectively, with significant differences among the four subgroups ($P < .0001$). The same tendency as grade A was recognized in liver damage grades B and C ($P < .0001$). On the other hand, 5-year survival rates in TNM stage I through liver damage grades A, B, and C were 52%, 43%, and 24%, respectively, with significant differences ($P < .0001$). The same results were recognized in stages II, III, and IV-A through the liver damage grades A, B, and C ($P < .0001$) (Table 6).

A prospective cohort study of cTACE for 99 patients with unresectable HCC (median maximum tumor diameter, 3.6 cm; single [n = 34], multiple [n = 65]) in an Asian cooperative study between Japan and Korea showed that the 1-year and 2-year survival rate for all 99 patients were 89.9% and 75%, respectively. The median TTP was 7.8 months, and the median survival time (MST) was 3.1 years. Of the 99 patients, 42 (42%) achieved a complete response (CR), and 31 (31%) had a partial response (PR). The response rate was 73% using mRECIST [121]. This report indicates that cTACE and the Asian TACE strategy (performance on demand as selectively as possible) has sufficient therapeutic effects compared with previous RCTs that were carried out in other countries.

8.1.2. Impact of Technical Aspects on Patient Survival

The technical aspect of TACE may be an important factor that influences the patient survival; however, the details have not been described in most reports. Yamakado et al. [122] first reported that TACE techniques impacted on patient survival. In 815 patients with HCC ≤7 cm (mean maximum tumor diameter, 3.1 ± 1.5 cm) and less than 5 lesions treated with TACE, the survival rates of patients who underwent selective/superselective TACE (n = 706) were significantly higher than those of patients who underwent nonselective TACE (n = 109) ($P = .0034$).

Selective/superselective TACE can improve the prognosis owing not only to enhancement of local therapeutic effects but also to avoidance of damage to the nontumorous liver parenchyma. However, the superiority of superselctive TACE compared with selective TACE on patient survival has not been proven. Takaki et al. [123] analyzed the survival rates between the selective TACE and superselective TACE in 199 patients (stage I [n = 30], II [n = 108], and III [n = 61]).

Survival rates at 1, 3, 5, 7, and 10 years in the superselective TACE and selective TACE groups were 90.3% and 92.5%, 62.9% and 66.9%, 48.4% and 30.5%, 22.5% and 18.3%, and 12.9% and 6.1%, respectively, and the MST of each group was 4.4 and 3.7 years, respectively. The survival rates did not differ significantly between the two groups ($P = .4521$), even although those at 5 and 7 years tended to be better for superselective TACE than for selective TACE as did the MST. They speculated that HCC-unrelated deaths at <2 years in the superselective TACE group might be attributed to the outcomes. They also mentioned that selective/superselective TACE was safe for HCC patients with Child-Pugh C class.

Table 6. Survival rates in a prospective cohort study of 8510 patients with unresectable HCC treated by cTACE

Grading/staging	n	Survival (%)						Median (month)	P value
		1-yr	2-yr	3-yr	4-yr	5-yr	7-yr		
Overall survival	8510	82	63	47	34	16	16	34	
Degree of liver damage (n = 7827)									
A	4008	87	71	56	42	33	21	41	
B	3053	80	59	41	29	21	12	12	.0001
C	766	63	37	23	15	8		17	
TNM stage (n = 7311)									
I	927	96	86	72	57	47	30	56	
II	2934	90	73	57	43	32	22	42	.0001
III	2949	78	56	39	26	20	11	29	
IV-A	501	49	27	16	10	10	—	12	
Combination of degree of liver damage and TNM Stage									
Liver damage A (n = 3499)									
I	489	98	92	78	64	52	38	62	
II	1439	94	80	66	52	39	26	50	.0001
III	1358	84	64	47	33	27	14	35	
IV-A	213	59	34	24	12	10	—	15	
Liver damage B (n = 2667)									
I	309	98	92	78	64	52	38	62	
II	1068	88	70	52	38	28	16	38	.0001
III	1116	79	54	32	22	15	8	26	
IV-A	174	45	21	13	10	10	—	15	
Liver damage C (n = 648)									
I	59	94	69	52	37	24	—	39	
II	224	72	49	29	19	11	—	24	.0001
III	282	66	30	23	14	9	—	17	
IV-A	83	27	16	3	—	—		11	

Table 7. Survival rates of 176 patients with Child-Pugh A or B class with HCC≤6 cm less than 5 lesions without PVTT treated by superselective TACE

Staging	n	Survival (%)					MST (months)
		1-yr	3-yr	5-yr	7-yr	9-yr	
Overall survival	176	97	82	55	34	22	65
TNM stage							
I	42	95	88	69	44	25	83
II	97	97	81	56	36	26	69
III	37	97	76	32	20	10	50

Stage I vs. Stage II = N.S.; Stage I vs. Stage III = .0085; Stage II vs. Stage III = .0136.

We retrospectively evaluated the efficacy of subsegmental TACE and ultraselective TACE for localized tumors [124]. In 176 patients with HCC ≤6 cm (mean maximum tumor diameter, 2.7 ± 1.2 cm) less than 5 lesions (single [n = 105], 2-3 [n = 64], 4-5 [n = 7]) without portal vein tumor thrombus (PVTT), survival rates at 1, 3, 5, 7, and 10 years were 97%, 82%,

55%, 34%, and 10%, respectively. During follow-up, 118 patients died including 26 (14.8%) who died of liver-unrelated causes. According to the TNM staging system, survival rates at 1, 3, 5, and 7 years in stage I patients (n = 42) were 95%, 88%, 69%, and 44%, respectively, and those in stage II (n = 97) and III (n = 37) patients were 97% and 97%, 81% and 76%, 56% and 32%, and 36% and 20%, respectively. The survival rates in stage III patients were significantly inferior to those in stage I and II patients ($P = .0085$ and $P = .0136$, respectively) (Table 7). Our results suggest that subsegmental/ultraselective TACE has excellent therapeutic effects for relatively small tumors, almost equal to those of other curative therapeutic options.

8.1.3. Impact of Anticancer Agents on Patient Survival

With regard to comparison of the different anticancer agents, no prospective studies or RCTs have shown to support the superiority of some kinds of anticancer agents. Several retrospective studies have shown that TACE using cisplatin shows better overall survival rates than TACE with doxorubicin or epirubicin [125, 126], although cisplatin requires pre- and post-hydration and has severe side effects, including hypersensitivity reactions [40]. In a report by Yodono et al. [125], the survival rates of the DDP-H (n = 96) and epirubicin (n = 106) groups at 1, 2, and 3 years were 88.5 % and 83%, 71.8% and 57.9%, and 62.4% and 36.5%, respectively, with statistical significance ($P = .0052$). Miriplatin is safe and has less side effects; however, it has significantly inferior local control rates as compared with epirubicn ($P < .0001$) or epirubicin plus mitomycin C ($P < .0001$) [44-46].

Switching the TACE anticancer agents may be a feasible option for advanced HCC, especially when the tumor becomes resistant to the initial form of TACE. Maeda et al. [127] treated 51 patients with advanced HCC resistant to TACE with epirubicin (median maximum tumor diameter, 38 mm; single [n = 7], single with satellite [n = 2], 2-3 [n = 7], and >3 [n = 35]; with PVTT [n = 36], hepatic venous tumor invasion [n = 2], and biliary duct tumor thrombus [n = 2]). Response rates were 11.8% and 27.5% by RECIST and European Association for the Study of the Liver (EASL) criteria, respectively. The overall survival rates were 61.9%, 48.2%, and 28.9% at 1, 2, and 3 years, respectively, and the MST was 15.4 months. Although it is difficult to judge whether second-line TACE using cisplatin can improve the prognosis because there are no reports regarding the prognosis of patients with HCC resistant to epirubicin-TACE, their results are superior to those of best supportive care in the previous RCT trials [2, 3]. The role of anticancer agents in superselective TACE is also unknown because the main antitumor effect of superselective TACE is thought to be ischemia rather than chemotherapeutic effects. However, it is clinically obvious that one chemotherapeutic agent has weak therapeutic effects as compared with others even in superselective TACE [45]. Kojiro et al. [128] presumed that sarcomatous change of HCC may be caused by the phenotypic change of HCC cells caused by anticancer therapy, or that a number of factors, including anticancer therapy, may accelerate the proliferation of the sarcomatous cells existing in the original tumors as one of the histological components. This suggests that the use of anticancer agents in TACE has a risk of rapid tumor progression.

8.1.4. Therapeutic Effects on Large HCC

Treatment for unresectable large HCCs is challenging. For small unresectable HCCs ≤3 cm, several local therapeutic options, such as RF ablation and ethanol injection, are available, as well as ultraselective TACE. However, local therapies may have limited effects on medium and large HCCs [96]. Chemotherapeutic agents have been effective for small HCC with good survival rates, whereas TACE with Lipiodol for large HCC carries the risk of adverse effects [62, 129]. We introduced stepwise superselective cTACE for the treatment of localized large HCC lesions >6 cm [84]. According to the angiographic findings, 2 to 3 TACE sessions are scheduled depending on the vascular anatomy. Each TACE session is performed in a superselective fashion at 3 to 10 week intervals according to the patient and tumor condition, and a maximum dose of Lipiodol used in a single TACE session is limited to less than 10 mL (Figures 7, 9). We reported the outcomes of 30 patients with tumors >5 cm (mean maximum tumor diameter; 7.7 ± 2.4 cm, range, 5.1-14 cm) but with less than 3 lesions (single [n = 25], multiple [n = 5]) without PVTT treated with cTACE, including stepwise TACE. The cumulative overall survival rates at 1, 2, 3, 4, 5, and 6 years were 82.3%, 78.5%, 73.9%, 73.9%, 49.3%, and 32.9%, respectively, and the MST was 4.5 ± 0.5 years [84]. In this cohort, however, TACE through the extrahepatic collaterals was necessary in 47% at the initial TACE and in 70% of patients during the treatment course, and this might be a key to improve the prognosis of patients with large HCC. Our results are superior to those of patients with large tumors treated with combination of TACE and RF ablation reported by Takaki et al. (the 1-, 3-, and 5-year overall survival rates were 100%, 62%, and 41%, respectively) [130]. However, our cohort is highly selected because large tumors generally produce multiple intrahepatic metastases and/or PVTT in the clinical setting. Therefore, our study evaluated the efficacy of cTACE in only a minority of patients with large HCCs. Yoon et al. [131] reported the outcomes of 163 patients with tumors ≥5 cm (single [n = 84], 2-3 [n = 21], >3 [n = 58]; median tumor diameter, 8.6 cm; PVTT in 58 [36%]; invading the main portal trunk [Vp4] [n = 10], first-order branch [Vp3] [n = 17], and second-order branch [Vp2] [n = 31]) treated with cisplatin-based cTACE as well as radiation therapy for PVTT. The patient survival rates were 60% at 1 year, 21% at 3 years, and 9% at 5 years and Child–Pugh class (P = .001), surgical resection (P = .003) or RF ablation (P = .018) after TACE, and tumor response (P = .002) were significant factors for patient survival on multivariate analysis. Their results indicate that the treatment of large HCC with PVTT and intrahepatic metastases is still difficult; however, TACE is considered to be the only therapeutic option, especially in patients with multiple tumors. Comparative studies with other therapeutic options, such as DEB-TACE, intraarterial infusion chemotherapy, and administration of antiangiogenic agents, are necessary.

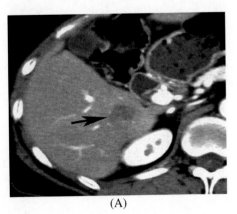

(A)

Figure 19. (Continued).

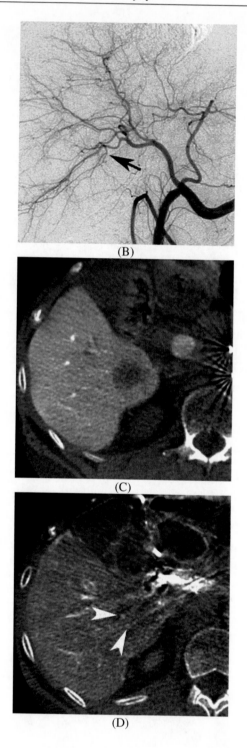

Figure 19. (Continued).

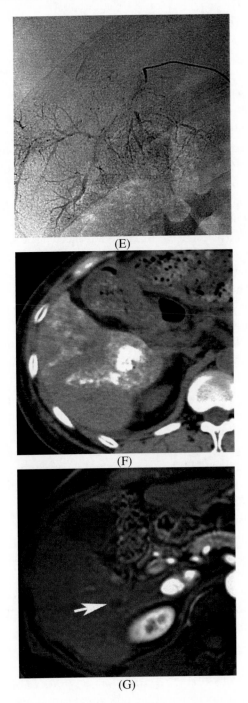

(E)

(F)

(G)

Figure 19. Ultraselective TACE for hypovascular HCC. **(A)** Arterial-phase CT shows a hypovascular tumor 2.4 cm in diameter in the right hepatic lobe (arrow). **(B)** Common hepatic arteriogram shows no tumor stains. **(C)** CBCTAP shows decreased intratumoral portal blood. **(D)** CBCTHA shows small hypervascular foci (arrowheads) in the hypovascular tumor. **(E)** Ultraselective TACE of a branch of A6 (arrow on **A**) was performed. **(F)** Unenhanced CT obtained 1 week after TACE shows dense Lipiodol accumulation in the tumor. **(G)** Arterial-phase gadoxetic acid-enhanced MR image obtained 2 years and 2 months after TACE shows complete tumor response (arrow).

8.1.5. Therapeutic Effects on Early-Stage HCC with Hypovascular Tumor Portion

TACE has limited efficacy for treating early-stage HCC lesions because these generally have less hypervascularity than overt HCC. Golfieri et al. [96] reported that there was a significant direct relationship between necrosis after TACE and tumor diameter: the greater the tumor diameter, the greater the percentage of necrosis, because more than 15% of 1 to 3-cm HCC nodules were still nourished by a limited portal blood supply. Takayasu et al. [132] also reported that the frequencies of tumor stain on arteriogram and retention of Lipiodol within the tumor were 84% and 94% in 31 overt HCCs, 23% and 69% in 22 early-advanced HCCs (a central nodule consists of moderately-differentiated HCC and the surrounding area consists of well-differentiated HCC), and 9% and 9% in 13 early HCCs (well-differentiated HCC), respectively. Histologically, the amount of necrosis areas in each tumor induced by TACE was 55% in overt HCCs, 14% in early advanced HCCs, and 0% in early HCCs. Significant differences ($P < .01$) in the mean necrosis rate were seen between overt HCCs and early advanced HCCs, between early advanced HCCs and early HCCs, and between overt HCCs and early HCCs. This study indicates that the difference in response to TACE seems to depend mainly on the development of tumor vessels; namely, whether the tumor appears hypervascular or hypovascular on the angiogram.

Ultraselective TACE is an alternative technique for the treatment of early-stage HCC (Figure 19). We performed ultraselective TACE for 47 early HCC lesions (mean diameter, 2 ± 0.8 cm) with obvious hypervascular foci and a hypovascular tumor portion comprising ≥50% of the area on the maximal axial tumor section of the CT image. The portal blood flow in the hypovascular portion was decreased in 32 lesions and preserved in 15 lesions on CTAP. After performing ultraselective TACE, dense accumulation of Lipiodol within almost the entire tumor, including the hypovascular tumor portion, was observed in 32 (68.1%) of our tumors with decreased portal blood (n = 23) and preserved portal blood (n = 9), and in total, 25 tumors (53.2%) were well controlled during the mean follow-up of 15.8 months [113]. This suggests that Lipiodol injected at the distal level of the hepatic artery simply does not reach the tumor sinusoids according to the arterial tumor vascularity. In ultraselective TACE, Lipiodol can be injected forcefully through the thinner microcatheter inserted into the tiny feeding artery, and therefore, it may be more widely distributed even in the hypovascular tumor portion, through arterioarterial and/or arterioportal communications via the peribiliary vascular plexus and/or the drainage route from the hypervascular tumor portion. We consider that ultraselective TACE may also play an important part in the treatment of early-stage HCC, especially in cases contraindicated for RF ablation, although the indication and timing of treatment may be controversial.

8.1.6. Therapeutic Effects on Intravascular Tumor Thrombus

Intravascular tumor invasion is one of the unfavorable prognostic factors for patients with HCC. According to the BCLC staging system, HCC with vascular invasion is contraindicated for TACE [79]. However, cTACE is effective for the selected patients with tumor thrombus (Figures 9, 14, 18, 20), and several reports have indicated the usefulness of TACE for intravascular tumor thrombus. Uraki et al. [133] treated 61 patients of HCC with PVTT (Vp$_2$ [n = 13], Vp$_3$ [n = 25], and Vp$_4$ [n = 23]) with cTACE. The 1-, 3- and 5-year survival rates were 42%, 11%, and 3%, respectively, with MST of 15 months. With regard to the relationship between the degrees of the PVTT and prognosis, Higashihara and Okazaki [12] reported that the 5-year survival rates and MST of the Vp_2 (n = 77), Vp_3 (n = 63), and Vp_4 (n = 81) groups treated with cTACE were 7.7% and 475 days, 8.6% and 406 days, and 6.2% and 350 days, respectively, and an extended survival could be obtained when tumor extent was limited to one lobe and the hepatic function was well preserved. However, the treatment effect of cTACE on PVTT is limited compared with surgical resection. In a report by Peng et al. [134], the 1-, 3-, and 5-year overall survivals of patients with PVTT tumors for the hepatectomy and cTACE groups were 42% and 37.8%, 14.1% and 7.3%, and 11.1% and 0.5%, respectively ($P < .001$). On subgroup analysis, the overall survivals for the hepatectomy group were better than for the TACE group for Vp_2, Vp_3, single tumor, and tumor size >5 cm ($P < .001$, $P = .002$, $P < .001$, and $P < .001$, respectively).

Lee at al. [135] analyzed the prognosis and angiographic finings of 82 patients with IVC tumor thrombi treated with cTACE. Overall cumulative survival rates, calculated from times of the detection of IVC tumor thrombi, were 62.1% at 6 months, 35.8% at 1 year, 24.3% at 2 years, and 17.2% at 3 years. Fifty-four (65.9%) patients had extrahepatic collateral artery supply: 47 from the right IPA, four from the right adrenal artery, two from the right IMA, and one from the right renal artery. The presence of extrahepatic collateral supply to IVC tumor thrombi showed a significant relationship with a history of chemoembolization ($P < .001$) and distension of IVC by tumor thrombi ($P < .005$). Their results indicate that TACE for IVC tumor thrombi is one of the effective therapeutic options. However, TACE for IVC tumor thrombi has a risk of pulmonary embolism induced by embolic agents passing through the arteriovenous shunting and disrupted necrotic tumor itself [92]. According to a report by Chern et al. [136], 47- to 180-μm PVA particles could be trapped by tumors and not passed through the lung. In addition, the surfaces of IVC and right atrium tumors were mostly covered with epithelium and this endothelial barrier might prevent the tumor from disrupting into the IVC. For these reasons, they concluded that TACE for IVC and right atrium tumor thrombi was safe. However, Lipiodol can pass through the arteriovenous shunting and causes severe pulmonary oil embolism when a large volume is injected [137].

For bile duct tumor thrombi, the usefulness of cTACE is also reported in a few cases. All intraductal tumor thrombi were dropped into the common bile duct after superselective cTACE and necrotic tumor casts could be removed endoscopically [138, 139]. These reports suggest that intraductal tumor thrombus without hyperbilirubinemia may not be a terminal illness, but rather, can be successfully managed by cTACE in the selected patients.

8.1.7. Hemostatic Effects for Ruptured HCC

In a report by Kung et al. [81], hemostasis of ruptured HCC with TAE and stabilization of hemodynamic status for $\geq$48 hours were achieved in 99% of the 167 patients. The cumulative survival rates at 30, 60, 120, and 360 days were 69%, 57%, 40%, and 23%, respectively and the 30-day mortality rate was 31%. In a literature review of 15 studies comprising 835 patients with ruptured HCC [140], the average 30-day mortality rates among patients undergoing conservative treatment, emergency operation, and TAE are 71%, 50%, and 48%, respectively. Emergency TAE can be effective for achieving hemostasis of ruptured HCC in patients in a hemodynamically unstable condition with minimal invasiveness (Figure 8). However, among patients with PVTT, a high serum creatinine level, acute respiratory failure, impaired neurologic status, and hyperbilirubinemia (>2.7 mg/dL), the mortality rate remains high [81]. In addition, peritoneal dissemination that frequently develops in patients who survive more than 3 months shortens the prognosis [82].

Advanced HCC also ruptures into the biliary system and causes hemobilia. Selective/superselective TACE is safe and effective for stopping hemobilia in the selected patients with even far-advanced HCC [141]. This suggests that TACE/TAE should be performed without hesitation even in patients with hyperbilirubinemia when uncontrolled massive hemobilia from an intraductal tumor occurs.

8.1.8. Efficacy of Preoperative TACE

Although TACE is indicated for inoperable HCC, preoperative TACE has been expected to be useful for reducing perioperative blood loss and improving survival. However, the efficacy of preoperative embolization for HCC is controversial, and the scientific evidence is insufficient to conclude whether preoperative TACE improves the survival of patients [142-144]. Although Lu et al. [144] did not identify any advantage of using preoperative TACE for improving either overall or recurrence-free survival in patients with HCCs measuring 2 to 8 cm in their maximum diameter, they found a survival benefit in a patient group with HCCs >8 cm. This suggests that tumor shrinkage by preoperative TACE can facilitate safe and curative surgical resection, especially in large tumors as well as in tumors with PVTT [131].

8.2. Outcomes of DEB-TACE

DEB has only recently been introduced into HCC treatment; therefore, only a few reports are available regarding the long-term results of DEB-TACE. In a prospective cohort study of 173 HCC patients (maximum tumor diameter, 7.6 ± 2.1 cm; 1 dominant ≤5 cm [22%], 1 dominant >5 cm [41.6%], multifocal ≤5 [26%], and multifocal >5 [10.4%]) treated with DEB-TACE using DC Bead, the overall survival rates at 1, 2, 3, 4, and 5 years were 93.6%, 83.8%, 62%, 41%, and 22.5%, respectively, and the MST was 43.8 months [145]. Burrel et al. [146] evaluated the outcomes of 104 HCC patients treated with TACE using DC Bead by the tumor stage. The 1, 3, 4 and 5-year survival for BCLC-A patients (n = 41) was 89.7%, 67.8%, 50.8% and 33.9%, with MST of 54.2 months, while for BCLC-B patients (n = 63), it was 88.2%, 64.4%, 47.3% and 39.4%, with MST of 47.7 months. Regarding the therapeutic effect of DEB-TACE using Hepasphere, the 1- and 2-year overall survival rates of 64 HCC patients (median maximum tumor diameter, 4.9 cm; single [n = 9], 2-3 [n = 20], and >3 lesions [n = 35]) were 72% and 43%, respectively, and the MST in the entire patient cohort was 20.5 months, and by stage was 24 months in BCLC-A, 20.5 months in BCLC-B, and 15.5 months in BCLC-C [147].

These outcomes of DEB-TACE show great variability in survival, because of the heterogeneity in patient selection, the etiology of the underlying cirrhosis, the embolization technique, or the choice of the particle size, as well as the relatively short-term follow-up. Direct comparisons of the outcomes between DEB-TACE and cTACE may also be impossible. Furthermore, no comparisons are available of the long-term prognosis after DEB-TACE between each embolic agent, DC Bead, Hepasphere, and Embozene-TANDEM.

8.3. Efficacy Results from Comparative Studies between cTACE and DEB-TACE

The PRECISION V study was an international, multicenter, prospective, randomized, single-blind, and phase II study to compare cTACE with DEB-TACE with DC Bead [89]. A total of 201 patients with unresectable HCC (BCLC-A or B, without PVTT or extrahepatic spread) underwent DEB-TACE (n = 93) or cTACE (n = 108). The primary efficacy endpoint was the 6-month tumor objective response (OR) rate (CR + PR) and it was 51.6% vs. 43.5% in the DC Bead vs. cTACE arm, respectively (P = .11). The disease control rates (OR + SD) were 63.4% vs. 51.9%, respectively (two-sided P = .11). Supplementary analyses showed that in the 67% of patients with more advanced disease (Child-Pugh B class, PS 1, bilobar or recurrent disease), the incidence of OR and disease control rates were statistically higher (P = .038 and P = .026, respectively) in the DC Bead group than the cTACE group. With regard to the systemic side effects of doxorubicin (alopecia, skin discoloration, mucositis, and marrow suppression), there was a significant benefit in favor of DC Bead over cTACE (P = .012).

Sacco et al. [53] conducted a prospective, randomized, single-center study to evaluate the short-term and long-term technical and clinical results of cTACE (n = 34) and DEB-TACE using DC Bead (n = 33). No statistically significant differences between the cTACE and DEB-TACE groups were found in the early tumor response at 1 month (CR : PR = 70% : 29.4% vs. 51.5% : 48.5%; P = .1), cumulative recurrence-free rate at 24 months (37.4% vs. 42.4%; P = .99), cumulative local recurrence-free rate at 24 months (35.3% vs. 36%; P = .46), cumulative disease-free rate at 24 months (80.1% vs. 82.5%; P = .64), and cumulative survival rate at 24 months (83.6% vs. 86.8%; P = .96).

On the other hand, Song et al. [148] retrospectively compared the therapeutic effects of the DEB-TACE group (n = 60) with the cTACE group (n = 69). The treatment response at 3 months in the DEB-TACE groups was significantly higher than that in the cTACE group (CR/PR/SD/progressive disease [PD] = 33/16/9/2 vs. 16/18/21/14, P < .001) and the median TTP of the DEB-TACE group was significantly better than that of the cTACE group (11.7 vs. 7.6 months, P = .018). Furthermore, subgroup analysis according to BCLC stage showed that the TTP was significantly longer in the DEB-TACE group than in the cTACE group (P = .038) in BCLC-B, while in BCLC-A, there was no significant difference in tumor progression between the two groups (P = .373). The MSTs in the DEB-TACE and cTACE groups were 32.2 ± 1.9 and 24.7 ± 1.7 months, respectively. The cumulative survival rates at 6, 12, and 18 months were 93%, 88%, and 88% in the DEB-TACE group and 80%, 67%, and 61% in the cTACE group (P = .005). Subgroup analysis showed that the difference between the two groups was more significant only in patients with BCLC-B than in patients with BCLC-A (P = .02 and P = .186, respectively).

It is impossible to directly compare each study as well as the results of cTACE from Asia because of the heterogeneity in patient background and embolization technique. However, DEB-TACE may not have obvious advantages against cTACE and it may be more suitable for intermediate-stage HCC. Early-stage HCC frequently has well-differentiated tumor portions [96, 113]; therefore, superselective cTACE may be more effective because it can also embolize the portal side.

8.4. Outcomes of Bland TAE

It is obvious that bland TAE has lesser damage to the liver than cTACE and DEB-TACE on the basis of the histopathological findings after bland TAE [62]. However, reports regarding the long-term results of bland TAE are also insufficient. Osuga et al. [62] embolized 9 HCC lesions ≥5 cm (mean, 8.2 cm) using Hepashere particles of 53 to 212 μm in a dry state. On CT obtained 1 month after TAE, complete necrosis was observed in 3 tumors, near-total necrosis (90%–99%) in 3, and partial necrosis (0%–90%) in 3. Two tumors were resected after TAE, and microscopic study showed a homogeneous distribution of Hepashere particles inside and at the margin of the tumor. These particles occluded the intratumoral vessels tightly with mild foreign body reactions and did not migrate into the hepatic sinusoids, peribiliary plexus, portal vein, or hepatic vein. No ischemic damage was observed in the adjacent hepatic parenchyma. According to their subsequent report regarding the long-term effect of bland TAE using the same-sized Hepashere, the 1- and 2-year survival rates of 59 naïve HCC patients with a mean largest tumor diameter of 4 cm (range, 1.2–14.7 cm) were 100% and 83%, respectively, and the MST was 30 months [91]. Bonomo et al. [92] reported the outcomes of bland TAE with 40- and/or 100-μm Embozene microspheres. They treated 74 HCC lesions (range, 12–122 mm) and local results at 1-month, 3- to 6-month, and 6- to 12-month follow-up by RECIST criteria were 62%, 37%, and 16%, respectively, for SD, and 35%, 56%, and 51%, respectively, for PR. CR has been observed only at late follow-up (3 lesions; 7%). However, one patient died of tumor rupture and pulmonary embolism within 24 hours of TAE. Maluccio et al. [93] also used small particles (50-μm PVA and 40-120-μm tris-acryl gelatin microspheres [Embosphere; Biosphere Medical]) for 322 HCC patients. One hundred nine patients without PVTT or extrahepatic disease had an MST of 40 months and 1-, 2-, and 3-year survival rates of 84%, 66%, and 51%, respectively. However, four patients died of acute hepatic failure and two died of pulmonary embolism. Fatal pulmonary embolism by TAE with 40- to 120-μm Embosphere in three of more than 850 patients was also reported by another author [94]. Small particles have strong therapeutic effects because these can impart terminal vessel blockage within the tumor; however, the risk of unexpected complications caused by migrated particles, such as hepatic infarction and pulmonary embolism, may increase. In the use of small-sized particles, a superselective approach and careful observation of pulmonary shunting is recommended.

Bland TAE may be useful for patients with large tumors or elderly patients because the procedure-related complications are generally mild compared with cTACE and DEB-TACE [62].

8.5. Outcomes of Y90-Microspheres

In a structured meta-analysis, the responses rate of glass microspheres and resin microspheres were 78% and 89%, respectively [149]. Using comparative effectiveness analysis, Salem et al. [73] reported longer TTP after Y90-radioembolization (n = 123) than after TACE (n = 122) (13.3 vs. 8.4 months, respectively [$P < .046$]), and similar MST (20.5 vs. 17.4 months, respectively) in patients without vascular invasion or extrahepatic spread. In BCLC-B patients, the MST was also similar between the two groups: 17.2 months for radioembolization vs. 17.5 months for TACE. Radioembolization can be safely performed in patients with PVTT; therefore, it might be a treatment option in intermediate-stage patients and also in patients with PVTT. Radioembolization is also better tolerated than TACE with statistically significant differences in terms of abdominal pain, length of hospital stay, and post-embolization symptoms [73, 150]. However, their TACE technique using high doses of anticancer drugs and PVA particles is quite different from the cTACE performed in Asia.

9. Technical Tips to Improve the Therapeutic Effects of TACE

9.1. Security of a Safety Margin for the Treatment

To perform an effective TACE for localized HCC, the tumor should be completely embolized as selectively as possible. On the other hand, the smaller the area embolized, the more likely TACE will be insufficient without an adequate safety margin. Sasaki et al. [13] reported that microsatellite lesions were detected in 46% of tumors ≤5 cm, and all but one were located within 5 mm of a main tumor <25 mm. Therefore, we suppose that the minimum safety margin is 5 mm for a tumor <25 mm and 10 mm for a tumor ≥25 mm, and tumors located outside of a 10-mm wide margin should be managed as multi-centrically developed tumors [32, 117]. This safety margin may correspond to corona enhancement around the tumor demonstrated on the late phase of CTHA or CBCTHA [28]. It is important to monitor whether the safety margin is included in the embolized area during the TACE procedure (Figure 4). We compared the technical success and local tumor control of TACE between tumors embolized using DSA alone (n = 98; mean diameter, 22.2 ± 10.1 mm) and tumors embolized using DSA and CBCT (n = 109; mean diameter, 19.9 ± 9.1 mm). There was a significant difference in technical success between the DSA and CBCT groups ($P < .001$) and the 1-, 2-, and 3-year local recurrence rates in the DSA and CBCT groups were 33.3% and 22.3%, 41.3% and 26.8%, and 48% and 30.6%, respectively ($P = .0217$) [117]. Iwazawa et al. [151] also reported that patients receiving CBCT-assisted TACE had significantly higher overall and local progression-free survival rates than those receiving TACE with DSA alone ($P = .005$ and $P = .003$, respectively).

Security of a circumferential safety margin is ideal; however, it is sometimes invasive for patients with poor liver function when the vascular territory of the residual feeder is large. Performing additional TACE should be determined according to a good balance of the vascular territory of the feeding branch and the hepatic function reserve of each patient. In addition, the tumor also recurs at a site where an adequate safety margin is obtained [117]. This is a limitation of TACE and suggests that it may not consistently achieve complete tumor necrosis even when it is successfully performed.

9.2. TACE-Guidance Software

In small tumors, identification of the tumor feeders, as well as tumor staining, is more difficult on DSA because these tumors are usually less hypervascular. Therefore, TACE can fail to embolize the target tumors completely when it is performed using DSA alone.

Recently, TACE-guidance software using CBCT data has been developed [33, 34]. We reported the usefulness of TACE-guidance software (EmboGuide; Philips Healthcare, Best, The Netherlands) including automated tumor-feeders detection (AFD) software [33] (Figure 4). This software is used on the workstation and the "virtual target lesion" segmented on the 1st-phase CBCTHA images referencing the CBCTAP and 2nd-phase CBCTHA images (including a safety margin approximately 5-mm-wide for tumors <25 mm, and 10-mm-wide for tumors ≥25 mm) is automatically superimposed on the 3D arteriogram. After decision of the start position of the vessel tracking on the 3D arteriogram, all potential feeders are automatically traced from the start position of the vessel tracking to all segmented tumors and highlighted on the display within a few seconds. In our preliminary study [33], 88 of 100 tumor-feeding subsubsegmental arteries in 68 tumors ≤30 mm (mean, 15.3 ± 5.2 mm) could be detected by AFD. When AFD software cannot identify the tumor feeder, the branches in the vicinity of the target lesion are determined as the tumor-feeding branches by careful observation while turning the 3D arteriogram, and it can also be highlighted on the display.

Iwazawa et al. [34] also evaluated the performance of AFD software produced by another company (FlightPlan for Liver; GE Healthcare, Waukesha, WI, USA). They found 65 tumor feeders of 59 HCC nodules during TACE, and the sensitivity of the software to detect tumor feeders was significantly higher than that of the manual assessment using DSA (87.7% vs. 71.8%, $P < 0.001$).

As mentioned above, the security of the safety margin is another key to achieving good local control; however, recognition of a minor feeding branch mainly supplying the safety margin using DSA may be difficult because obvious tumor staining is not usually demonstrated even on selective DSA. AFD can help to identify the branches suspected of being tumor feeders among all branches toward the tumor and can reduce the physicians' work during the TACE procedure [33]. Furthermore, this software may improve the local tumor control and reduce the procedural time, the total dose of contrast material, and radiation exposure.

9.3. Special Techniques to Embolize Vessels That are Difficult to Catheterize

Despite the advancement of catheter-guidewire technologies, small branch arteries, such as some extrahepatic collateral pathways and the caudate hepatic artery, are infrequently still impossible to catheterize [98, 100, 152-158]. Several useful techniques are available to embolize vessels that are difficult to catheterize.

9.3.1. A Catheter with a Large Side Hole

A catheter with a large side hole is useful to select a branch arising at an acute angle from the major vessel [152] (Figure 21). A large hole approximately 3 to 5 mm in length, enough to advance a microcatheter, is created near the tip of a shepherd hook catheter with a surgical scalpel. This catheter is mainly used to select the IPA derived from the proximal portion of the celiac artery. We first used a 5-F catheter to create a large side hole, but now we create it on a 4-F catheter. After the catheter is introduced into the celiac artery, the side hole is controlled in position at the orifice of the IPA by the injection of contrast material. A microguidewire is introduced into the IPA through the side hole and then a microcatheter is advanced. Catheters with a large side hole have an advantage in seeking the orifice of the IPA located in the proximal portion of the celiac trunk, in that the catheter tip is introduced deep into the celiac artery, which stabilizes the catheter, making the positioning of the side hole easy. The side hole is larger than the end hole, so the injected contrast material can flow through and be easily recognized. This catheter is also useful for selective catheterization of small branches arising from the proximal portion of the major artery, such as the inferior adrenal artery and renal capsular artery arising from the renal artery or the left gastric artery arising from the celiac artery. This technique can also be applied for selective catheterization into the small vessel arising from the distal portion of the large vessel at an acute angle, such as the right IPA or right renal capsular artery, because the catheter shaft as far as the side hole can support the microcatheter-guidewire manipulation (Figure 22). For this purpose, the side hole is created on a twisted or curved catheter at the desired site.

As an additional advantage, because this catheter does not have a special form, it can be easily made from a common angiographic catheter during the procedure.

9.3.2. A Catheter with a Cleft

The small artery arising from the aorta with an acute angle at the orifice may also infrequently be impossible to catheterize, because the tip of a conventional angiographic catheter frequently hits the vessel wall at the angled portion, and a microcatheter-guidewire system cannot be advanced into the vessel lumen. A catheter with a cleft is useful to select such vessels [153] (Figure 23). During the procedure, a cleft approximately 3 mm in length is created with a surgical scalpel at the tip of a 4-F shepherd hook catheter. The cleft is created at the desired site of the catheter tip according to the direction of the vessel angulation on the basis of the CT and angiographic findings. For example, if the desired artery sharply turns right at the orifice, the cleft is created on the right side of the catheter when seated in the artery. This catheter can also easily be created during the procedure; however, there is a potential risk of intimal injury in the use of this catheter because the catheter tip becomes sharp. Therefore, careful catheter manipulation during the procedure is recommended.

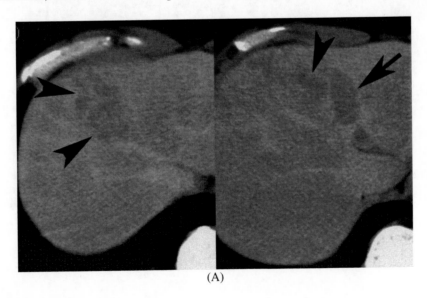

(A)

Figure 20. (Continued).

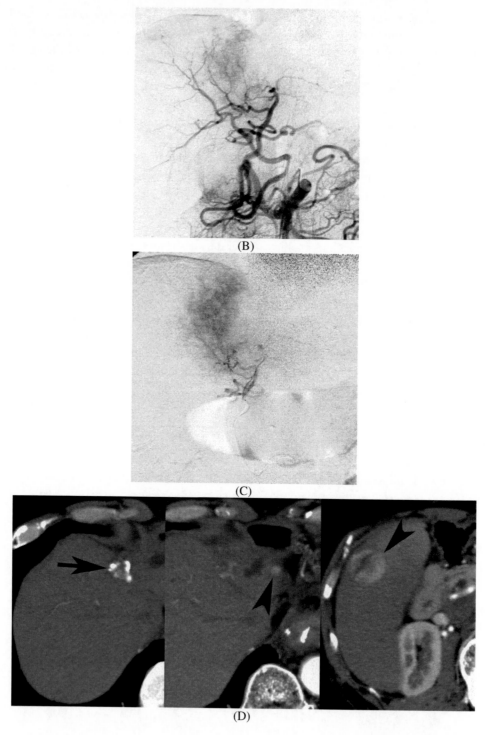

Figure 20. (Continued).

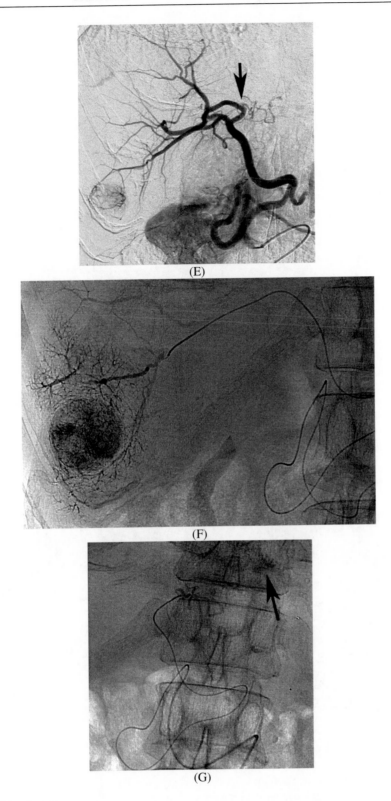

(E)

(F)

(G)

Figure 20. (Continued).

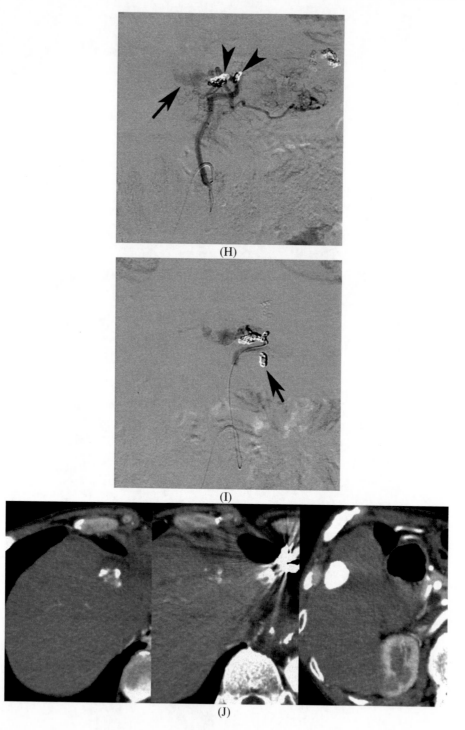

(H)

(I)

(J)

Figure 20. TACE for massive type HCC invading the left portal vein. (**A**) Delayed-phase CT shows an irregular-shaped tumor 6.5 cm in diameter (arrowheads) invading the left portal vein (arrow). (**B**) This patient has celiac artery stenosis. Superior mesenteric arteriogram shows a tumor supplied by the left hepatic artery. (**C**) TACE of the left hepatic artery was repeated 6 times. (**D**) Arterial-phase CT obtained 10 years and 9 months after the initial TACE shows good control of the primary tumor (arrow) but development of two new lesions (arrowheads). (**E**) Superior mesenteric arteriogram demonstrates one tumor, but the other is unclear. **(F)** First, TACE of a branch of A5 was performed. **(G)** Second, TACE was performed through A1 (arrow on **E**). The arrow indicates the tumor. Thereafter, the tumor in S1 recurred and two TACE sessions were added via the left gastric artery and the left hepatic artery (not shown). **(H)** However, the S1 tumor recurred 15 years and 2 months after the initial TACE. At that time, the tumor (arrow) was completely supplied by the left gastric artery. The arrowheads indicate the metallic coils deployed during the previous TACE. **(I)** TACE was performed after coil embolization of the gastric branches. **(J)** Arterial-phase CT obtained 15 years and 7 months after the initial TACE shows that all tumors are well controlled. However, the patient died of pneumonia 16 years and 1 month after the initial TACE.

9.3.3. Combined Use of a Metallic Coil

Combined use of embolization with a metallic coil makes it possible to perform effective TACE through unselectable tumor-feeding branches arising from the extrahepatic collateral pathways [100] (Figure 20). This technique is mainly used in TACE through an artery supplying the alimentary tract or the pancreas. After coil embolization distal to the unselectable tumor-feeding branch to prevent inflow of the embolic agents, the microcatheter is pulled back until the proximal site of the tumor-feeding branch and TACE can be safely performed. In our experience, Tornado Embolization Microcoils (Cook) can be deployed through a microcatheter with a tip ≤2-F using a 0.016-inch guidewire as the pusher wire in almost all cases [154]. However, the trial of this coil embolization through a thinner microcatheter should be performed with the personal responsibility of each operator, because coil deployment is not accepted by most thinner microcatheters.

Coil embolization, mostly combined with GS embolization, is also performed for hemostasis of ruptured HCC [81] and occlusion of arterioportal shunts [154].

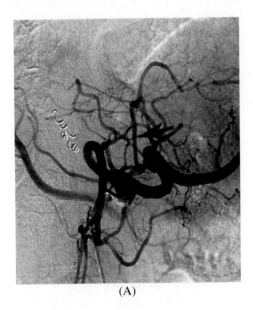

(A)

Figure 21. (Continued).

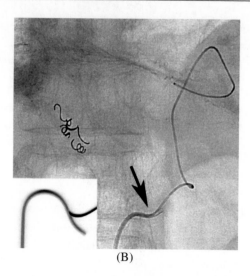

(B)

Figure 21. A catheter with a large side hole. **(A)** Celiac arteriogram shows the left IPA arising from the proximal portion (arrow). **(B)** The vessel was successfully selected through the side hole created near the catheter tip (arrow).

9.3.4. Combined Use of a Microballoon Catheter

This technique makes it possible to perform selective TACE through unselectable tumor-feeding hepatic arterial branches, such as the caudate artery (Figure 24). Two sites of the femoral artery are punctured and a microballoon catheter is advanced distal to the tumor feeder. Then, another microcatheter is introduced into the proximal site of the tumor feeder through the second access. TACE can be performed through the microcatheter under occlusion of the artery distal to the tumor feeder by balloon inflation. Now, a microballoon catheter with a side hole is commercially available in Japan and this technique can be completed through one access route [23]. The combined use of a balloon catheter and metallic coil embolization is also useful to embolize a tiny branch arising from the celiac axis [155].

9.3.5. Other Useful Techniques for Selective Catheterization

The turn-back technique was reported by Kiyosue et al. [156] to select an artery originating at an acute angle. A J-shaped microcatheter is introduced into the artery neighboring the target artery with the use of the guidewire technique. The microguidewire is pulled back approximately 10 cm from the microcatheter tip. The microcatheter is then pushed and bent in the parent artery. Further pushing of the microcatheter results in withdrawal of the tip from the neighboring artery into the parent artery. The tip of the microcatheter is directed into or adjacent to the orifice of the target artery by pushing and/or pulling the microcatheter. The microguidewire is advanced into the target artery distally, and the microcatheter is then advanced into the target artery over the wire. They could catheterize into the middle hepatic artery, right gastric artery, right IPA, and tracheal artery using this technique after failed catheterization by conventional techniques. A similar technique was reported by Kwon et al. [157] as the "microcatheter loop technique" to select the proper hepatic artery via the pancreaticoduodenal arcade route from the superior mesenteric artery in a case with celiac artery occlusion.

Shaping a microcatheter by steam-heating is simple but useful for selective catheterization into the vessel arising at an acute angle. For this purpose, a non-braded microcatheter (Microferret-18; Cook) is suitable. When the tip of the microcatheter faces the orifice of the target vessel, a guidewire is inserted into it, and the microcatheter is then advanced into the branch. This microcatheter has less flexibility and a 2.4-F tip; therefore, advancement into the angled vessel, such as the caudate artery, is frequently difficult. In such circumstances, an over-the-wire technique to exchange the shaped microcatheter for a flexible one is required [158]. We routinely use a 180-cm-long microguidewire and 105- or 110-cm-long microcatheter through a 65 or 70-cm-long 4-F catheter. While keeping the microguidewire in the target vessel, the microcatheter is withdrawn. When the proximal end of the microcatheter is pulled back as far as the distal end of the guidewire, the tip of the microcatheter is located in the 4-F catheter but outside the sheath. So, the 4-F catheter and microguidewire are clamped by a surgical forceps outside of the sheath. Then, the microcatheter is withdrawn and another flexible microcatheter with a tip <2-F is advanced over the wire. When the tip of the microcatheter is reached at the clamped site, the distal end of the microguidewire is usually outside the microcatheter and can be grasped by hand. The surgical forceps is opened, and then the microcatheter can be advanced into the target branch over the wire. This technique is complicated; however, it can be applied for selective catheterization of many vessels that are impossible to catheterize by conventional catheter techniques.

9.4. Combination of TACE and Percutaneous Local Therapy

Combination therapy of TACE and percutaneous ethanol injection (PEI) is effective for achieving more complete necrosis of large tumors. TACE performed 1 to 2 weeks before PEI makes the texture of the tumor parenchyma necrotic, making diffusion of the ethanol easier and washout of the ethanol to the nontumorous area more difficult. As a result, ethanol can infiltrate the entire tumor and provide complete necrosis of the tumor. In a report by Tanaka et al. [159], complete tumor necrosis could be achieved in all 11 tumors ≥3 cm (mean, 4.8 ± 1.8 cm; range, 3-8.2 cm) treated with combined therapy.

TACE is also combined with RF ablation to increase the extent of the ablative areas, confirm the tumor margin by accumulated Lipiodol on CT, and decrease the risk of neoplastic seeding caused by intraprocedural bleeding from the tumor [7]. Fujimori et al. [8] reported excellent long-term outcomes of this combination therapy. They treated 382 naïve HCCs (mean diameter, 2.8 ± 1.4 cm; range, 1-12 cm) of 277 patients. The initial complete response rate within 1 week of RF ablation was 100% by mRECIST and local tumor progression rate was 5.4%. The overall and recurrence-free survival rates were 56.3% and 22.5% at 5 years, and 23.5% and 9.3% at 10 years. In 210 Child-Pugh A class patients, the 5- and 10-year overall survival rates were 64.4% and 30.6%, respectively. Since they routinely used CT-fluoroscopy to navigate the RF needle, complete ablation of tumors located in the subphrenic areas could be done with a transpulmonary approach. For such occasions, pneumothorax was the most frequent complication (32/59 complications of 488 procedures). No death related to the procedure was reported. This combination therapy is safe and repeatable, and their results are almost equal to those of hepatectomy.

9.5. Combined Use of Molecular Targeted Agents

TACE interrupts the blood supply to HCC, and tumor cells that survive treatment upregulate the oxygen-sensitive transcription factor hypoxia-inducible factor-1α and its downstream target, the angiogenic agent VEGF [160]. An increase in plasma VEGF levels after TACE has been well documented and may be a potential cause of recurrent disease [161]. Indeed, HCC tumor samples from patients previously treated with TACE contain significantly more VEGF-positive cells than tumor samples from patients undergoing liver resection without TACE ($P < .01$) [162].

Sorafenib (Nexavar: Beyer Schering Pharma, Leverkusen, Germany) is a multikinase inhibitor with antiangiogenic and antiproliferative properties, targeting multiple pathways. Two large randomized phase III studies demonstrated that sorafenib significantly improves overall survival in patients with advanced HCC [163, 164].

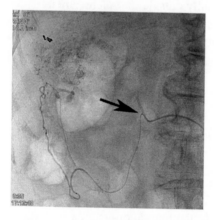

Figure 22. A catheter with a large side hole. The right renal capsular artery arising from the distal portion of right renal artery at an acute angle is successfully selected through the side hole (arrow) on the curved catheter.

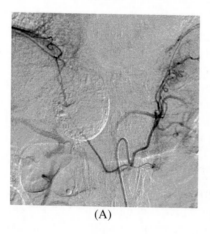

(A)

Figure 23. (Continued).

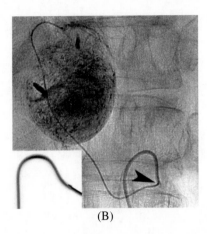

(B)

Figure 23. A catheter with a cleft. (A) The bilateral IPAs arise from the proximal portion of the celiac artey at an acute angle. The catheter tip hit the angled portion and the microguidewire could not be advanced into the right IPA. (B) The righ IPA was successfully selected using a catheter with a cleft created on the right side of the catheter (arrow).

Theoretically, combination of antiangiogenic agents with TACE can decrease post-TACE angiogenesis and improve the efficacy of locoregional therapy, as well as possibly decreasing the incidence of systemic disease. According to the randomized, controlled phase III trial, assessing the efficacy and safety of sorafenib after response to cTACE in Japanese and Korean patients with unresectable HCC, sorafenib did not significantly improve the median TTP of patients who were administered sorafenib after TACE (n = 229) and patients who underwent TACE alone (n = 227) (5.4 vs. 3.7 months; hazard ratio, 0.87; $P = .252$) [47]. The relatively long interval between the last TACE and randomization (median time, 9.3 weeks; range, 5.6–13.3 weeks) and the inconsistent administration of low doses of sorafenib (400 mg/day) were speculated as the main causes of this negative outcome.

The SPACE study was a global phase II study evaluating scheduled DEB-TACE with continuous sorafenib (800 mg/day) (n = 154)/placebo (n = 153) in BCLC-B HCC patients. However, the median TTP was similar in the sorafenib and placebo groups (169 vs. 165 days, hazard ratio, 0.797, $P = .072$) [165].

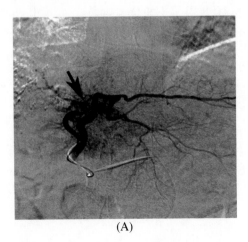

(A)

Figure 24. (Continued).

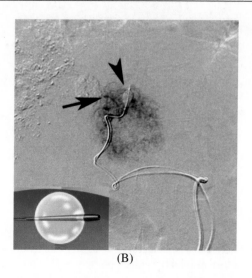

(B)

Figure 24. Combined use of a microballoon catheter. (A) The caudate artery (arrow) could not be selected using a coaxial technique. (B) Left hepatic arteriogram under balloon occlusion (arrowhead) shows only the caudate artery (arrow) and tumor stain and TACE was successfully performed.

On the other hand, Sansonno et al. [166] reported the promising results of prospective, single-center, placebo-controlled, randomized, double-blind clinical study to evaluate the effectiveness of cTACE combined with sorafenib as a sequential treatment regimen. They performed cTACE for hepatitis virus C (HCV) infected patients with BCLC-B. And sorafenib (800 mg/day) or placebo was administered in step with the diagnosis of a tumor CR on CT image evaluation 30 days after TACE treatment. The median TTP was 9.2 months in the sorafenib group (n = 31) and 4.9 months in the placebo group (n = 31) (hazard ratio, 2.5; $P <$ .001). In addition, fewer patients in the sorafenib group than in the placebo group experienced intrahepatic tumor recurrence at 6 months after TACE (22% vs. 71%, respectively, $P = .005$). Their study suggests that early administration of high doses of sorafenib after TACE may contribute to improvement in the TTP. It also suggests that patients with HCV may exhibit an improved overall survival with sorafenib as compared with HCC of other etiologies.

Furthermore, the combination of TACE and another antiangiogenic agent, TSU-68 (a dual VEGF receptor-2 [VEGFR-2] and platelet-derived growth factor receptor-β [PDGFR-β] inhibitor) [167], is now being evaluated in a multicenter phase III study (ORIENTAL study).

Since plasma VEGF and other angiogenic factors increase 1 to 2 days after TACE therapy [168], initiating an antiangiogenic agent before TACE theoretically suppresses TACE-hypoxia induced angiogenesis more effectively. Pawlik et al. [169] reported that a phase II trial of sorafenib combined with concurrent DEB-TACE (800 mg/day of sorafenib initiation 1 week before TACE) was safe and provided promising tumor control (disease control rate of 92% by RECIST criteria and 100% by EASL criteria).

Administration of antiangiogenic agents may also make it possible to expand the indication of TACE for BCLC-C patients with extrahepatic metastases. Establishment of such treatment strategies is urgent and it may be good news for BCLC-C patients with Child-Pugh A class.

10. TACE-Refractory HCC

10.1. Concepts of TACE-Refractory HCC

Repetitive TACE treatments become less effective in patients with recurrent HCC [170], and such cases are clinically considered as TACE-refractory. According to the HCC treatment manual proposed by the Japan Society of Hepatology [171], the definition of TACE-refractory HCC includes four conditions: (1) more than two consecutive insufficient Lipiodol depositions in the tumor (<50% of tumor areas) or rapid progression of new tumors on CT obtained at least 1 month after TACE that was adequately performed; (2) development of vascular invasion; (3) development of extrahepatic disease; and (4) an upward trend of tumor markers only by a transient decrease after TACE.

The causes of TACE-refractory HCC may be wide-ranging. We speculate that the main causes can be divided into four factors: a technical factor of TACE of which physicians are not aware during the procedure (for example, missing of a small feeder including one arising from the extrahepatic collaterals and incomplete blockage of the tumor feeders); chemosensitive factor; tumor morphology; and changes in the tumor nature and/or intratumoral hemodynamics. Generally, nonnodular HCC lesions, such as multinodular and infiltrative HCC lesions, are resistant to TACE, as well as to RF ablation [7, 172]. In addition, cholangiolar, glandular, or spindle cell areas suggestive of a mixed hepatocholangiocellular phenotype are frequently seen in local recurrent tumors after TACE [173]. Furthermore, the portal blood supply to a recurrent tumor is another cause of resistance to TACE (Figure 3) [15].

10.2. Treatment Strategy for TACE-Refractory HCC

Antiangiogenic agents are recommended for the treatment of HCC refractory to TACE; however, the therapeutic effect is not satisfactory. If the recurrent tumor is hypervascular and shown as having ordinary HCC features on imaging, additional TACE with switched anticancer drugs, performed at a more distal level or through the extrahepatic collaterals if necessary, should be attempted. DEB-TACE is also effective for some cTACE-refractory HCCs, even with use of the same anticancer drug [174, 175]; therefore, changing the embolic agent may be another option. If changes in the tumor characteristics and/or intratumoral blood supply are suspected on imaging, therapeutic options other than TACE, such as local ablation therapy, intraarterial infusion chemotherapy, radiation therapy, or sorafenib therapy, should be selected.

The combined use of antiangiogenic agents and TACE may also be effective for some TACE-refractory HCC (Figure 25). The tumor vasculature is structurally and functionally abnormal, and collectively these vascular abnormalities lead to an abnormal tumor microenvironment characterized by interstitial hypertension, hypoxia, and acidosis [176]. An impaired blood supply and interstitial hypertension interfere with the drug delivery to the tumor. If the antiangiogenic agent can down-regulate VEGF signaling in tumors, then the vasculature might revert back to a more normal state. These morphological changes are accompanied by functional changes: decreased interstitial fluid pressure, increased tumor oxygenation, and improved penetration of the drugs into the tumor. As a result, TACE-refractory HCC can change to TACE-effective HCC. It is an urgent need to evaluate which types of TACE-refractory HCCs can be successfully treated with this combination therapy.

11. Complications

Several complications develop after TACE [1-3, 83, 92-94, 98, 177-196]. These include post-embolization syndrome, acute hepatic failure, infectious complications, ischemic complications, acute tumor lysis syndrome, systemic embolization, and vascular injuries. The incidences for individual types of complications are highly dependent on the patient selection, the chemoembolic agent, and the procedure itself.

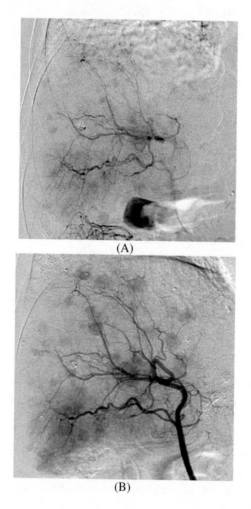

(A)

(B)

Figure 25. (Continued).

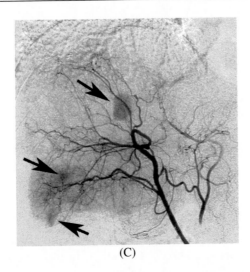

(C)

Figure 25. TACE-refractory HCC treated with combined sorafenib with TACE . (A) Right hepatic arteriogram at the 8th TACE with miriplatin (4 years and 7 months after the initial TACE) shows multiple tumors in the right hepatic lobe. Three months later, the 9th TACE with miriplatin was performed on the left hepatic lobe (not shown). (B) Five months later, sorafenib (800 mg/day) therapy was started; however, the tumors rapidly progressed. Right hepatic arteriogram obtained 7 months after the 8th TACE shows tumor progression despite previous TACE and sorafenib administration. The 10th TACE with miriplatin was performed. Surprisingly, the tumors became well controlled thereafter. (C) The 11th TACE was performed 3 years and 2 months after the 8th TACE. At that time, only 3 tumors were seen (arrows). These were superselectively embolized, and to date (3 years and 4 months after the 8th TACE), no tumor recurrence has been detected (not shown).

11.1. Post-Embolization Syndrome

Post-embolization syndrome is defined as pain, fever, nausea, and vomiting [179]. Post-embolization syndrome itself is not considered a complication but rather an expected outcome of embolotherapy. A large embolized liver volume, either tumorous tissues or nontumorous tissues, may be associated with an increased risk of post-embolization syndrome [179, 180]. Embolization of the cystic artery is also considered the cause of post-procedural pain [179]. Opioid analgesics are widely used for the control of TACE/TAE-related pain [85]. Prochlorperazine is also added as a further antiemetic option on an as needed basis after the procedure. Post-embolization syndrome is generally mild after bland TAE with microspheres compared with cTACE [62].

11.2. Acute Liver Failure

Acute liver failure related to TACE may develop when a large volume of the normal liver is embolized, especially in patients with Child-Pugh B or C class. The reported incidences of acute hepatic failure are 1.7 to 2.3% [178, 180]; however, these are strongly influenced by the patient background and extent of embolization. After introduction of a microcatheter in TACE, development of TACE/TAE-related acute liver failure becomes rare. Chung et al. [181] speculated that acute hepatic failure may occur in patients who have at least two of the following risk factors: poor liver function (Child-Pugh B or C class), major portal vein occlusion, biliary obstruction, and TACE with an excessive amount (≥20 mL) of Lipiodol. Intensive treatment should be performed according to the clinical symptoms and disorders.

11.3. Infectious Complications

Liver abscess is a severe infectious complication of TACE and is well known to cause procedure-related mortality as well as irreversible hepatic failure. In a large series by Song et al. [83], the incidence of cTACE-related liver abscess was 0.2% (15/6225 procedures) and the mortality rate was 13.3% (2/14 patients). Their incidence is similar to the reported incidence by Sakamoto et al. [177]. In DEB-TACE, liver abscess developed in 6/237 (2.5%) patients, 50% of which were fatal [180]. Use of smaller embolic particles is also known to cause biliary necrosis and to predispose abscess formation. In the group with hepatic metastasis, previous endoscopic papillotomy or bilioenteric anastomosis, or gastrointestinal mucosal malignancy, the absolute value of the incidence of liver abscess was more than 10 times higher than that in the corresponding control group. Preexisting percutaneous transhepatic biliary drainage (PTBD) may play a role in abscess formation and the presence of PVTT may also increase the chance of post-embolic liver abscess [83]. Combined treatment with parenteral antibiotics and percutaneous catheter drainage with or without surgical drainage should be promptly performed.

11.4. Ischemic Complications

The incidences and grades of ischemic complications generally depend on catheter positioning, particle size, and magnitude of embolization.

Hepatic infarction develops after TACE, and major portal vein obstruction is a well-known risk factor [177]. An arterioportal shunt is another risk factor and the areas where a large amount of Lipiodol is injected overflowing into the portal vein may also undergo infarction [112]. Therefore, the embolized areas should be kept to a minimum in ultraselective TACE [18].

Gallbladder infarction develops owing to inadvertent occlusion of the cystic artery. Takayasu et al. [182] reported that necrotizing ulcerative cholecystitis was histologically found in the gallbladder after TACE. It is very important to advance the catheter distal to the cystic artery and avoid reflux of the embolic agents into the cystic artery. Cholecystectomy or percutaneous cholecystostomy should be performed in patients with serious conditions.

Makuuchi et al. [183] reported that the intrahepatic and extrahepatic bile ducts would become necrotic if small GS particles <250 μm (GS powder) were used in TACE. We speculated that selective TACE of the caudate artery (A1) and/or medial subsegmental artery (A4) presented a risk of developing bile duct stricture regardless of the size of the GS particles because the proximate branches of A1 and/or A4 supplied the main bile duct [184, 185]. This suggests that deep advancement of a microcatheter is recommended in superselective TACE of A1 and A4. In addition, careful observation is required to check for overflow of the embolic materials into the proximate branches. If the microcatheter cannot be deeply advanced, complete blockage of A1 and A4 should be avoided. Main bile duct stenosis typically develops at the right or left hepatic ducts or at the common hepatic duct, reflecting the poor collateral vascular supply, as compared with a denser arterial network and a relatively high proportion of supply to the lower common bile duct [186]. Optimal management of main bile duct stricture following TACE has not yet been established. Surgical resection or PTBD is performed when jaundice develops. Plastic stent placement is also recommended, provided that the patient consents and is thought likely to be compliant with repeat intervention.

Intrahepatic biloma formation (bile duct necrosis) also develops after TACE. The intrahepatic bile ducts do not have a dual blood supply and are fed exclusively from the hepatic arterial branches that give off a vascular plexus around the bile ducts. The possible mechanism of biloma formation after TACE is considered to be the development of peripheral bile duct necrosis with bile leakage caused by microvascular damage of the peribiliary capillary plexus. Sakamoto et al. [187] reported that the incidence of intrahepatic biloma formation after TACE was 3.6% and it was statistically higher in patients with a main tumor size ≤5 cm and in those with the presence of intrahepatic bile duct dilatation. Technique-related risk factors such as catheter positioning, repeated TACE with frequency of less than 3 months, and regimen of chemoembolization also influence the incidence of biloma formation. In addition, biloma formation more frequently occurs after TACE of the normal liver because the perivascular plexus is dilated in the cirrhotic liver and can act as a portoarterial shunt to compensate for the decreased arterial flow to the bile duct. In our previous analysis, the incidence of biloma formation after subsegmental TACE was 3.1% [188].

Additional ischemic complications, pancreatitis, gastrointestinal mucosal lesions, and splenic infarction have been reported [189, 190]. These complications can be avoided by using a microcatheter; however, the risk remains through a fine retroperitoneal network between the hepatic artery and extrahepatic collaterals [101, 105].

11.5. Acute Tumor Lysis Syndrome

Acute tumor lysis syndrome (ATLS) tends to occur more frequently in hematological malignancies with high proliferative fractions and large bulky tumors, such as Burkitt's lymphoma and other high grade non-Hodgkin's lymphomas, and with acute and chronic leukemia. ATLS is characterized by severe hyperuricemia, hyperphosphatemia, hyperkalemia, hypocalcemia, and acute renal failure [191]. These symptoms usually occur as a result of chemotherapy-induced electrolyte and metabolic disturbance. Although ATLS is less likely to occur in patients with solid tumors, several cases of ATLS related to HCC treatment, including TACE, RF ablation, and sorafenib administration, have been reported [129, 192-196]. TACE-induced ATLS rarely develops in huge HCCs including chemosensitive tumors, a large number of ischemic areas within the tumor, high serum potassium level, high serum phosphate level, elevated uric acid level, high lactate levels, high lactate dehydrogenase (LDH) level, impaired renal function, volume depletion, and drugs that block the tubular reabsorption of uric acid [129]. For this reason, we recommend stepwise TACE for large HCC [84], although partial embolization of the tumor has a risk of high VEGF expression. ATLS is a hematological emergency and its management depends on anticipation, prevention, early recognition, and prompt treatment of the metabolic abnormalities.

11.6. Systemic Embolization

Pulmonary oil embolism develops after cTACE. Chung et al. [137] reported six cases of pulmonary oil embolism after TACE using Lipiodol >20 mL (average, 28.3 mL). The symptoms were dyspnea and hemoptysis associated with chest radiographic abnormalities. The respiratory symptoms and chest radiographic abnormalities were most severe 2 to 10 days after TACE and slowly disappeared thereafter, except in one patient who died 10 days later because of respiratory arrest. They recommended that the maximum dose of Lipiodol be limited to less than 20 mL. In TACE, at least some proportion of Lipiodol injected into the hepatic artery leaves the liver through the normal hepatic vasculature or an arteriovenous shunt for HCC and embolizes the pulmonary vascular network. Whenever a large amount of Lipiodol is delivered to the hepatic artery, massive pulmonary embolism can occur. Fatal pulmonary complications also develop when small-sized microspheres are used [92-94].

Cerebral embolism of Lipiodol, a rare but severe complication of cTACE, has been reported during the injection of high doses of Lipiodol (mean, 25.9 ± 14.7 mL; maximum, 50 mL) [197, 198]. In an experimental study in the rat liver, Lipiodol injected into the hepatic artery rapidly entered the portal branches through the arterioportal communications, passed through the sinusoids from the portal into the hepatic veins and then into the systemic circulation [199]. As mentioned above, pulmonary oil embolism develops in humans when high doses of Lipiodol are injected into the hepatic artery [137]. The patent foramen ovale may serve as a persistent tunnel that allows Lipiodol to pass from the right to the left atrium and to enter the cerebrovascular system. Patients with advanced liver disease are likely to have a pulmonary arteriovenous shunt; a right-to-left shunt from the IPA to the pulmonary vasculature is another possible route causing systemic embolization [200]. In TACE of the IPA, therefore, careful observation is recommended during the injection of the embolic agents. Treatment for cerebral Lipiodol embolism is similar to that for acute cerebral infarction and includes preventing cerebral edema, mediating blood pressure, improving the cerebral blood circulation, and general supportive measures [198]. However, the mortality rate is high (4/13, 30.8%) [198]. This complication may occur in bland-TAE with smaller-sized microspheres.

11.7. Vascular Injuries

Iatrogenic arterial injury may occur during catheter-guidewire manipulation. Iatrogenic dissection heals spontaneously in the majority of patients; however, permanent occlusion or extensive stenosis may develop in some cases and causes the development of extrahepatic collaterals. The guidewire-induced vessel perforation can also heal spontaneously; however, embolization with metallic coils is required when continuous bleeding is seen on repeat arteriogram [177].

TACE injures the hepatic artery by arteritis; therefore, repeated TACE procedures leads to deterioration in the liver function. Arai et al. [201] reported that a major drawback of nonselective TACE therapy is the decrease in survival rates after 2 years due to hepatic failure even in patients with small tumors. In addition, further treatment is frequently difficult in patients whose hepatic artery is attenuated by previous TACE. It is feasible that damage to the hepatic artery by TACE can be kept to a minimum so as to prolong the duration of transcatheter management. For these reasons, superselective catheterization is essential for TACE of localized tumors [18].

TACE also induces arterioportal shunts. Arterioportal shunts are not severe complications; however, they frequently disturb additional TACE. In our previous analysis, the incidence of development of arterioportal shunts after superselective TACE was 13.2% [188]. The incidence may be strongly influenced by the types of chemoembolic agents and is significantly lower in TACE with miriplatin than in TACE with other chemotherapeutics [45]. Significant arterioportal shunts should be blocked by metallic coils and/or GS particles before performing TACE. Bland TAE using a large-sized particle without Lipiodol may be a less risky alternative, although it has a weak therapeutic effect on tumors. Murata et al. [202] reported the usefulness of TACE under temporary occlusion of the arterioportal shunts from the portal side using a balloon catheter that is percutaneously introduced into the portal vein. However, this technique has not been widely distributed because of its invasiveness and complexity.

11.8. Miscellaneous Complications

Variceal bleeding, tumor rupture, disseminated intravascular coagulation, and complications related to anticancer drugs and contrast material may also develop after TACE [2, 3, 177, 178, 181]. In TACE through the extrahepatic collaterals, spinal cord injury may occur after TACE of the intercostal or lumbar arteries [181], skin necrosis after TACE of the IMA or intercostal artery [98, 104], and pleural effusion and weakness of the diaphragm after TACE of the IPA [203]. Careful observation is needed during TACE through the extrahepatic collaterals to avoid unexpected procedure-related complications [105].

In the PRECISION V trial, alopecia occurred in 20.4% of the patients of the cTACE group because 100 to 150 mg of doxorubicin was used in the cTACE group of the PRECISION V patient series [89]. In the daily practice of cTACE in Asia, however, alopecia may not occur because such high doses of doxorubicin have never been used.

Conclusion

Although TACE is classified as a palliative therapy, it plays an important role in the treatment for HCC. Because of the high incidence of tumor recurrence, TACE may be required during the subsequent course in the majority of HCC patients who were initially treated by some therapeutic options other than TACE. Therefore, advances in TACE technology remains critical. There is a wide variety of TACE techniques including the choice of chemoembolic agents, as well as the combined use of an antiangiogenic agent and percutaneous local therapy. Therefore, it is necessary to make proper use of each technique according to the patient and tumor background. In addition, we should be well aware that TACE may also damage the liver and cause several severe complications.

References

[1]   Yamada, R; Sato, M; Kawabata, M; Nakatsuka, H; Nakamura, K; Takashima, S. Hepatic artery embolization in 120 patients with unresectable hepatoma. *Radiology,* 1983, 148(2), 397-401.

[2]   Lo, CM; Ngan, H; Tso, WK; Liu, CL; Lam, CM; Poon, RT; et al. Randomized controlled trial of transarterial lipiodol chemoembolization for unresectable hepatocellular carcinoma. *Hepatology,* 2002, 35(5), 1164-71.

[3]   Llovet, JM; Real, MI; Montaña, X; Planas, R; Coll, S; Aponte, J; et al. Arterial embolisation or chemoembolisation versus symptomatic treatment in patients with unresectable hepatocellular carcinoma: a randomised controlled trial. *Lancet,* 2002, 359(9319), 1734-9.

[4]   Cammà, C; Schepis, F; Orlando, A; Albanese, M; Shahied, L; Trevisani, F; et al. Transarterial chemoembolization for unresectable hepatocellular carcinoma: meta-analysis of randomized controlled trials. *Radiology,* 2002, 224(1), 47-54.

[5]   Marelli, L; Stigliano, R; Triantos, C; Senzolo, M; Cholongitas, E; Davies, N; et al. Transarterial therapy for hepatocellular carcinoma: which technique is more effective? A systematic review of cohort and randomized studies. *Cardiovasc Intervent Radiol,* 2007, 30(1), 6-25.

[6]   Kudo, T; Arii, Y; Ikai, I; Omata, K; Kojiro, M; Sakamoto, M; et al. Report of the 18th nationwide follow-up survey of primary liver cancer in Japan (2004-2005). *Kanzo,* 2010, 51(8), 460-84 (in Japanese).

[7]   Yamakado, K; Nakatsuka, A; Ohmori, S; Shiraki, K; Nakano, T; Ikoma, J; et al. Radiofrequency ablation combined with chemoembolization in hepatocellular carcinoma: treatment response based on tumor size and morphology. *J Vasc Interv Radiol,* 2002, 13(12), 1225-32.

[8]   Fujimori, M; Takaki, H; Nakatsuka, A; Uraki, J; Yamanaka, T; Hasegawa, T; et al. Survival with up to 10-year follow-up after combination therapy of chemoembolization and radiofrequency ablation for the treatment of hepatocellular carcinoma: single-center experience. *J Vasc Interv Radiol,* 2013, 24(5), 655-66.

[9]   Matsui, O; Kadoya, M; Kameyama, T; Yoshikawa, J; Takashima, T; Nakanuma, Y; et al. Benign and malignant nodules in cirrhotic livers: distinction based on blood supply. *Radiology,* 1991, 178(2), 493-7.

[10]   Ekelund, L; Lin, G; Jeppsson, B. Blood supply of experimental liver tumors after intraarterial embolization with Gelfoam powder and absolute ethanol. *Cardiovasc Intervent Radiol,* 1984, 7(5), 234-9.

[11]   Goseki, N; Nosaka, T; Endo, M; Koike, M. Nourishment of hepatocellular carcinoma cells through the portal blood flow with and without transcatheter arterial embolization. *Cancer,* 1995, 76(5), 736-42.

[12] Higashihara, H; Okazaki, M. Transcatheter arterial chemoembolization of hepatocellular carcinoma: a Japanese experience. *Hepatogastroenterology,* 2002, 49(43), 72-8.

[13] Sasaki, A; Kai, S; Iwashita, Y; Hirano, S; Ohta, M; Kitano, S. Microsatellite distribution and indication for locoregional therapy in small hepatocellular carcinoma. *Cancer,* 2005, 103(2), 299-306.

[14] Choi, SH; Chung, JW; Lee, HS. Hepatocellular carcinoma supplied by portal flow after repeated transcatheter arterial chemoembolization. *AJR Am J Roentgenol,* 2003, 181(3), 889-90.

[15] Miyayama, S; Matsui, O; Zen, Y; Yamashiro, M; Hattori, Y; Orito, N; et al. Portal blood supply to locally progressed hepatocellular carcinoma after transcatheter arterial chemoembolization: observation on CT during arterial portography. *Hepatol Res,* 2011, 41(9), 853-66.

[16] Nakao, N; Miura, K; Takahashi, H; Ohishi, M; Mirura, T; Okamoto, E; et al. Hepatocellular carcinoma: combined hepatic, arterial, and portal venous embolization. *Radiology,* 1986, 161(2), 303-7.

[17] Yamakado, K; Hirano, T; Kato, N; Takeda, K; Nakagawa, T; Takase, K; et al. Hepatocellular carcinoma: treatment with a combination of transcatheter arterial chemoembolization and transportal ethanol injection. *Radiology,* 1994, 193(1), 75-80.

[18] Miyayama, S; Matsui, O; Yamashiro, M; Ryu, Y; Kaito, K; Ozaki, K; et al. Ultraselective transcatheter arterial chemoembolization with a 2-F tip microcatheter for small hepatocellular carcinomas: relationship between local tumor recurrence and visualization of the portal vein with iodized oil. *J Vasc Interv Radiol,* 2007, 18(3), 365-76.

[19] Irie, T; Kuramochi, M; Takahashi, N. Dense accumulation of Lipiodol emulsion in hepatocellular carcinoma nodule during selective balloon-occluded transarterial chemoembolization: measurement of balloon occluded arterial stump pressure. *Cardiovasc Intervent Radiol,* 2013, 36(3), 706-13.

[20] Uchida, H; Ohishi, H; Matsuo, N; Nishimine, K; Ohue, S; Nishimura, Y; et al. Transcatheter hepatic segmental arterial embolization using Lipiodol mixed with an anticancer drug and Gelfoam particles for hepatocellular carcinoma. *Cardiovasc Intervent Radiol,* 1990, 13(3), 140-5.

[21] Matsui, O; Kadoya, M; Yoshikawa, J; Gabata, T; Arai, K; Demachi, H; et al. Small hepatocellular carcinoma: treatment with subsegmental transcatheter arterial embolization. *Radiology,* 1993, 188(1), 79-83.

[22] Shimohira, M; Ogino, H; Kawai, T; Kushita, A; Watanabe, M; Kawaguchi, T; et al. Use of the triaxial microcatheter method in super-selective transcatheter arterial chemoembolization for hepatocellular carcinoma. *Br J Radiol,* 2011, 84(998), 184-7.

[23] Koganemaru, M; Abe, T; Anai, H; Tanaka, N; Nonoshita, M; Iwamoto, R; et al. A newly developed double lumen microballoon catheter with a side hole: initial experience of intraarterial infusion chemotherapy and/or embolization. *Jpn J Radiol,* 2012, 30(10), 870-4.

[24] Matsui, O; Miyayama, S; Sanada, J; Kobayashi, S; Khoda, W; Minami, T; et al. Interventional oncology: new options for interstitial treatments and intravascular approaches. *J Hepatobiliary Pancreat Sci,* 2010, 17(4), 407-9.

[25] Ueda, K; Matsui, O; Kawamori, Y; Nakanuma, Y; Kadoya, M; Yoshikawa, J; et al. Hypervascular hepatocellular carcinoma: evaluation of hemodynamics with dynamic CT during hepatic arteriography. *Radiology*, 1998, 206(1), 161-6.

[26] Ueda, K; Matsui, O; Kawamori, Y; Kadoya, M; Yoshikawa, J; Gabata, T; et al. Differentiation of hypervascular hepatic pseudolesions from hepatocellular carcinoma: value of single-level dynamic CT during hepatic arteriography. *J Comput Assist Tomogr*, 1998, 22(5), 703-8.

[27] Miyayama, S; Yamashiro, M; Okuda, M; Yoshie, Y; Nakashima, Y; Ikeno, H; et al. Detection of corona enhancement of hypervascular hepatocellular carcinoma by C-arm dual-phase cone-beam CT during hepatic arteriography. *Cardiovasc Intervent Radiol*, 2011, 34(1), 81-6.

[28] Miyayama, S; Yamashiro, M; Hattori, Y; Orito, N; Matsui, K; Tsuji, K; et al. Efficacy of cone-beam computed tomography during transcatheter arterial chemoembolization for hepatocellular carcinoma. *Jpn J Radiol*, 2011, 29(6), 371-7.

[29] Takayasu, K; Muramatsu, Y; Maeda, T; Iwata, R; Furukawa, H; Muramatsu, Y; et al. Targeted transarterial oily chemoembolization for small foci of hepatocellular carcinoma using a unified helical CT and angiography system: analysis of factors affecting local recurrence and survival rates. *AJR Am J Roentgenol*, 2001, 176(3), 681-8.

[30] Hirota, S; Nakao, N; Yamamoto, S; Kobayashi, K; Maeda, H; Ishikura, R; et al. Cone-beam CT with flat-panel-detector digital angiography system: early experience in abdominal interventional procedures. *Cardiovasc Intervent Radiol*, 2006, 29(6), 1034-8.

[31] Miyayama, S; Matsui, O; Yamashiro, M; Ryu, Y; Takata, H; Takeda, T; et al. Detection of hepatocellular carcinoma by CT during arterial portography using a cone-beam CT technology, comparison with conventional CTAP. *Abdom Imaging*, 2009, 34(4), 502-6.

[32] Miyayama, S; Yamashiro, M; Okuda, M; Yoshie, Y; Sugimori, N; Igarashi, S; et al. Usefulness of cone-beam computed tomography during ultraselective transcatheter arterial chemoembolization for small hepatocellular carcinomas that cannot be demonstrated on angiography. *Cardiovasc Intervent Radiol*, 2009, 32(2), 255-64.

[33] Miyayama, S; Yamashiro, M; Hashimoto, M; Hashimoto, N; Ikuno, M; Okumura, K; et al. Identification of small hepatocellular carcinoma and tumor-feeding branches with cone-beam CT guidance technology during transcatheter arterial chemoembolization. *J Vasc Interv Radiol*, 2013, 24(4), 501-8.

[34] Iwazawa, J; Ohue, S; Hashimoto, N; Muramoto, O; Mitani, T. Clinical utility and limitations of tumor-feeder detection software for liver cancer embolization. *Eur J Radiol*, 2013, 82(10), 1665-71.

[35] Tan, C; Etcubanas, E; Wollner, N; Rosen, G; Gilladoga, A; Showel, J; et al. Adriamycin—an antitumor antibiotic in the treatment of neoplastic diseases. *Cancer*, 1973, 32(1), 9-17.

[36] Verma, D; O'Brien, S; Thomas, D; Faderl, S; Koller, C; Pierce, S; et al. Therapy-related acute myelogenous leukemia and myelodysplastic syndrome in patients with acute lymphoblastic leukemia treated with the hyperfractionated cyclophosphamide, vincristine, doxorubicin, and dexamethasone regimens. *Cancer*, 2009, 115(1), 101-6.

[37] Italia, C; Paglia, L; Trabattoni, A; Luchini, S; Villas, F; Beretta, L; et al. Distribution of 4' epi-doxorubicin in human tissues. *Br J Cancer*, 1983, 47(4), 545-7.

[38] Hata, T; Hoshi, T; Kanamori, K; Matsumae, A; Sano, Y; Shima, T; et al. Mitomycin, a new antibiotic from Streptomyces. I. *J Antibiot (Tokyo),* 1956, 9(4), 141-6.

[39] Lippman, AJ; Helson, C; Helson, L; Krakoff, IH. Clinical trials of cis-diamminedichloroplatinum (NSC-119875). *Cancer Chemother Rep,* 1973, 57(2), 191-200.

[40] Kawaoka, T; Aikata, H; Katamura, Y; Takaki, S; Waki, K; Hiramatsu, A; et al. Hypersensitivity reactions to transcatheter chemoembolization with cisplatin and Lipiodol suspension for unresectable hepatocellular carcinoma. *J Vasc Interv Radiol,* 2010, 21(8), 1219-25.

[41] Curt, GA; Grygiel, JJ; Corden, BJ; Ozols, RF; Weiss, RB; Tell, DT; et al. A phase I and pharmacokinetic study of diamminecyclobutane-dicarboxylatoplatinum (NSC 241240). *Cancer Res,* 1983, 43(9), 4470-3.

[42] Kishimoto, S; Noguchi, T; Yamaoka, T; Fukushima, S; Takeuchi, Y. In vitro release of SM-11355, cis[((1R,2R)-1,2-cyclohexanediamine-N,N')bis(myristato)] platinum(II) suspended in lipiodol. *Biol Pharm Bull,* 2000, 23(5), 637-40.

[43] Kora, S; Urakawa, H; Mitsufuji, T; Osame, A; Higashihara, H; Yoshimitsu, K. Warming effect on miriplatin-lipiodol suspension as a chemotherapeutic agent for transarterial chemoembolization for hepatocellular carcinoma: preliminary clinical experience. *Cardiovasc Intervent Radiol,* 2013, 36(4), 1023-9.

[44] Iwazawa, J; Ohue, S; Hashimoto, N; Mitani, T. Local tumor progression following lipiodol-based targeted chemoembolization of hepatocellular carcinoma: a retrospective comparison of miriplatin and epirubicin. *Cancer Manag Res,* 2012, 4, 113-9.

[45] Miyayama, S; Yamashiro, M; Shibata, Y; Hashimoto, M; Yoshida, M; Tsuji, K; et al. Comparison of local control effects of superselective transcatheter arterial chemoembolization using epirubicin plus mitomycin C and miriplatin for hepatocellular carcinoma. *Jpn J Radiol,* 2012, 30(3), 263-70.

[46] Handa, T; Imai, Y; Sugawara, K; Chikayama, T; Nakazawa, M; Ando, S; et al. Transcatheter arterial chemoembolization for hepatocellular carcinoma: comparison of the therapeutic efficacies between miriplatin and epirubicin. *Hepatol Res,* 2013 (Epub ahead of print).

[47] Kudo, M; Imanaka, K; Chida, N; Nakachi, K; Tak, WY; Takayama, T; et al. Phase III study of sorafenib after transarterial chemoembolisation in Japanese and Korean patients with unresectable hepatocellular carcinoma. *Eur J Cancer,* 2011, 47(14), 2117-27.

[48] Iwai, K; Maeda, H; Konno, T. Use of oily contrast medium for selective drug targeting to tumor: enhanced therapeutic effect and X-ray image. *Cancer Res,* 1984, 44(5), 2115-21.

[49] Nakakuma, K; Tashiro, S; Hiraoka, T; Uemura, K; Konno, T; Miyauchi, Y; et al. Studies on anticancer treatment with an oily anticancer drug injected into the ligated feeding hepatic artery for liver cancer. *Cancer,* 1983, 52(12), 2193-200.

[50] Ohishi, H; Uchida, H; Yoshimura, H; Ohue, S;, Ueda, J; Katsuragi, M; et al. Hepatocellular carcinoma detected by iodized oil. Use of anticancer agents. *Radiology,* 1985, 154(1), 25-9.

[51] Nakamura H; Hashimoto T; Oi H; Sawada S. Iodized oil in the portal vein. *Radiology,* 1988, 167(2), 415-7.

[52] Terayama, N; Matsui, O; Gabata, T; Kobayashi, S; Sanada, J; Ueda, K; et al. Accumulation of iodized oil within the nonneoplastic liver adjacent to hepatocellular carcinoma via the drainage routes of the tumor after transcatheter arterial embolization. *Cardiovasc Intervent Radiol,* 2001, 24(6), 383-7.

[53] Sacco, R; Bargellini, I; Bertini, M; Bozzi, E; Romano, A; Petruzzi, P; et al. Conventional versus doxorubicin-eluting bead transarterial chemoembolization for hepatocellular carcinoma. *J Vasc Interv Radiol,* 2011, 22(11), 1545-52.

[54] Lewis, AL; Gonzalez, MV; Lloyd, AW; Hall, B; Tang, Y; Willis, SL; et al. DC Bead: in vitro characterization of a drug-delivery device for transarterial chemoembolization. *J Vasc Interv Radiol,* 2006, 17(2 Pt 1), 335-42.

[55] Demachi, H; Matsui, O; Abo, H; Tatsu H. Simulation model based on non-newtonian fluid mechanics applied to the evaluation of the embolic effect of emulsions of iodized oil and anticancer drug. *Cardiovasc Intervent Radiol,* 2000, 23(4), 285-90.

[56] Imaeda, T; Yamawaki, Y; Seki, M; Goto, H; Iinuma, G; Kanematsu, M; et al. Lipiodol retention and massive necrosis after lipiodol-chemoembolization of hepatocellular carcinoma: correlation between computed tomography and histopathology. *Cardiovasc Intervent Radiol,* 1993, 16(4), 209-13.

[57] Kan, Z; McCuskey, PA; Wright, KC; Wallace, S. Role of Kupffer cells in iodized oil embolization. *Invest Radiol,* 1994, 29(11), 990-3.

[58] Kloeckner, R; Otto, G; Biesterfeld, S; Oberholzer, K; Dueber, C; Pitton, MB. MDCT versus MRI assessment of tumor response after transarterial chemoembolization for the treatment of hepatocellular carcinoma. *Cardiovasc Intervent Radiol,* 2010, 33(3), 532-40.

[59] Boucher, E; Bouguen, G; Garin, E; Guillygomarch, A; Boudjema, K; Raoul, JL. Adjuvant intraarterial injection of ^{131}I-labeled lipiodol after resection of hepatocellular carcinoma: progress report of a case-control study with a 5-year minimal follow-up. *J Nucl Med,* 2008, 49(3), 362-6.

[60] Loffroy, R; Guiu, B; Cercueil, JP; Krausé, D. Endovascular therapeutic embolization: an overview of occluding agents and their effects on embolised tissues. *Curr Vasc Pharmacol,* 2009, 7(2), 250-63.

[61] Sato, M; Yamada, R. Experimental and clinical studies on the hepatic artery embolization for treatment of hepatoma. *Nippon Acta Radiologica,* 1983, 43, 977-1005 (in Japanese).

[62] Osuga, K; Khankan, AA; Hori, S; Okada, A; Sugiura, T; Maeda, M; et al. Transarterial embolization for large hepatocellular carcinoma with use of superabsorbent polymer microspheres: initial experience. *J Vasc Interv Radiol,* 2002, 13(9 Pt 1), 929-34.

[63] Tadavarthy, SM; Moller, JH; Amplatz, K. Polyvinyl alcohol (Ivalon)—a new embolic material. *Am J Roentgenol Radium Ther Nucl Med,* 1975, 125(3), 609-16.

[64] Vaidya, S; Tozer, KR; Chen, J. An overview of embolic agents. *Semin Intervent Radiol,* 2008, 25(3), 204-15.

[65] Soo, CS; Chuang, VP; Wallace, S; Charnsangavej, C; Carrasco, H. Treatment of hepatic neoplasm through extrahepatic collaterals. *Radiology,* 1983, 147(1), 45-9.

[66] Jordan, O; Denys, A; De Baere, T; Boulens, N; Doelker, E. Comparative study of chemoembolization loadable beads: in vitro drug release and physical properties of DC Bead and Hepasphere loaded with doxorubicin and irinotecan. *J Vasc Interv Radiol,* 2010, 21(7), 1084-90.

[67] Maeda, N; Osuga, K; Higashihara, H; Mikami, K; Tomoda, K; Hori, S; et al. In vitro characterization of cisplatin-loaded superabsorbent polymer microspheres designed for chemoembolization. *J Vasc Interv Radiol,* 2010, 21(6), 877-81.

[68] Blümmel, J; Reinhardt, S; Schäfer, M; Gilbert, C; Sun, L; Ren, J. Drug-eluting beads in the treatment of hepatocellular carcinoma and colorectal cancer metastases to the liver. *European Oncology and Haematology,* 2012, 8(3), 162-6.

[69] Namur, J; Wassef, M; Millot, JM; Lewis, AL;, Manfait, M; Laurent, A. Drug-eluting beads for liver embolization: concentration of doxorubicin in tissue and in beads in a pig model. *J Vasc Interv Radiol,* 2010, 21(2), 259-67.

[70] Padia, SA; Shivaram, G; Bastawrous, S; Bhargava, P; Vo, NJ; Vaidya, S; et al. Safety and Efficacy of drug-eluting bead chemoembolization for hepatocellular carcinoma: comparison of small-versus medium-size particles. *J Vasc Interv Radiol,* 2013, 24(3), 301-6.

[71] Park, JH; Han, JK; Chung, JW; Choi, BI; Han, MC; Kim, YI. Superselective transcatheter arterial embolization with ethanol and iodized oil for hepatocellular carcinoma. *J Vasc Interv Radiol,* 1993, 4(3), 333-9.

[72] Yu, SC; Hui, JW; Hui, EP; Mo, F; Lee, PS; Wong, J; et al. Embolization efficacy and treatment effectiveness of transarterial therapy for unresectable hepatocellular carcinoma: a case-controlled comparison of transarterial ethanol ablation with Lipiodol–ethanol mixture versus transcatheter arterial chemoembolization. *J Vasc Interv Radiol,* 2009, 20(3), 352-9.

[73] Salem, R; Lewandowski, RJ; Kulik, L; Wang, E; Riaz, A; Ryu, RK; et al. Radioembolization results in longer time-to-progression and reduced toxicity compared with chemoembolization in patients with hepatocellular carcinoma. *Gastroenterology,* 2011, 140(2), 497-507.

[74] McWilliams, JP; Kee, ST; Loh, CT; Lee, EW; Liu, DM. Prophylactic embolization of the cystic artery before radioembolization: feasibility, safety, and outcomes. *Cardiovasc Intervent Radiol,* 2011, 34(4), 786-92.

[75] Gunji, T; Kawauchi, N; Ohnishi, S; Ishikawa, T; Nakagama, H; Kaneko, T; et al. Treatment of hepatocellular carcinoma associated with advanced cirrhosis by transcatheter arterial chemoembolization using autologous blood clot: a preliminary report. *Hepatology,* 1992, 15(2), 252-7.

[76] Gunji, T; Kawauchi, N; Akahane, M; Watanabe, K; Kanamori, H; Ohnishi, S. Long-term outcomes of transcatheter arterial chemoembolization with autologous blood clot for unresectable hepatocellular carcinoma. *Int J Oncol,* 2002, 21(2), 427-32.

[77] Ishida, K; Hirooka, M; Hiraoka, A; Kumagai, T; Uehara, T; Hiasa, Y; et al. Treatment of hepatocellular carcinoma using arterial chemoembolization with degradable starch microspheres and continuous arterial infusion of 5-fluiriuracil. *Jpn J Clin Oncol,* 2008, 38(9), 596-603.

[78] Loewe, C; Cejna, M; Schoder, M; Thurnher, MM; Lammer, J; Thurnher, SA. Arterial embolization of unresectable hepatocellular carcinoma with use of cyanoacrylate and lipiodol. *J Vasc Inter Radiol,* 2002, 13(1), 61-9.

[79] Llovet, JM; Di Bisceglie, AM; Bruix, J; Kramer, BS; Lencioni, R; Zhu, AX; et al. for the Panel of Experts in HCC-Design Clinical Trials. Design and endpoints of clinical trials in hepatocellular carcinoma. *J Natl Cancer Inst,* 2008, 100(10), 698-711.

[80] Arii, S; Sata, M; Sakamoto, M; Shimada, M; Kumada, T; Shiina, S; et al. Management
      of hepatocellular carcinoma: report of consensus meeting in the 45th annual meeting of
      the Japan Society of Hepatology (2009). *Hepatol Res,* 2010, 40(7), 667-85.
[81] Kung, CT; Liu, BM; Ng, SH; Lee, TY; Cheng, YF; Chen, MC; et al. Transcatheter
      arterial embolization in the emergency department for hemodynamic instability due to
      ruptured hepatocellular carcinoma: analysis of 167 cases. *AJR Am J Roentgenol,* 2008,
      191(6), W231-9.
[82] Okazaki, M; Higashihara, H; Koganemaru, F; Nakamura, T; Kitsuki, H; Hoashi, T; et
      al. Intraperitoneal hemorrhage from hepatocellular carcinoma: emergency
      chemoemboli-zation or embolization. *Radiology,* 1991, 180(3), 647-51.
[83] Song, SY; Chung, JW; Han, JK; Lim, HG; Koh, YH; Park, JH; et al. Liver abscess after
      transcatheter oily chemoembolization for hepatic tumors: incidence, predisposing
      factors, and clinical outcome. *J Vasc Interv Radiol,* 2001, 12(3), 313-20.
[84] Miyayama, S; Yamashiro, M; Okuda, M; Yoshie, Y; Sugimori, N; Igarashi, S; et al.
      Chemoembolization for the treatment of large hepatocellular carcinoma. *J Vasc Interv
      Radiol,* 2010, 21(8), 1226-34.
[85] Zhou, B; Wang, J; Yan, Z;, Shi, P; Kan, Z. Liver cancer: effects, safety, and cost-
      effectiveness of controlled-release oxycodone for pain control after TACE. *Radiology,*
      2012, 262(3), 1014-21.
[86] Satake, M; Uchida, H; Arai, Y; Anai, H; Sakaguchi, H; Nagata, T; et al. Transcatheter
      arterial chemoembolization (TACE) with Lipiodol to treat hepatocellular carcinoma:
      survey results from the TACE study group of Japan. *Cardiovasc Intervent Radiol,* 2008,
      31(4), 756-61.
[87] Takayasu, K; Arii, S; Kudo, M; Ichida, T; Matsui, O; Izumi, N; et al. Superselective
      transarterial chemoembolization for hepatocellular carcinoma. Validation of treatment
      algorithm proposed by Japanese guidelines. *J Hepatol,* 2012, 56, 886-92.
[88] Lu, W; Li, YH; He, XF; Zhao, JB; Chen, Y; Mei, QL. Necrosis and apoptosis in
      hepatocellular carcinoma following low-dose versus high-dose preoperative
      chemoembolization. *Cardiovasc Intervent Radiol,* 2008, 31(6), 1133-40.
[89] Lammer, J; Malagari, K; Vogl, T; Pilleul, F; Denys, A; Watkinson, A; et al. Prospective
      randomized study of doxorubicin-eluting-bead embolization in the treatment of
      hepatocellular carcinoma: results of the PRECISION V study. *Cardiovasc Intervent
      Radiol,* 2010, 33(1), 41-52.
[90] Lencioni, R; de Baere, T; Burrel, M; Caridi, JG; Lammer, J; Malagari, K; et al.
      Transcatheter treatment of hepatocellular carcinoma with Doxorubicin-loaded DC Bead
      (DEBDOX): technical recommendations. *Cardiovasc Intervent Radiol,* 2012, 35(5),
      980-5.
[91] Osuga, K; Hori, S; Hiraishi, K; Sugiura, T; Hata, Y; Higashihara, H; et al. Bland
      embolization of hepatocellular carcinoma using superabsorbent polymer microspheres.
      Cardiovasc Intervent Radiol, 2008, 31(6), 1108-16.
[92] Bonomo, G; Pedicini, V; Monfardini, L; Della Vigna, P; Poretti, D; Orgera, G; et al.
      Bland embolization in patients with unresectable hepatocellular carcinoma using
      precise, tightly size-calibrated, anti-inflammatory microparticles: first clinical
      experience and one-year follow-up. *Cardiovasc Intervent Radiol,* 2009, 33(3), 552-9.

[93] Maluccio, MA; Covey, AM; Porat, LB; Schubert, J; Brody, LA; Sofocleous, CT; et al. Transcatheter arterial embolization with only particles for the treatment of unresectable hepatocellular carcinoma. *J Vasc Interv Radiol*, 2008, 19(6), 862-9.

[94] Brown, KT. Fatal pulmonary complications after arterial embolization with 40-120-μm tris-acryl gelatin microspheres. *J Vasc Interv Radiol*, 2004, 15(2 Pt 1), 197-200.

[95] Malagari, K; Pomoni, M; Kelekis, A; Pomoni, A; Dourakis, S; Spyridopoulos, T; et al. Prospective randomized comparison of chemoembolization with doxorubicin-eluting beads and bland embolization with BeadBlock for hepatocellular carcinoma. *Cardiovasc Intervent Radiol*, 2010, 33(3), 541-51.

[96] Golfieri, R; Cappelli, A; Cucchetti, A; Piscaglia, F; Carpenzano, M; Peri, E; et al. Efficacy of selective transarterial chemoembolization in inducing tumor necrosis in small (<5 cm) hepatocellular carcinomas. *Hepatology*, 2011, 53(5), 1580-9.

[97] Kim, HC; Chung, JW; Lee, W; Jae, HJ; Park, JH. Recognizing extrahepatic collateral vessels that supply hepatocellular carcinoma to avoid complications of transcatheter arterial chemoembolization. *Radiographics*, 2005, 25 Suppl 1, S25-39.

[98] Miyayama, S; Matsui, O; Taki, K; Minami, T; Ryu, Y; Ito, C; et al. Extrahepatic blood supply to hepatocellular carcinoma: angiographic demonstration and transcatheter arterial chemoembolization. *Cardiovasc Intervent Radiol*, 2006, 29(1), 39-48.

[99] Chung, JW; Kim, HC; Yoon, JH; Lee, HS; Jae, HJ; Lee, W; et al. Transcatheter arterial chemoembolization of hepatocellular carcinoma: prevalence and causative factors of extrahepatic collateral arteries in 479 patients. *Korean J Radiol*, 2006, 7(4), 257-66.

[100] Miyayama, S; Yamashiro, M; Okuda, M; Yoshie, Y; Nakashima, Y; Ikeno, H; et al. The march of extrahepatic collaterals: analysis of blood supply to hepatocellular carcinoma located in the bare area of the liver after chemoembolization. *Cardiovasc Intervent Radiol*, 2010, 33(3), 513-22.

[101] Miyayama, S; Matsui, O; Taki, K; Minami, T; Ito, C; Shinmura, R; et al. Transcatheter arterial chemoembolization for hepatocellular carcinoma fed by the reconstructed inferior phrenic artery: anatomical and technical analysis. *J Vasc Interv Radiol*, 2004, 15(8), 815-23.

[102] Miyayama,, S; Matsui,, O; Nishida,, H; Yamamori,, S; Minami,, T; Shinmura,, R; et al. Transcatheter arterial chemoembolization for unresectable hepatocellular carcinoma fed by the cystic artery. *J Vasc Interv Radiol*, 2003, 14(9 Pt 1), 1155-61.

[103] Miyayama, S; Yamashiro, M; Shibata, Y; Hashimoto, M; Yoshida, M; Tsuji, K; et al. Arterial blood supply to the caudate lobe of the liver from the proximal branches of the right inferior phrenic artery in patients with recurrent hepatocellular carcinoma after chemoembolization. *Jpn J Radiol*, 2012, 30(1), 45-52.

[104] Kajiwara, K; Kakizawa, H; Takeuchi, N; Toyota, N; Hieda, M; Ishikawa, M; et al. Cutaneous complications after transcatheter arterial treatment for hepatocellular carcinoma via the internal mammary artery: how to avoid this complication. *Jpn J Radiol*, 2011, 29(5), 307-15.

[105] Miyayama, S; Yamashiro, S; Okuda, M; Aburano, H; Shigenari, N; Morinaga, K; et al. Anastomosis between the hepatic artery and the extrahepatic collateral or between extrahepatic collaterals: observation on angiography. *J Med Imag Radiat Oncol*, 2009, 53(3), 271-82.

[106] Miyayama S; Yamashiro, M; Hashimoto, M; Yoshida, M; Hashimoto, N; Ikuno, M; et al. Clinical features of hepatocellular carcinoma supplied by the left internal mammary artery. *Jpn J Radiol,* 2012, 30(10), 798-805.

[107] Miyayama, S; Yamashiro, M; Okuda, M; Yoshie, Y; Sugimori, N; Igarashi, S; et al. Hepatocellular carcinoma supplied by the right lumbar artery. *Cardiovasc Intervent Radiol* 2010, 33(1), 53-60.

[108] Komatsu, T; Matsui, O; Kadoya, M; Yoshikawa, J; Gabata, T; Takashima, T. Cystic artery origin of the segment V hepatic artery. *Cardiovasc Intervent Radiol,* 1999, 22(2), 165-7.

[109] Kanazawa, S; Wright, KC; Kasi, LP; Charnsangavej, C; Wallace, S. Preliminary experimental evaluation of temporary segmental hepatic venous occlusion: angiographic, pathologic, and scintigraphic findings. *J Vasc Interv Radiol,* 1993, 4(6), 759-66.

[110] Miyayama, S. TAE. *Jpn J Clin Radiol,* 2009, 54(3), 380-90 (in Japanese).

[111] Miyayama, S; Matsui, O; Taki, K; Minami, T; Ryu, Y;, Ito, C; et al. Arterial blood supply to the posterior aspect of segment IV of the liver from the caudate branch: demonstration at CT after iodized oil injection. *Radiology,* 2005, 237(3), 1110-4.

[112] Miyayama, S; Mitsui, T; Zen, Y; Sudo, Y; Yamashiro, M; Okuda, M; et al. Histopathological findings after ultraselective transcatheter arterial chemoembolization for hepatocellular carcinoma. *Hepatol Res,* 2009, 39(4), 374-81.

[113] Miyayama, S; Matsui, S; Yamashiro, M; Ryu, Y; Takata, H; Takeda, T; et al. Iodized oil accumulation in the hypovascular tumor portion of early-stage hepatocellular carcinoma after ultraselective transcatheter arterial chemoembolization. *Hepatol Int,* 2007, 1(4), 451-9.

[114] Sakon, M; Nagano, H; Nakamori, S; Dono, K; Umeshita, K; Murakami, T; et al. Intrahepatic recurrences of hepatocellular carcinoma after hepatectomy: analysis based on tumor hemodynamics. *Arch Surg,* 2002, 137(1), 94-9.

[115] Miyayama, S; Matsui, O; Yamashiro, M; Ryu, Y; Takata, H; Takeda, T; et al. Visualization of hepatic lymphatic vessels during transcatheter arterial chemoembolization for hepatocellular carcinoma. *J Vasc Interv Radiol,* 2007, 18(9), 1111-7.

[116] Arai, H; Kobayashi, T; Nagashima, T; Takizawa, D; Toyoda, M; Takayama, H; et al. Balloon-occluded transcatheter arterial chemoembolization using miriplatin for hepatocellular carcinoma. *Kanzo,* 2013, 54(1), 81-3 (in Japanese).

[117] Miyayama, S; Yamashiro, M; Hashimoto, M; Hashimoto, N; Ikuno, I; Okumura, K; et al. Comparison of local control in transcatheter arterial chemoembolization of hepatocellular carcinoma ≤6 cm with or without intraprocedural monitoring of the embolized area using cone-beam computed tomography. *Cardiovasc Intervent Radiol,* 2013 (Epub ahead of print).

[118] Loffroy, R; Lin, M; Yenokyan, G; Rao, PP; Bhagat, N; Noordhoek, N; et al. Intraprocedural C-arm dual-phase cone-beam CT: can it be used to predict short-term response to TACE with drug-eluting beads in patients with hepatocellular carcinoma? *Radiology,* 2013, 266(2), 636-48.

[119] Lencioni, R; Llovet, JM. Modified RECIST (mRECIST) assessment for hepatocellular carcinoma. *Semin Liver Dis,* 2010, 30(1), 52-60.

[120] Takayasu, K; Arii, S; Ikai, I; Omata, M; Okita, K; Ichida, T; et al. Prospective cohort study of transarterial chemoembolization for unresectable hepatocellular carcinoma in 8510 patients. *Gastroenterology*, 2006, 131(2), 461-9.

[121] Ikeda, M; Arai, Y; Park, SJ; Takeuchi, Y; Anai, H; Kim, JK; et al. Prospective study of transcatheter arterial chemoembolization for unresectable hepatocellular carcinoma: an Asian cooperative study between Japan and Korea. *J Vasc Interv Radiol*, 2013, 24(4), 490-500.

[122] Yamakado, K; Miyayama, S; Hirota, S; Mizunuma, K; Nakamura, K; Inaba, Y; et al. Hepatic arterial embolization for unresectable hepatocellular carcinomas: do technical factors affect prognosis? *Jpn J Radiol*, 2012, 30(7), 560-6.

[123] Takaki, S; Sakaguchi, H; Anai, H; Tanaka, T; Yamamoto, K; Morimoto, K; et al. Long-term outcome of transcatheter subsegmental and segmental arterial chemoembolization using lipiodol for hepatocellular carcinoma. *Cardiovasc Intervent Radiol*, 2012, 35(3), 544-54.

[124] Miyayama, S. Transcatheter arterial chemoembolization for hepatocellular carcinoma: current status and future. *J Kyoto Pref Univ Med*, 2012, 121(6), 313-22 (in Japanese).

[125] Yodono, H; Matsuo, K; Shinohara, A. A retrospective comparative study of epirubicin-lipiodol emulsion and cisplatin-lipiodol suspension for use with transcatheter arterial chemoembolization. *Anticancer Drugs*, 2011, 22(3), 277-82.

[126] Kamada, K; Nakanishi, T; Kitamoto, M; Aikata, H; Kawakami, Y; Ito, K; et al. Long-term prognosis of patients undergoing transcatheter arterial chemoembolization for unresectable hepatocellular carcinoma: comparison of cisplatin lipiodol suspension and doxorubicin hydrochloride emulsion. *J Vasc Interv Radiol*, 2001, 12(7), 847-54.

[127] Maeda, N; Osuga, K; Higashihara, H; Tomoda, K; Mikami, K; Nakazawa, T; et al. Transarterial chemoembolization with cisplatin as second-line treatment for hepatocellular carcinoma unresponsive to chemoembolization with epirubicin-Lipiodol emulsion. *Cardiovasc Intervent Radiol*, 2012, 35(1), 82-9.

[128] Kojiro, M; Sugihara, S; Kakizoe, S; Nakashima, O; Kiyomatsu, K. Hepatocellular carcinoma with sarcomatous change: a special reference to the relationship with anticancer therapy. *Cancer Chemother Pharmacol*, 1989, 23, S4-8.

[129] Sakamoto, N; Monzawa, S; Nagano, H; Nishizaki, H; Arai, Y; Sugimura, K. Acute tumor lysis syndrome caused by transcatheter oily chemoembolization in a patient with a large hepatocellular carcinoma. *Cardiovasc Intervent Radiol*, 2007, 30(3), 508-11.

[130] Takaki, H; Yamakado, K; Uraki, J; Nakatsuka, A; Fuke, H; Yamamoto, N; et al. Radiofrequency ablation combined with chemoembolization for the treatment of hepatocellular carcinomas larger than 5 cm. *J Vasc Interv Radiol*, 2009, 20(2), 217-24.

[131] Yoon, HM; Kim, JH; Kim, EJ; Gwon, DI; Ko, GY; Ko, HK. Modified cisplatin-based transcatheter arterial chemoembolization for large hepatocellular carcinoma: multivariate analysis of predictive factors for tumor response and survival in a 163-patient cohort. *J Vasc Interv Radiol*, 2013, 24(11), 1639-46.

[132] Takayasu, K; Wakao, F; Moriyama, N; Muramatsu, Y; Sakamoto, M; Hirohashi, S; et al. Response of early-stage hepatocellular carcinoma and borderline lesions to therapeutic arterial embolization. *AJR Am J Rentgenol*, 1993, 160(2), 301-6.

[133] Uraki, J; Yamakado, K; Nakatsuka, A; Takeda, K. Transcatheter hepatic arterial chemoembolization for hepatocellular carcinoma invading the portal veins: therapeutic effects and prognostic factors. *Eur J Radiol*, 2004, 51(1), 12-8.

[134] Peng, ZW; Guo, RP; Zhang, YJ;, Lin, XJ; Chen, MS; Lau, WY. Hepatic resection versus transcatheter arterial chemoembolization for the treatment of hepatocellular carcinoma with portal vein tumor thrombus. *Cancer*, 2012, 118(19), 4725-36.

[135] Lee, IJ; Chung, JW; Kim, HC; Yin, YH; So, YH; Jeon, UB; et al. Extrahepatic collateral artery supply to the tumor thrombi of hepatocellular carcinoma invading inferior vena cava: the prevalence and determinant factors. *J Vasc Interv Radiol*, 2009, 20(1), 22-9.

[136] Chern, MC; Chuang, VP; Cheng, T;, Lin, ZH;, Lin, YM. Transcatheter arterial chemoembolization for advanced hepatocellular carcinoma with inferior vena cava and right atrial tumors. *Cardiovasc Intervent Radiol*, 2008, 31(4), 735-44.

[137] Chung, JW; Park, JH; Im, JG; Han, JK; Han, MC. Pulmonary oil embolism after transcatheter oily chemoembolization of hepatocellular carcinoma. *Radiology*, 1993, 187(3), 689-93.

[138] Okuda, M; Miyayama, S; Yamashiro, M; Yoshie, Y; Sugimori, N; Igarashi, S; et al. Sloughing of intraductal tumor thrombus of hepatocellular carcinoma after transcatheter arterial chemoembolization. *Cardiovasc Intervent Radiol*, 2010, 33(3), 619-23.

[139] Hiraki, T; Sakurai, J; Gobara, H; Kawamoto, H; Mukai, T; Hase, S; et al. Sloughing of intraductal tumor thrombus of hepatocellular carcinoma after transcatheter chemoembolization causing obstructive jaundice and acute pancreatitis. *J Vasc Interv Radiol*, 2006, 17(7), 583-5.

[140] Chen, WK; Chang, YT; Chung, YT; Yang, HR. Outcomes of emergency treatment in ruptured hepatocellular carcinoma in the ED. *Am J Emerg Med*, 2005, 23(6), 730-6.

[141] Kitagawa, K; Yamakado, K; Nakatsuka, A; Tanaka, N; Fujii, A; Takano, K; et al. Selective transcatheter hepatic arterial chemoembolization for hemobilia from hepatocellular carcinoma: report of three cases. *J Vasc Interv Radiol*, 1999, 10(10), 1357-60.

[142] Yamasaki, S; Hasegawa, H; Kinoshita, H; Furukawa, M; Imaoka, S; Takasaki, K; et al. A prospective randomized trial of the preventive effect of pre-operative transcatheter arterial embolization against recurrence of hepatocellular carcinoma. *Jpn J Cancer Res*, 1996, 87(2), 206-11.
Paye, F; Jagot, P; Vilgrain, V; Farges, O; Borie, D; Belghiti, J. Preoperative chemoembolization of hepatocellular carcinoma: a comparative study. *Arch Surg*, 1998, 133(7), 767-72.

[143] Lu, CD; Peng, SY; Jiang, XC; Chiba, Y; Tanigawa, N. Preoperative transcatheter arterial chemoembolization and prognosis of patients with hepatocellular carcinomas: retrospective analysis of 120 cases. *World J Surg*, 1999, 23(3), 293-300.

[144] Malagari K; Pomoni M; Moschouris H; Bouma E; Koskinas J; Stefaniotou A; et al. Chemoembolization with doxorubicin-eluting beads for unresectable hepatocellular carcinoma: five-year survival analysis. *Cardiovasc Intervent Radiol* 2012, 35(5), 1119-28.

[145] Burrel, M; Reig, M; Forner, A; Barrufet, M; de Lope, CR; Tremosini, S; et al. Survival of patients with hepatocellular carcinoma treated by transarterial chemoembolization (TACE) using drug-eluting beads. Implications for clinical practice and trial design. *J Hepatol*, 2012, 56(6), 1330-5.

[146] Dekervel, J; van Malenstein, H; Vandecaveye, V; Nevens, F; van Pelt, J; Heye, S. Transcatheter arterial chemoembolization with doxorubicin-eluting superabsorbent

polymer microspheres in the treatment of hepatocellular carcinoma: midterm follow-up. *J Vasc Interv Radiol*, 2014, 25(2), 248-255.e1.

[147] Song, MJ; Chun, HJ; Song do, S; Kim, HY; Yoo, SH; Park, CH; et al. Comparative study between doxorubicin-eluting beads and conventional transarterial chemoembolization for treatment of hepatocellular carcinoma. *J Hepatol*, 2012, 57(6), 1244-50.

[148] Vente, MA; Wondergem, M; van der Tweel, I; van den Bosch, MA; Zonnenberg, BA; Lam, MG; et al. Yttrium-90 microsphere radioembolization for the treatment of liver malignancies: a structured meta-analysis. *Eur Radiol*, 2009, 19(4), 951-9.

[149] Goin, JE; Dancey, JE; Roberts, CA; Sickles, CJ; Leung, DA; Soulen, MC. Comparison of post-embolization syndrome in the treatment of patients with hepatocellular carcinoma: trans-catheter arterial chemo-embolization versus yttrium-90 glass microspheres. *World J Nucl Med*, 2004, 3(1), 49-56.

[150] Iwazawa, J; Ohue, S; Hashimoto, N. Survival after C-arm CT-assisted chemoembolization of unresectable hepatocellular carcinoma. *Eur J Radiol*, 2012, 81(12), 3985-92.

[151] Miyayama, S; Matsui, O; Akakura, Y; Yamamoto, T; Fujinaga, Y; Koda, W; et al. Use of a catheter with a large side hole for selective catheterization of the inferior phrenic artery. *J Vasc Interv Radiol*, 2001, 12(4), 497-9.

[152] Miyayama, S; Yamashiro, M; Okuda, M; Aburano, H; Shigenari, N; Morinaga, K; et al. Creation of a cleft in an angiography catheter to facilitate catheterization of branches of the aorta arising at an acute angle. *J Vasc Interv Radiol*, 2008, 19(12), 1769-71.

[153] Miyayama, S; Yamashiro, M; Hattori, Y; Orito, N; Matsui, K; Tsuji, K; et al. Microcoil embolization during abdominal vascular interventions through microcatheters with a tip of 2 French or less. *Jpn J Radiol*, 2011, 29(4), 286-90.

[154] Miyayama, S; Matsui, O; Taki, K; Minami, T; Ito, C; Shinmura, R; et al. Combined use of an occlusion balloon catheter and a microcatheter for embolization of the unselectable right inferior phrenic artery supplying hepatocellular carcinoma. *Cardiovasc Intervent Radiol*, 2004, 27(6), 677-81.

[155] Kiyosue, H; Matsumoto, S; Hori, Y; Okahara, M; Sagara, Y; Mori, H. Turn-back technique with use of a shaped microcatheter for superselective catheterization of arteries originating at acute angles. *J Vasc Interv Radiol*, 2004, 15(6), 641-3.

[156] Kwon, JW; Chung, JW; Song, SY; Lim, HG; Myung, JS; Choi, YH; et al. Transcatheter arterial embolization for hepatocellular carcinomas in patients with celiac axis occlusion. *J Vasc Interv Radiol*, 2002, 13(7), 689-94.

[157] Miyayama, S; Yamashiro, M; Yoshie, Y; Nakashima, Y; Ikeno, H; et al. Hepatocellular carcinoma in the caudate lobe of the liver: variations of its feeding branches on arteriography. *Jpn J Radiol*, 2010, 28(8), 555-62.

[158] Tanaka, K; Okazaki, H; Nakamura, S; Endo, O;, Inoue, S; Takamura, Y; et al. Hepatocellular carcinoma: treatment with a combination therapy of transcatheter arterial embolization and percutaneous ethanol injection. *Radiology*, 1991, 179(3), 713-7.

[159] Virmani, S; Rhee, TK; Ryu, RK; Sato, KT; Lewandowski, RJ; Mulcahy, MF; et al. Comparison of hypoxia-inducible factor-1alpha expression before and after transcatheter arterial embolization in rabbit VX2 liver tumors. *J Vasc Interv Radiol*, 2008, 19(10), 1483-9.

[160] Sergio, A; Cristofori, C; Cardin, R; Pivetta, G; Ragazzi, R; Baldan, A; et al. Transcatheter arterial chemoembolization (TACE) in hepatocellular carcinoma (HCC): the role of angiogenesis and invasiveness. *Am J Gastroenterol*, 2008, 103(4), 914-21.

[161] Wang, B; Xu, H; Gao, ZQ; Ning, HF; Sun, YQ; Cao, GW. Increased expression of vascular endothelial growth factor in hepatocellular carcinoma after transcatheter arterial chemoembolization. *Acta Radiol*, 2008, 49(5), 523-9.

[162] Llovet, JM; Ricci, S; Mazzaferro, V; Hilgard, P; Gane, E; Blanc, JF; et al. Sorafenib in advanced hepatocellular carcinoma. *N Engl J Med*, 2008, 359(4), 378–90.

[163] Cheng, AL; Kang, YK; Chen, Z; Tsao, CJ; Qin, S; Kim, JS; et al. Efficacy and safety of sorafenib in patients in the Asia-Pacific region with advanced hepatocellular carcinoma: a phase III randomised, double-blind, placebo-controlled trial. *Lancet Oncol*, 2009,10(1), 25–34.

[164] Lencioni, R. Chemoembolization for hepatocellular carcinoma. *Semin Oncol*, 2012, 39(4), 503-9.

[165] Sansonno, D; Lauletta, G; Russi, S; Conteduca, V; Sansonno, L; Dammacco, F. Transarterial chemoembolization plus sorafenib: a sequential therapeutic scheme for HCV-related intermediate-stage hepatocellular carcinoma: a randomized clinical trial. *Oncologist*, 2012, 17(3), 359-66.

[166] Laird, AD; Vajkoczy, P; Shawver, LK; Thurnher, A; Liang, C; Mohammadi, M; et al. SU6668 is a potent antiangiogenic and antitumor agent that induces regression of established tumors. *Cancer Res*, 2000, 60(15), 4152-60.

[167] Shim, JH; Park, JW; Kim, JH; An, M; Kong, SY; Nam, BH; et al. Association between increment of serum VEGF level and prognosis after transcatheter arterial chemoembolization in hepatocellular carcinoma patients. *Cancer Sci*, 2008, 99(10), 2037-44.

[168] Pawlik, TM; Reyes, DK; Cosgrove, D; Kamel, IR; Bhagat, N; Geschwind, JF. Phase II trial of sorafenib combined with concurrent transarterial chemoembolization with drug-eluting beads for hepatocellular carcinoma. *J Clin Oncl*, 2011, 29(30), 3960-7.

[169] Golfieri, R; Renzulli, M; Mosconi, C; Forlani, L; Giampalma, E; Piscaglia, F; et al. Hepatocellular carcinoma responding to superselective transarterial chemoemboli-zation: an issue of nodule dimension? *J Vasc Interv Radiol*, 2013, 24(4), 509-17.

[170] Kudo, M. TACE-refractory HCC. In. The Japan Society of Hepatology, editor. Kangan Shinryo Manual. 2nd ed. Tokyo: *Igaku Shoin*, 2010, 118-20.

[171] Hashimoto, T; Nakamura, H; Hori, S; Tomoda, K; Nakanishi, K; Murakami, T; et al. Hepatocellular carcinoma: efficacy of transcatheter oily chemoembolization in relation to macroscopic and microscopic patterns of tumor growth among 100 patients with partial hepatectomy. *Cardiovasc Intervent Radiol*, 1995, 18(2), 82-6.

[172] Zen, C; Zen, Y; Mitry, RR; Corbeil, D; Karbanova´, J; O'Grady, J; et al. Mixed phenotype hepatocellular carcinoma after transarterial chemoembolization and liver transplantation. *Liver Transpl*, 2011, 17(8), 943-54.

[173] Seki, A; Hori, S; Kobayashi, K; Narumiya, S. Transcatheter arterial chemoembolization with epirubicin-loaded superabsorbent polymer microspheres for 135 hepatocellular carcinoma patients: single-center experience. *Cardiovasc Intervent Radiol*, 2011, 34(3), 557-65.

[174] Song do, S; Choi, JY; Yoo, SH; Kim, HY; Song, MJ; Bae, SH; et al. DC bead transarterial chemoembolization is effective in hepatocellular carcinoma refractory to

conventional transarterial chemoembolization: a pilot study. *Gut and Liver*, 2013, 7(1), 89-95.

[175] Jain, RK. Normalization of tumor vasculature: an emerging concept in antiangiogenic treatment. *Science*, 2005, 307(5706), 58-62.

[176] Sakamoto, I; Aso, N; Nagaoki, K; Matsuoka, Y; Uetani, M; Ashizawa, K; et al. Complications associated with transcatheter arterial embolization for hepatic tumors. *Radiographics* 1998, 18(3), 605-19.

[177] Brown, DB; Cardella, JF; Sacks, D; Goldberg, SN; Gervais, DA; Rajan, D; et al. Quality improvement guidelines for transhepatic arterial chemoembolization, embolization, and chemotherapeutic infusion for hepatic malignancy. *J Vasc Interv Radiol*, 2009, 20(7 Suppl), S219-S226, S226.e1-10.

[178] Leung, DA; Goin, JE; Sickles, C; Raskay, BJ; Soulen, MC. Determinants of postembolization syndrome after hepatic chemoembolization. *J Vasc Interv Radiol*, 2001, 12(3), 321-6.

[179] Malagari, K; Pomoni, M; Spyridopoulos, TN; Moschouris, H; Kelekis, A; Dourakis, S; et al. Safety profile of sequential transcatheter chemoembolization with DC Bead™, results of 237 hepatocellular (HCC) patients. *Cardiovasc Intervent Radiol*, 2011, 34(4), 774-85.

[180] Chung, JW; Park, JH; Han, JK; Choi, BI; Han, MC; Lee, HS; Kim, CY. Hepatic tumors: predisposing factors for complications of transcatheter oily chemoembolization. *Radiology*, 1996, 198(1), 33-40.

[181] Takayasu, K; Moriyama, N; Muramatsu, Y; Shima, Y; Ushio, K; Yamada, T; et al. Gallbladder infarction after hepatic artery embolization. *AJR Am J Roentgenol*, 1985, 144(1), 135-8.

[182] Makuuchi, M; Sukigara, M; Mori, T; Kobayashi, J; Yamazaki, S; Hasegawa, H; et al. Bile duct necrosis: complication of transcatheter hepatic arterial embolization. *Radiology*, 1985, 156(2), 331-4.

[183] Miyayama, S; Yamashiro, M; Okuda, M; Yoshie, Y; Nakashima, Y; Ikeno, H; et al. Main bile duct stricture occurring after transcatheter arterial chemoembolization for hepatocellular carcinoma. *Cardiovasc Intervent Radiol*, 2010, 33(6), 1168-79.

[184] Miyayama, S; Yamashiro, M; Hashimoto, M; Hashimoto, N; Ikuno, M; Okumura, K; et al. Blood supply of the main bile duct from the caudate artery and medial subsegmental artery of the hepatic artery: evaluation using images obtained during transcatheter arterial chemoembolization for hepatocellular carcinoma. *Hepatol Res*, 2013, 43(11), 1175-81.

[185] Chen, WJ; Ying, DJ; Liu, ZJ; He, ZP. Analysis of the arterial supply of the extrahepatic bile ducts and its clinical significance. *Clin Anat*, 1999, 12(4), 245-9.

[186] Sakamoto, I; Iwanaga, S; Nagaoki, K; Matsuoka, Y; Ashizawa, K; Uetani, M; et al. Intrahepatic biloma formation (bile duct necrosis) after transcatheter arterial chemoembolization. *AJR Am J Roentgenol*, 2003, 181(1), 79-87.

[187] Miyayama, S; Matsui, O. Subsegmental TAE. In: Kudo M, editor. Shokakibyo Seminar 97; Tokyo: *Herusu Shuppan*, 2004, 45-53 (in Japanese).

[188] Kishimoto, W; Nakao, A; Takagi, H; Hayakawa, T. Acute pancreatitis after transcatheter arterial embolization (TAE) for hepatocellular carcinoma. *Am J Gastroenterol*, 1989, 84(11), 1396-9.

[189] Kuribayashi, S; Phillips, DA; Harrington, DP; Bettmann, MA; Garnic, JD; Come, SE; et al. Therapeutic embolization of the gastroduodenal artery in hepatic artery infusion chemotherapy. *AJR Am J Roentgenol*, 1981, 137(6), 1169-72.

[190] Chasty, RC; Liu-Yin, JA. Acute tumour lysis syndrome. *Br J Hosp Med*, 1993, 49(7), 488-92.

[191] Burney, IA. Acute tumor lysis syndrome after transcatheter chemoembolization of hepatocellular carcinoma. *South Med, J,* 1998, 91(5), 467-70.

[192] Hsieh, PM; Hung, KC; Chen, YS. Tumor lysis syndrome after transarterial chemoembolization of hepatocellular carcinoma: case reports and literature review. *World J Gastroenterol*, 2009, 15(37), 4726-8.

[193] Katiman, D; Manikam, J; Goh, KL; Abdullah, BJ; Mahadeva, S. Tumour lysis syndrome: a rare complication of trans-arterial chemo-embolisation with doxorubicin beads for hepatocellular carcinoma. *J Gastrointest Cancer*, 2012, 43(1 suppl), 187-190.

[194] Lehner, SG; Gould, JE; Saad, WE; Brown, DB. Tumor lysis syndrome after radiofrequency ablation of hepatocellular carcinoma. *AJR Am J Roentgenol*, 2005, 185(5), 1307-9.

[195] Huang, WS; Yang, CH. Sorafenib induced tumor lysis syndrome in an advanced hepatocellular carcinoma patient. *Word J Gastroenterol*, 2009, 15(35), 4464-6.

[196] Matsumoto, K; Nojiri, J; Takase, Y; Egashira, Y; Azama, S; Kato, A; et al. Cerebral Lipiodol embolism: a complication of transcatheter arterial chemoembolization for hepatocellular carcinoma. *Cardiovasc Intervent Radiol*, 2007, 30(3), 512-4.

[197] Li, Z; Ni, RF; Busireddy, KK; Jin, YH; Zhao, X; Li, MM; et al. Cerebral lipiodol embolism following transcatheter arterial chemoembolization for hepatocellular carcinoma, a report of two cases and literature review. *Chin Med J (Engl)*, 2011, 124(24), 4355-8.

[198] Kan, Z; Ivancev, K; Hägerstrand, I; Chuang, VP; Lunderquist, A. In vivo microscopy of the liver after injection of Lipiodol into the hepatic artery and portal vein in the rat. *Acta Radiol*, 1989, 30(4), 419-25.

[199] Miyayama, S; Yamashiro, M; Yoshie, Y; Okuda, M; Nakashima, Y; Ikeno, H; et al. Inferior phrenic arteries: angiographic anatomy, variations, and catheterization techniques for transcatheter arterial chemoembolization. *Jpn J Radiol*, 2010, 28(7), 502-11.

[200] Arai, K; Matsui, O; Takashima, T; Kadoya, M; Yoshikawa, J; Gabata, T; et al. Efficacy of transcatheter arterial embolization therapy for small hepatocellular carcinomas: comparison with other treatments. *Radiat Med*, 1990, 8(5), 191-8.

[201] Murata, S; Tajima, H; Nakazawa, K; Onozawa, S; Kumita, S; Nomura, K. Initial experience of transcatheter arterial chemoembolization during portal vein occlusion for unresectable hepatocellular carcinoma with marked arterioportal shunts. *Eur Radiol*, 2009, 19(8), 2016-23.

[202] Lee, DH; Chung, JW; Kim, HC; Jae, HJ; Yoon, CJ; Kang, SG; et al. Development of diaphragmatic weakness after transcatheter arterial chemoembolization of the right inferior phrenic artery: frequency and determinant factors. *J Vasc Interv Radiol*, 2009, 20(4), 484-9.

Chapter 7

Proton Beam Therapy for Hepatocellular Carcinoma

Hideyuki Sakurai*, Toshiyuki Okumura, Nobuyoshi Fukumitsu,
Hitoshi Ishikawa, Kayoko Ohnishi, Masashi Mizumoto,
Toshiyuki Terunuma, Hiroaki Kumada and Takeji Sakae*
Proton Medical Research Center, University of Tsukuba, Tsukuba, Ibaraki, Japan

Abstract

Radiation therapy has been continuously advancing and evolving. It has been a challenge to reduce unnecessary radiation doses for normal tissue while increasing radiation doses for targets. Since the dose distribution of proton beam therapy is excellent, it is possible to achieve intense treatment of the hepatocellular carcinoma while protecting the normal liver. Local control rate of hepatocellular carcinoma by proton is reported about 85-90% at 3 years and 80-90% at 5 years, and overall survival rate is about 55-65% at 2 years and 20-50% at 5 years with very few side effects. Clinical data with proton beam therapy have been accumulating and are expected to be incorporated into the standard treatment of hepatocellular carcinoma in the future. In this chapter, we explain radiation therapy, which is currently performed for liver cancers, particularly focusing on proton beam therapy.

1. Introduction

Many technological advances have been made in radiation therapy. Historically, it has been a challenge to reduce unnecessary radiation doses for normal tissue while increasing radiation doses for targets.

Computed tomography (CT) was not available until the 1970s, and treatment plans were designed based on 2-dimensional images. Since it was difficult to accurately identify the

---

* Corresponding author: Email: hsakurai@pmrc.tsukuba.ac.jp. tsakae@md.tsukuba.ac.jp.

location of liver tumors within the liver, radiation therapy has not been performed for hepatocellular carcinoma (HCC). Normal liver tissue is highly sensitive to radiation. Considering the tolerance dose for normal liver tissue, radiation therapy could only be performed with palliative intent, using techniques that were available at that time.

However, in the 1980s, CT appeared as part of the treatment plan, and it became easy to focus on all cancer targets, which facilitated radiation therapy, while reducing normal tissue damage employing various irradiation techniques (i.e., 3-dimensional dose calculation and treatment planning, highly reproducible treatment techniques, and technical advances in the precision of the treatment system). For HCC, it became possible to reduce the unnecessary exposure of the normal liver volume to irradiation, and, at the same time, quantitative evaluation and prediction of the risk of liver damage became possible using the dose-volume histogram (DVH). Using these techniques, 3-dimensional conformal radiation therapy (3DCRT) was performed mainly for cases in which the application of other treatment options would be difficult, such as portal vein tumor thrombosis.

Today, radiation therapy has been continuously advancing and evolving, and technologies far beyond 3DCRT have been realized with regard to concentrating doses to cancers, such as stereotactic body radiation therapy (SBRT) and particle therapy. These advanced radiation therapies have been proposed for the initial stage of cancer treatment, similar to surgery, and have become performed widely.

The advantages of radiation therapy are its low invasiveness, broad indications, and high therapeutic efficacy. On the other hand, attention should be paid to potential adverse effects. Treatment planning with sufficient consideration of the influence on organs around the cancers is essential. SBRT and particle therapy for HCC may cause liver damage, stomach & intestinal damage, and skin damage as complications, depending on the treatment field. To perform these high-precision radiation therapies, institutions must maintain a system safely and provide the latest technology.

Particle therapy is the application of ions that are accelerated to a high speed for cancer treatment. Proton beam therapy is performed using hydrogen. In conventional radiation therapy, X-rays enter through the body surface, penetrate the cancer target, and pass through to the other side of the body surface, which exposes normal tissue other than the cancer target to a high radiation dose. In contrast, in particle therapy, particles enter through the body surface and stop at the position of the cancer target, forming a peak, and do not pass through to deeper regions. This peak, representing the dose distribution of particle therapy, is termed the Bragg peak. Since the dose distribution of particle therapy is better than that of X-ray, it is possible to achieve intense treatment of the target while protecting the surrounding normal tissue.

Proton beam therapy, which is covered in this chapter, is currently the most popular particle therapy in Western countries and Asian countries, mainly in Japan. Since it is difficult to perform a randomized clinical trial to compare proton beam therapy with other local treatment methods, such as surgery, sufficient consensus for proton beam therapy has not been reached with regard to the efficacy and safety, but also the appropriate criteria to judge indications. But clinical treatment data with proton beam therapy have been accumulating and are expected to be incorporated into the standard treatment of HCC in the future.

In this chapter, we explain radiation therapy, which is currently performed for liver cancers, particularly focusing on proton beam therapy.

2. History of Particle Beam Therapy

About 100 years ago, Ernst Rutherford discovered α and β radiation from uranium in 1899, and demonstrated the presence of protons in 1919 [1, 2].

The medical application of particle beam therapy was initially proposed by Robert Wilson of Harvard University [3]. Considering radiation therapy for cancer, he suggested that protons or heavier ions could exhibit beneficial effects on the normal tissue. Early studies focused on the characteristic dose distribution curve of proton beams in the deeper regions. The dose distribution of protons reaches a relatively low dose plateau at entry and forms a sharp dose peak, termed the Bragg peak, at the end of the acceleration energy-specified range. Thereafter, the dose rapidly decreases to almost 0 within about 1 cm. Thus, the dose for tissues deeper than the target can be reduced to 0.

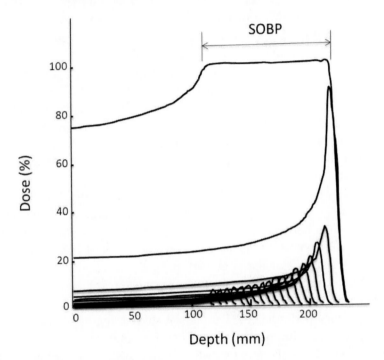

Figure 1. Spread-out Bragg peak (SOBP) is built up by superimposing Bragg peaks of different intensity and range for yielding suitable depth dose for irradiation of a thick, deep-seated target. By the appropriate number of peaks and their intensities, the narrow peak of the natural accelerator beam can be broadened and flattened as required.

To realize the clinical application, it is necessary to adjust the depth of the Bragg peak and create a flat dose distribution throughout the depth in order to homogenously irradiate the target tumor. This method is termed the spread-out Bragg Peak (SOBP), and it can be created by superimposing proton beams with different energies [4] (Figure 1). By contrast, the regions posterior and proximal to the target are exposed to higher doses in photon beam therapy. Thus, proton beam therapy is superior with respect to the dose distribution, excluding the shallow regions directly beneath the skin. The principle of radiation therapy is to apply a high dose to the target while minimizing the exposure of normal tissue around the target. Indeed, proton beams have properties that are appropriate to the realization of this objective.

The acquisition of proton beams for medical applications became possible using an accelerator when research facilities for high-energy physics were constructed after World War II, and the world's first study on their medical use was performed at a facility constructed in Berkeley in 1954, followed by Uppsala, Sweden, in 1957 and Harvard in 1961. In order to translate the application of proton beams to human medical care, the biological properties of proton beams have been investigated in various experiments using animals and cells. The level of biological responses induced by irradiation varies between protons, heavy particles, and X-ray radiation, although these are applied at physically the same dose, and differences are described as the relative biological effectiveness (RBE). In 1952, Tobias investigated the biological effects of proton, and reported that the RBE for the LD_{50} (50% lethal dose; radiation dose to produce lethality on 50 % of animals) of "white mice" was approximately 1 for whole-body irradiation by 315±15 MeV protons relative to 180 kVp X-rays [5]. At the outset, differences of radiation effect in the several end points, such as cell death, gene mutation, and carcinogenesis, were evaluated using kVp x-irradiation as the standard [6, 7]. Over time, evaluations have been made based on the higher-energy photon of cobalt 60 and megavoltage x-ray as the standards. The RBE varies depending on the end point, but the RBE of charged particles is considered to be almost equivalent to or greater than 1.0. It has been elucidated that RBE varies not only between megavoltage x-ray and charged particles, but also among particles with different weights, and among the same particles with different energies [8, 9]. Consensus has been reached that the RBE of proton beams is 1.1 in clinical application.

J. Lawrence at Lawrence Berkeley Laboratory (LBL) and C. Huggins of the University of Chicago drew attention to the phenomenon that surgical resection of the pituitary gland dramatically reduces the hormone levels, and they considered the use of irradiation of the pituitary gland with proton beams in the treatment of advanced breast cancer [10, 11]. J. Laurence, C. Tobias, and C. Huggins et al. performed a collaborative investigation in which they examined the time-course of the reduction of hormone secretion from the pituitary after proton beam irradiation at 200 to 300 Gy [12].

Lawrence et al. then performed the first human study using protons as part of a phase I clinical study. Proton beam irradiation was applied 3 times per week for a total cumulative dose of 140 to 300 Gy. Thus, the first irradiation of humans was performed at LBL in 1954 [13]. However, the irradiation method at that time was different from the current method using the Bragg peak. They applied a plateau part of 340 MeV proton beam dose distribution, generating the dose distribution using multi-field irradiation passing through the pituitary. LBL subsequently switched the subject of their investigations from protons to heavier particles, i.e., helium, carbon, and neon, with the modification of the accelerator in 1957. In 1992, clinical trials were completed as operation of the Bevalac accelerator for treatment was suspended, and the clinical data collected was summarized by J. Castro [14].

In Europe, fractionated irradiation (1-10 times) of cancer patients was performed at University of Uppsala, Sweden, in 1956 using proton beams supplied by a 185 MeV synchrocyclotron. Patients with glioblastoma multiforme and carcinomas of the cervix, nasopharynx, head & neck, and other sites were treated [15].

In Boston, the 160 MeV Harvard Cyclotron Laboratory (HCL) was built for nuclear physics research under the supervision of Robert Wilson in 1949, but it was soon used solely for studies of medical applications in 1961. In particular, Kjellberg et al. of the Neurosurgical Department of Massachusetts General Hospital (MGH) and the HCL team initiated a study of single irradiation of pituitary adenoma and intracranial arteriovenous malformation. They set the Bragg peak of the proton beam at the pituitary and were able to achieve clinically superior outcomes [16, 17].

Suit et al. aimed to achieve curative irradiation of cancers with proton beams using the same accelerator. In their therapeutic strategy, proton beam irradiation was applied at a dose equivalent to that of photon beams, i.e., at a daily single dose of 2 Gy [RBE] for 6-8 weeks [18]. In this proton beam therapy, which was begun in 1974, the total dose was set at a level higher than that of photon beams. Firstly, the target was limited to sarcoma at the skull base, and the indications were gradually expanded thereafter. Among these subsequent indications, melanoma of the uvea was particularly notable [19]. Constable et al. developed these techniques by performing irradiation experiments using monkeys [20]. Goitein et al. designed a 3-dimensional treatment planning [21] and achieved clinically superior outcomes [22]. During this period, several inventions that later became important therapeutic techniques, also for photon beam therapy, were made, i.e., the use of digitally reconstructed radiographs (DRRs), beam's eye-view, dose-volume histogram, and so on. [23, 24].

By 1984, six additional treatment facilities become operational worldwide: Dubna in 1967, Moscow in 1969, and St Petersburg in 1975 in the Soviet Union, Chiba in 1979 and Tsukuba in 1983 in Japan, and Villigen, Switzerland, in 1984.

Proton beam therapy for the liver was initiated in the 1980s in Tsukuba [25, 26]. They introduced a fluoroscopic device for positioning to accurately irradiate deep-seated targets that moved with respiration [27], and developed a technique to insert a fiducial marker in the liver to confirm positioning of the target [28] and a system to intermittently emit proton beams in synchronization with respiratory motion [29]. These are now used as basic treatment techniques for the liver. Currently, many particle beam facilities are available for treatment of the liver, and the clinical outcomes continue to accumulate.

3. Principle of Facility Design

In proton therapy, first, protons produced at the ion-source are accelerated until they become highly energized, and then the accelerated proton beam with narrow and mono-energy is transported close to the patient. The proton beams, which have been modulated to the proper energy and distribution by the beam delivery system, are emitted from the beam port to irradiate the patient. Using this methodology, therapeutic doses of the protons are finally delivered to the target region within the patient's body. Thus, facilities for proton therapy are comprised of several devices that can facilitate the required functions. Fundamentally, the facilities consist of (a) a particle accelerator, (b) a beam transport system including a gantry, (c) a beam delivery system and (d) patient positioning devices, etc. As a typical example of a hospital-based proton therapy facility comprised of these components, a schematic diagram of the synchrotron-based proton therapy facility installed in the Proton Medical Research Center (PMRC) at the University of Tsukuba Hospital is shown in Figure 2. The devices are installed in each room shielded by a thick concrete enclosure, and the accelerator and beam transport system are separated from the treatment rooms in order to protect the patient. The separation of the treatment room from the device also allows personnel to enter the treatment room freely while the proton beam is in use in another treatment room.

In the present section, details of the devices, such as the accelerator and the beam transport system are explained, respectively. Meanwhile, the beam delivery system can produce a broad and spread-out Bragg peak (SOBP) beam or a scanning beam, and allows beam shaping within the target region. Thus, because the both systems are important and complicated, these details are explained in next sections.

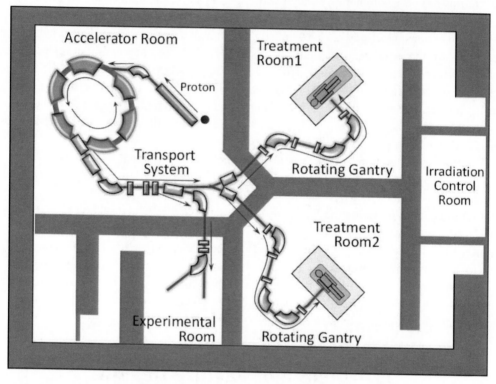

Figure 2. Schema of a typical hospital-based proton therapy facility.

3.1. Accelerator

Proton beams applied for proton therapy are produced by several types of particle accelerators. To deliver therapeutic doses of proton beams to treat several cancers in the human body, including adult patients, it is necessary that the beam penetration be greater than 30 cm in depth. Thus the accelerators must produce proton beams with energies of up to 250 MeV. Furthermore, the accelerators must also be able to change the energies from approximately 100 MeV to 250 MeV in a step-wise manner, in order to administer therapeutic doses to the deeper target regions, in addition to the treatment of superficial cancers. To treat ocular lesions, in particular, proton energies of 60-75 MeV are needed to achieve proton ranges of from 3.0 to 4.5 cm in depth. In addition, to perform the irradiation within a reasonable treatment time, a sufficient intensity of the beam is required. When a dose rate of 2 Gy/min is delivered in a volume of 1,000 cm^3 in the target region, $>5x10^{10}$ particles per second, equivalent to a beam current of approximately 10 nA, must be accelerated using the device.

To accelerate particles, including protons, straight accelerators (linear accelerator, linac) and circular type accelerators are normally used. At present, when proton therapy is performed in a hospital, either a synchrotron or a cyclotron, as a circular type accelerator, is usually applied. The application of each type of accelerator to the therapy has characteristics in terms of the structure, beam intensity and method of changing energy. The key features of each accelerator are introduced as below.

3.1.1. Linear Accelerator

Linear accelerators (linac) are generally characterized by a very high beam intensity. The linac has a number of accelerating cavities driven by a radio frequency (RF) power supply, and particles obtain their velocity by traversing the acceleration cavity only once. To accelerate the particles up to the target energy level, some linac units are connected in series, along a linear path. Thus, to produce high-energy proton beams, the linacs are logically long. When protons are accelerated to 200 MeV using a linac, the accelerator system can reach lengths of up to 40 meters. Problems in terms of the size of the device and construction costs, including its shielding facility, have impeded the adaptation of linacs to hospital-based proton therapy. Thus, linacs are usually used as an injector system for synchrotrons, as described below.

A major turning point in the production of a compact proton linear accelerator came about with the invention of a Radio Frequency Quadrupole (RFQ) by I. M. Kapchinsky and V. A. Teplyakov in 1969. The RFQ is a compact RF accelerating structure that can accelerate particles generated from an ion-source up to a few MeV. Four plates (electrodes called vanes) are set in the resonator tank and maintain axial symmetry. The beam passes through the center of the tank. The top-face of each vane facing into the center is machined to produce a fine slope (modulation), which generates a longitudinal electric field that accelerates the beam. The pitch of the modulation is adjusted in accordance with the particle velocity. A further advantage of the RFQ is the ability to implement a collecting and focusing function. The total length of the structure of the RFQ device is approximately 3 meters and can accelerate protons up to 3 MeV.

Proton beams accelerated by the RFQ up to a few MeV can be accelerated further using a Drift Tube Linac (DTL) system, which was developed by L. Alvarez. The centers of all drift tubes are aligned with the center of the tank to achieve optimal accuracy. The DTL tank is fed by high frequency and high-power RF to generate an accelerating voltage between the drift-tubes. A focusing magnet is installed in the drift-tube and its length is adjusted according to the increasing particle velocity. Thus, many DTL tanks must be set in a linear manner if it is necessary to accelerate the particles to higher energy.

3.1.2. Cyclotron

To resolve the problem of the length of the linac to produce high-energy energy beams, cyclic accelerators are being employed for hospital-based particle therapy. Cyclic accelerators use magnets to constrain the particles to move in a closed path and traverse a single RF-powered accelerating structure multiple times.

The original concept of the cyclotron was conceived by Lawrence in the early 1930s, based on a radio-frequency electric field linear accelerator with multiple accelerating gaps. Particles in the cyclotron are accelerated by a fixed magnetic field and a fixed RF between two D-shape electrodes (dees). Figure 3 shows the schema of a cyclotron. The dees are supported in a vacuum tank and are set in the gap between the poles of a large electromagnet. An ion-source is installed in the center of the magnet, and low-velocity ions injected from the ion-source begin to move toward the electrode and the particles enter the electric field-free space within the hollow electrode, continuing their path on a semi-circular arc. When the particles reach the gap between the electrodes, they gain further acceleration due to the synchrony between the RF and the orbital frequencies of the particles. The particles are accelerated spirally outward until they reach the radius of the magnet poles, and finally reach the maximum energy. Thus, the maximum energy of the particles as a result of acceleration by the cyclotron is determined by the dimension of the dees. The accelerated particles are extracted from the cyclotron at the periphery of the magnetic field by deflecting them from the circular path into the beam-transport system.

In classical cyclotrons, the magnetic field and the frequency of the RF field were constant, and they could only accelerate the protons to 10-15 MeV. The limit of the maximum energy was due to the relativistic mass increase of the proton. Therefore, using these systems, it was impossible to apply the therapy against deeper cancers, due to the lack of sufficient energy. This problem was overcome by the development of an isochronous cyclotron that compensated for the relativistic mass increase by increasing the radius of the magnetic field. In principle, the isochronous cyclotron causes the beam to stray from the median plane and to strike the magnet pole pieces due to axial defocusing of the beam when the magnetic field strength increases with the radius. To improve the tendency of the isochronous cyclotron, the azimuthally varying field (AVF) cyclotron, which allows for compensation of the defocusing by creating alternate high- and low-magnetic field sectors, has been developed. In contrast with the isochronous cyclotron that produces a constant orbital frequency, the synchrocyclotron, which allows the frequency of each field to be varied, has been also proposed. Modern cyclotrons have combined these methodologies and techniques in order to effectively produce huge energy beams [30]. Furthermore, using superconducting technologies, the cyclotron for hospital-based proton therapy is expected to become more compact.

The concept of the modern cyclotron was put into practical use as a 230 MeV cyclotron installed at Massachusetts General Hospital for proton therapy [31]. The diameter and height of the magnet are 4.34 meters and 2.1 meters, respectively. Moreover, an even more compact cyclotron combined with a superconducting magnet has also been proposed [32] for installation at the Rinecker Proton Therapy Center in Munich. The diameter of the magnet is 3.09 meters and the height is 1.65 meters.

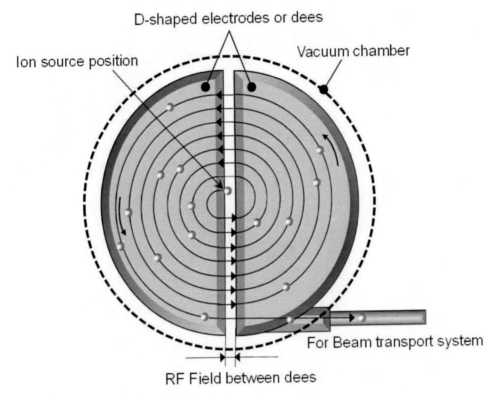

Figure 3. Schema of a classical cyclotron.

In Europe and the United States, many of the proton therapy facilities have employed cyclotrons for proton therapy. In Japan, the National Cancer Center Hospital East has installed a cyclotron-based proton therapy device. The hospital employs a normal conducting AVF cyclotron, the cyclotron can accelerate protons to 235 MeV and its beam current is 300nA. The diameter of the cyclotron is approximately 4 meters. Aizawa hospital has also employed a cyclotron-based treatment device, as noted later.

3.1.3. Synchrotron

The synchrotron has the same ability as the cyclotron to accelerate particles to higher energy. However, in contrast with the cyclotron, the synchrotron has some key features in terms of the application to particle radiotherapy. First, the synchrotron allows the beam energy to be altered in accordance with the intended use; and the energy spread of the beam can thus be minimized throughout the energy range. The former property works by modulation of the beam energy for dose depth control in place of using the range-shifting device with a variable thickness absorber. In particular, it can be used for the scanning irradiation methods necessary for precise modulation of the energy. Based upon these potential advantages, proton therapy facilities employing the synchrotron have recently increased.

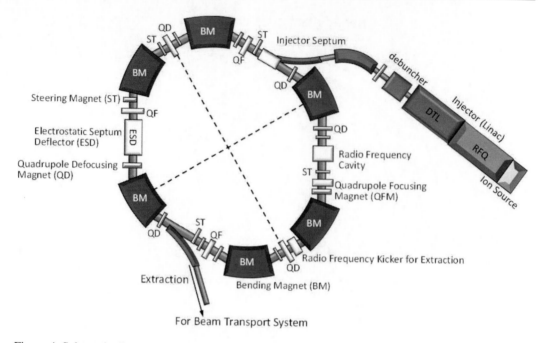

Figure 4. Schematic diagram of a typical hospital-based synchrotron system.

Figure 4 shows a schematic diagram of a typical hospital-based synchrotron system for proton therapy. This system is constructed mainly from two accelerators; a linac and a synchrotron ring. The linac, which serves as an injector for the synchrotron, accelerates particles up to a few MeV. The linac normally consists of an ion-source, a RFQ and a debuncher. However linacs for radiotherapy often combine a DTL just behind the RFQ in order to further increase the particle velocity. The low-velocity particles that are injected in to the synchrotron ring finally are accelerated further until they reach the target energy level of a few hundred MeV, while maintaining its orbit determined by the ring.

The shape of the synchrotron ring is usually a lattice structure comprised of several components: the septum magnet, RF cavity, bending magnet, quadrupole focusing/defocusing magnet, sextupole magnet, electrostatic septum deflector, steering magnet, RF kicker, etc. For typical synchrotrons for proton therapy that were manufactured until the 2000s, the ring was generally comprised of six sets of 60° sector bending magnets and a drift space. The diameter of the ring is approximately 7 meters. However more recent synchrotrons, manufactured in the 2010s have improved such that the ring is comprised of four sets of 90° sector bending magnets resulting in a smaller dimension than conventional rings.

When the particles pass through the RF cavity as a high-voltage acceleration system installed in the straight section between two bending magnets, their velocities increase directly with the frequency of the system. Furthermore, by increasing the magnetic field of the bending magnet in conjunction with increasing the frequency, a collection of particles is maintained in a fixed orbit of the ring during the acceleration cycle. Several magnets, i.e., the quadrupole focusing/defocusing magnet, sextupole magnets and steering magnets located at the drift space, control the optics of the beam on the orbit. The particles that reach the target velocity are finally extracted to the beam transport system at the septum magnet of the ring.

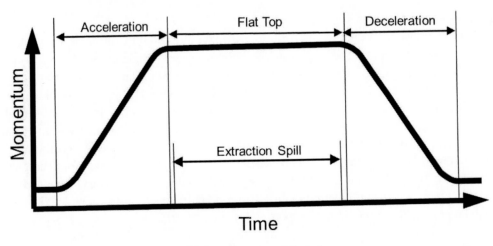

Figure 5. Operation pattern of synchrotron of University of Tsukuba.

Synchrotrons produce a pulsed output due to the finite time required for acceleration. The beam acceleration cycle can take from 0.2 to a few seconds. Hence, the pulse repetition rate is typically 0.5-2 Hz. Figure 5 shows a timing cycle of the beam on the orbit of the synchrotron of the PMRC at the University of Tsukuba Hospital, as a typical example of a hospital-based synchrotron [33]. For extraction of the beam from the ring, in case of the irradiation of organs that are not affected by respiratory motion, such as the prostate, repetition of the beam extraction follows with the properties of each synchrotron. On the other hand, during irradiation of organs that are susceptible to respiratory motion, such as the lung and liver, in the case of the PMRC at the University of Tsukuba and the M.D. Anderson Cancer Center, the timing of the extraction depends on respiration gating along with the breathing waveform of the patient. Thus, for the application of synchrotron to such therapy, the beam cycle or the extraction spill length must be maintained for as long as possible. Details of irradiation in consideration of respiration are described later.

The first hospital-based proton therapy facility was constructed at the Loma Linda University Medical Center, using a synchrotron accelerator [34]. In Japan, the first synchrotron for hospital-based proton therapy was installed in the PMRC at the University of Tsukuba Hospital [35]. The synchrotron consists of six sets of drift space and 60° sector magnets, and can accelerate the protons up to 250 MeV, which allows the production of four energy modulated beams of 155, 200, 230 and 250 MeV in accordance with the target depth. Most of the proton therapy facilities in Japan use synchrotron-based treatment systems. Furthermore, all heavy-ion (carbon) therapy facilities have applied synchrotron-based system. In the US, the M D Anderson Cancer Center has employed a synchrotron-based facility for proton therapy.

3.2. Beam Transport

The proton beams extracted from the each circular accelerator must be delivered to the patient with negligible beam loss while maintaining adequate optical parameters, which is achieved using the beam transport system. This section briefly describes the beam transport system. The gantry is also described as a component of the transport system.

3.2.1. Beam transport system

First, the transport system of a cyclotron-based facility is slightly different from that of a synchrotron-based facility. The cyclotron can only produce a single energy beam, as noted above. Thus in the transport system in combination with the cyclotron, a range shifting device that can modulate the energy of the extracted beams, is essential. The range-shifting device generally changes the energy roughly with a variable thickness absorber. In case of the proton facility installed in National Cancer Center Hospital East in Japan, the energy of the proton beams extracted from the AVF cyclotron is fixed at 235 MeV, and an energy absorber device made of graphite was installed behind the accelerator. By using the absorber, four energies of beam as 110, 150, 190 and 235 MeV are supplied to the beam delivery system. In the transport system, a beam collimator was installed just behind the absorber device and it works to maintain the optics of the beam transport.

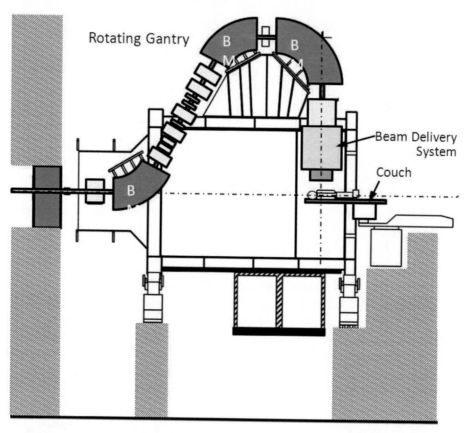

Figure 6. Schema of a typical gantry system for proton therapy.

The typical beam transport system is comprised of several magnets: the quadrupole magnets, steering magnets and bending magnets. The proton beams from the accelerator are delivered by the bending magnets to each treatment room. The quadrupole magnets and steering magnets control the condition of the beam optics, such as the orbit gradient and the beam position, and the beam slits downstream of the bending magnets, reduce the momentum width of the proton beams. Furthermore, some beam monitors installed at appropriate locations along the beam path measure the beam condition necessary to control the beam orbit. The beam condition changes, depending on the energy of each beam and the angle of the rotating gantry. Thus, fine-tuning and control for each device are necessary for each condition. Utilizing the system comprised of these devices enables adequate transport of the proton beams to each beam delivery system in the treatment rooms.

3.2.2. Rotating gantry

To allow beam transport with the greatest flexibility for irradiation of the patient, a rotating gantry mounting a beam delivery system was developed. Many hospital-based proton therapy facilities have employed the rotating gantry and a number of the gantries have been installed at these facilities. The rotating gantry allows the beam direction to rotate 360° around the patient on the treatment couch. A schematic diagram of the rotating gantry installed in the PMRC at the University of Tsukuba Hospital is shown in Figure 6. The typical gantry consists of several bending magnets, which can eventually bend the maximum energy beam in the direction toward the couch. In the case of PMRC, the beam is bent along the gantry through a total bend of 210°; one 60° bend followed by a 150° bend (60° + 90°), as shown in Figure 6. Some quadrupole focusing elements are also installed between the bending magnets. To perform accurate irradiation with the beam at any gantry angle, the heavy magnets must be tightly supported in order to constrain the discrepancy between the central beam axis and the axis of rotation of the gantry within a diameter sphere ± 1 mm, as the gantry rotates. The size of a conventional gantry can be as large as approximately 5 meters in radius, in order to mount the beam delivery system. Accordingly, the apparatus requires a rigid structure with a diameter of 10 m, a length of 10 m and with a total weight of up to 200 tons. The dimension also influences the size and cost of the shielded room containing the apparatus. To alleviate the concern regarding the dimensions of the gantry structure, a corkscrew-type gantry, which arranges the bending magnets in a spiral manner, was proposed by Koehler [36], and enables the overall length of the gantry to be reduced. Recent proton therapy facilities have begun to employ the corkscrew-type gantry, as described below. Furthermore, the Paul Scherrer Institute (PSI) has proposed a compact gantry system that only turns 190° [37], which only works in conjunction with a 180° couch rotation. The advanced gantry system allows a significant reduction of the footprint and the dimensions of the facility, and provides easy access to the patient in the treatment room. The concept of the half-turn gantry has been applied to the innovative compact proton therapy system described below.

3.3. Advanced Compact Facilities

The technologies for the particle therapy are continually being improved, and some innovative ideas and concepts are being put into practical use. The trends of these improvements, in terms of the facilities, appear to be the establishment of a "single treatment room" and "downsizing". There are important factors to facilitating the widespread implementation of proton therapy. The recently developed compact and advanced facilities are introduced.

3.3.1. Vertically structured single treatment room facility

In Japan, the use of single gantry-based proton therapy facilities is increasing. Several heavy industry manufacturers have designed and produced a compact vertically structured facility. A compact synchrotron or cyclotron is installed at the bottom floor of the hospital, and a rotating gantry enclosed within an irradiation room is located immediately above the accelerator. The beam transport system connecting the accelerator and the gantry is set up vertically. In the case of a synchrotron-based facility, the diameter of the accelerator is approximately 5 meters, due to the application of the modern ring structure, comprised of four sets of 90° sector bending magnets. Furthermore, the overall length of the gantry space is shortened by the application of the corkscrew-type gantry. Thus, a minimal footprint facility has been realized by the combination of these recent technologies.

A cyclotron-based vertically structured facility manufactured by Sumitomo Heavy Industry, Ltd. was installed in Aizawa hospital in Matsumoto, Japan in 2012. A compact synchrotron-based vertically structured proton therapy facility was also commercialized by Mitsubishi Electric Corporation in 2012.

3.3.2. Accelerator-mounted gantry based compact proton therapy device

Application of superconducting technology to the accelerator has enabled further downsizing of the radiotherapy facilities. Mevion Medical systems, Inc. and Massachusetts Institute of Technology (MIT) developed a compact synchrocyclotron for proton therapy using a double ring-superconducting magnet. The magnet has achieved a strong magnetic field of 10 Tesla in the superconducting state at 4 Kelvin. The synchrocyclotron generates a 250 MeV proton beam that can deliver therapeutic doses to 32 cm in depth. The beam current is 100 nA, and it is therefore possible to provide an absorbed dose of 10 Gy / min. The dimension of the superconducting-based synchrocyclotron is 1.8 meters in diameter and 18 tons in weight. It is noteworthy that the accelerator is mounted on the frame of a rotating gantry, allowing it to be compact and light. Furthermore, the extracted beam from the accelerator enters the beam nozzle directly, because the beam exit port of the accelerator is connected to the beam delivery system. This progressive approach has enabled the elimination of the need for the beam transport system to be situated between the accelerator and the beam delivery system but also removes the need for an accelerator room. Consequently, the amount of shielding and its space have also decreased. The absence of the transport system also contributes to eliminate the troubles caused by malfunction of the system. Furthermore, as the device also employs the half-turn gantry method, mentioned above, the gantry with the accelerator can only turn 190°. Therefore, the innovative application of a complex of several technologies for downsizing has allowed the dimensions of the facility to be reduced dramatically. The first such commercially-produced device has been installed in Barnes-Jewish Hospital in Washington University in Missouri, USA, and the first therapy using the device was performed at the end of 2013.

4. Beam Delivery

Proton beams that are delivered by an accelerator are narrow with mono-energy, and their Bragg peak is localized over a small region. In the nozzle of the gantry, the beam size and the energy distribution must be modified to achieve dose distribution covering the target volume within the patient's body.

4.1. Beam Modification Techniques

The proton beams must be modified to fulfill the following requirements.

(1) to expand the beam in a transverse plane to irradiate the whole tumor
(2) to adjust the proton energy according to the maximum depth of the tumor
(3) to increase the energy spread to uniformly irradiate a thick tumor
(4) to make corrections to take into account the shape of the tumor and any non-uniformity of the normal tissue, through which the proton beam passes.

To expand the beam in a transverse (lateral) plane, static and dynamic broadening methods have been applied in the beam delivery systems. Figure 7 shows a schematic view of beam broadening by a double scatterer [38]. This is one of the static broadening methods. On the first scatterer, which has the optimized thickness of metal for the incident energy of protons, a thin beam with diameter of less than 1 cm is expanded in the angular space. The second scatterer has a cylindrical structure with high Z (atomic number) material in the center region and low Z material in the outer region. The high Z material allows for additional broadening for the center region of the Gaussian shape of the broadened beam by the first scatterer. The water equivalent thickness of the low Z material should be the same as that of the material of the center region. Through the use of these two scatterers, the lateral shape of the beam is modified to a trapezoidal shape, with flatness in the center region. By collimating the flat intensity distribution, one can achieve a static and flat dosed area that covers the target in the lateral plane, crossing the iso-center, the center of rotation of the irradiation axis.

Figure 8 shows a schematic view of beam broadening using a wobbling magnet [39, 40]. While this is a dynamic broadening method, it is usually used for static beam delivery because it exhibits little interplay effect during the moving of the beam. In this method, the scatterer expands the thin beam in the angular space. As a typical case of beam wobbling, simple circular rotation is illustrated in the figure. By collimating the flat region of the intensity distribution, one can achieve a flat dosed area that covers the target in the lateral plane crossing the iso-center. In this method of beam broadening, the effective size of the source point on the scatterer is relatively small. This causes a small penumbra with the lateral dose distribution.

In the dynamic beam delivery system, beam broadening can be achieved by accumulating small dosed areas using spot scanning or continuous raster scanning, as shown in Figure 9.

To adjust the proton energy according to the maximum depth of the tumor, several types of range shifters or fine degraders have been applied in the beam delivery systems. Figure 10 shows a schematic view of energy degradation by binary- and wedge-type range shifters [39, 40]. This equipment can cause energy degradation by changing the thickness of the material. The binary-type range shifter uses plastic boards with thicknesses that change in a binary manner, such as 1, 2, 4, 8, 16, 32, 64 and 128 mm. Stacking boards, which are selected by the binary code, can achieve the required thickness with the resolution of the smallest thinnest board, 1mm.

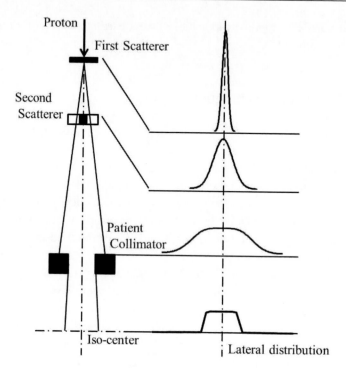

Figure 7. Beam broadening by the double scatterer.

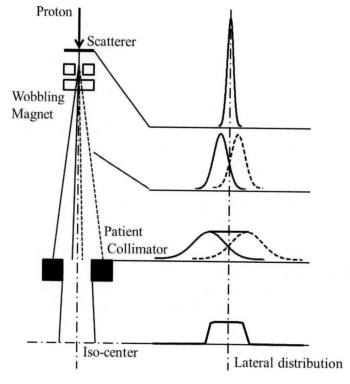

Figure 8. Beam broadening by the Wobbling magnet.

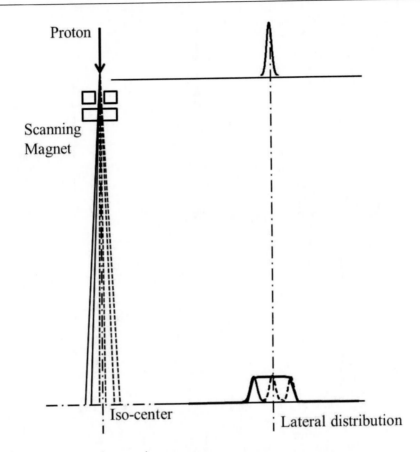

Figure 9. Beam broadening by the scanning magnet.

The spread out Bragg peak (SOBP) can be achieved by stacking the energy shifted Bragg peak with a ridge filter or rotating wheel [39, 40], as shown in Figure 11. The treatment planning system can estimate the water equivalent thickness of the target volume by using 3-dimensional data of the density calculated from the CT data. To achieve uniform irradiation of a thick tumor, mixing of the proton beam energy is optimized. The SOBP filters are designed to facilitate the energy mixing. By using the ridge filter, one can achieve a static field with flat spreading of the peak.

To obtain good conformity on the distal end of the target volume, it is necessary to take into account the shape of the tumor and non-uniformity of the normal tissue through which the proton beam passes.

The treatment planning system can estimate the water equivalent depth of the distal end of the target volume by using 3-dimensional data of the density calculated from the CT data.

In the static beam delivery system, the depth of the dosed area is controlled by changing the thickness of the bolus to achieve coverage of the distal end of the target, as shown in Figure 12(a). In the scanning method, coverage of the distal end of the target can be achieved by changing the energy for each spot or each layer of dose stacking, as shown in Figure 12 (b).

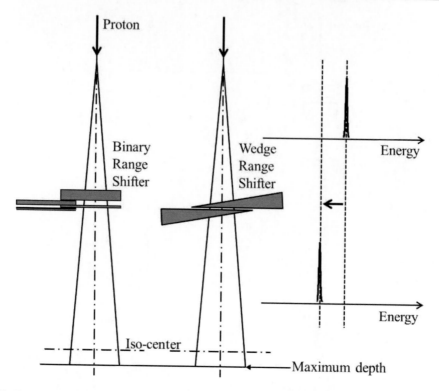

Figure 10. Energy degradation by binary-type and wedge-type range shifters.

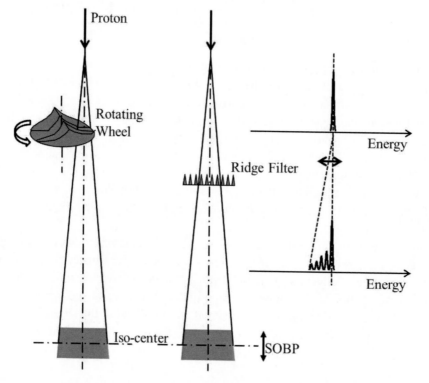

Figure 11. Energy modulation by the SOBP filters, rotating wheel and ridge.

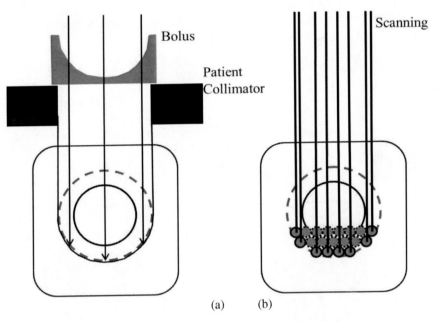

Figure 12. Energy compensation by the bolus (a) and energy stacking in the scanning method (b).

4.2. Characteristics of the Dose Distribution

Figure 13 shows a schematic view of the dose distribution by the static beam delivery system (a) and the dynamic beam delivery system (b). In the case of the static method, the SOBP is constant for any lateral position because of the characteristics of the SOBP filter, as described above. This causes expansion of 100% of the dosed volume in the upstream area of the beam incident. Compared with the static method, the dosed area is better controlled using the scanning method; thus, conformity of the dosed volume to the target volume can be achieved. Based upon the differences in the dose distribution between the two methods, a portion of the full (100%) dosed volume on the normal tissue in Figure 13 (a) is reduced to 90 or 80% of the dosed volume in Figure 13 (b).

Table 1 presents a comparison between the static and dynamic methods. The advantage of the static method is the motion tolerance due to minimization of the interplay effect between target movement and beam delivery. The effect will appear mainly as an increase in the lateral penumbra. Due to the preparation of the bolus and the patient collimator, adaptive therapy cannot be performed easily using the static method. Since there is no need for preparation of the filter, one characteristic advantage of the dynamic method in scanning is the easy achievement of the adaptive therapy to the changing situation around the target. Minimal generation of neutrons, as a secondary radiation, is also an attractive characteristic of the scanning method. The problem of the interplay effect between target motion and dynamic beam delivery is a considerable point. If a large size scanning pencil beam is adopted to suppress the interplay effect, we will get a large lateral penumbra, as indicated in the table. Repainting is also an effective approach to suppress the interplay effect. To achieve a practical system for the scanning method, it is necessary to optimize the motion tolerance, penumbra and time for the irradiation. One simple solution for such optimization is the use of fast scanning with small beam size and repainting.

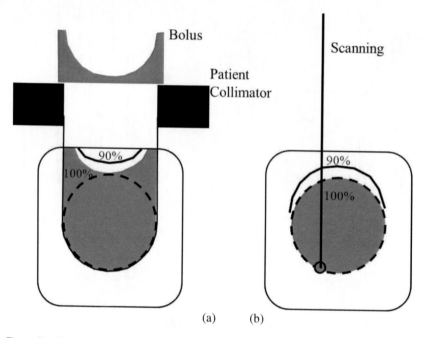

Figure 13. Dose distribution by the static method (a) and the dynamic method (b).

Table 1. Comparison between the static and dynamic methods

	Static method	Dynamic method
Conformal	not bad	good
Motion tolerance	good	requires repainting
IMPT	not able	able
Penumbra	5-10mm	5-20mm
Adaptive	not easy	easy
Secondary radiation	0.1-0.2%	<0.1%

4.3. Example of the Beam Delivery System

A schematic view of the beam delivery system used in the Proton Medical Research Center at the University of Tsukuba is shown as Figure 14. The static method is adopted in this case to achieve beam spread in the transverse plane. The double scattering method, described in [38], is applied to achieve sufficient beam spreading in the distance (3.2 m) from the first scatterer to the target position, which is illustrated as the iso-center. The thickness of the first scatterer and the type of the second scatterer can be set automatically for different respective energies. By using this method, the flatness of the irradiation field is sensitive to deviation of the beam position on the second scatterer. Therefore, we installed a flatness monitor to check the homogeneity of the dose at the target. The maximum usable irradiation field is a 15 cm square. The maximum depth covered is 31 g/cm^2. Accelerator energies of 155, 200, 230 and 250 MeV are used to cover the region to a wide depth. To make fine adjustments to the energy, a binary type range shifter (fine degrader) is installed in the beam preparation system. This can cause range shifts of 0 to 127 mm water equivalent lengths with a step size of 1 mm. A ridge filter expands the energy spread to an extent corresponding to the thickness of the tumor. This creates an appropriate spread of Bragg peaks (SOBP) for each tumor. A rotating changer can introduce a ridge filter into the beam, which is designed to produce the required spread of between 0 mm and 120 mm. A bolus (range compensator) is machined from an artificial wooden material (chemical wood), which is positioned above the final collimator to correct the maximum proton energy in the lateral plane, following the configuration of the tumor. The bolus and the collimator are identified by a 2-dimensional bar-code pattern.

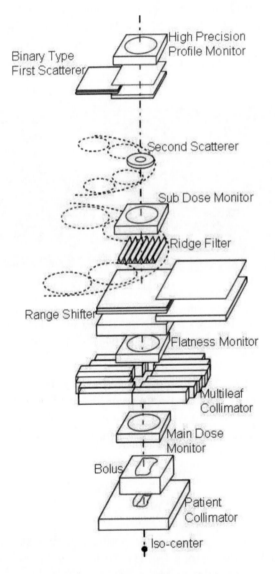

Figure 14. Schematic view of the beam delivery system with the double scatterer.

5. Method of Respiratory Control

The characteristic dose distribution of the proton beam, the Bragg-Peak (BP), is suitable to provide a good contrast of the dose distribution between tumor and normal tissue. This dose distribution is calculated by the treatment planning system (TPS) based on CT data. Therefore minimizing the positional reproducible error of tumor and normal tissue from the CT data is important to achieve the planned proton therapy. Although there are various factors to reduce the positional reproducibility of the tumor and normal tissue, error factors are categorized into two time-domain conceptions: inter-fractional error and intra-fractional error.

Inter-fractional error of tumor and normal tissue arises from daily differences of the patient immobilization and the volume of internal structure. This reproducibility is checked by comparison with the Digital Reconstructed Radiography (DRR) calculated by using CT image (Figure 15) and the kV X-ray image taken just before irradiation of treatment beam. The 3D reproducibility of tumor position is achieved principally by at least checking bi-planar X-ray images. This technique is described as Image Guided Radiotherapy (IGRT) and effectively reduces the inter-fraction error.

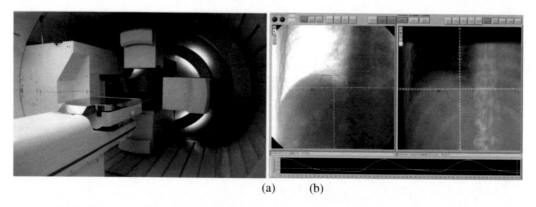

(a)   (b)

Figure 15. Display of the IGRT system at the University of Tsukuba (a). Left and right images represent a fluoroscopic image and the DRR (b), respectively. The waveform below is an external respiration signal. Red line indicates an outline of the target region. The small green square indicates the position of a metallic fiducial marker.

Intra-fractional error is mainly caused by respiratory motion during irradiation. This 4D reproducibility of the tumor position is important for treatment of tumors in the liver because the amplitude of the liver motion with respiration is generally larger than that of the inter-fractional motion. In the following sections, we focus on intra-fractional error and respiratory control methods.

5.1. Respiratory Motion of the Liver

A large number of studies of respiratory motion of tumors have been well summarized in the report of the AAPM Task Group 76 [41]. To identify the location of liver tumor, X-ray fluoroscopy is generally used, with a hi-Z metallic fiducial marker implanted in the liver, because the liver cannot be seen by fluoroscopy. Figure 16 shows some types of metallic fiducial markers. These metallic fiducial markers are implanted in the vicinity of the liver tumor in the patient before treatment in order to check the position of tumor during planning and for every fraction. Figure 17 shows a typical respiratory motion pattern of the liver. Although abdominal organ motion with respiration is very complex, the amplitude of motion is mainly in the superior-inferior (SI) direction. The amplitude of motion for the liver and diaphragm in the SI direction is 12-25 mm during shallow breathing and 35 - 55 mm during deep breathing. It is obvious that there is strong dependency of the breathing mode. The respiratory cycle is normally 3-4 s. While the amplitude and cycle of liver motion are not exactly regular, in general, the positional stability of the exhalation phase is better than that of the inhalation phase. This is because that the volume of air drawn into lung due to diaphragm motion is not consistent for every breath. Furthermore, it is also known that the exhalation phase generally lasts longer than the inhalation phase, as shown in Figure 17.

Table 2. Amplitude of motion of the liver and diaphragm. The mean range of motion and the (minimum-maximum) ranges in mm. The motion is in the superior- inferior (SI) direction. This table is modified from AAPM TG76 table 3

Site	observer	Breathing mode	
		Shallow	Deep
Liver	Weiss et al.	13 +/- 5	-
	Harauz et al.	14	-
	Suramo et al.	25 (10-40)	55 (30-80)
	Davies et al.	10 (5-17)	37 (21-57)
Diaphragm	Wade	17	101
	Korin et al.	13	39
	Davies et al.	12 (7-28)	43 (25-57)
	Weiss et al.	13 +/- 5	-
	Giraud et al.	-	35 (3-95)
	Ford et al.	20 (13-31)	-

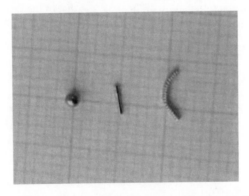

Figure 16. Metallic fiducial markers. Left : f2 mm gold sphere, Middle: f 0.6 mm, length 5 mm cylindrical platinum-coated iridium, Right: f 0.75 mm coil shape gold.

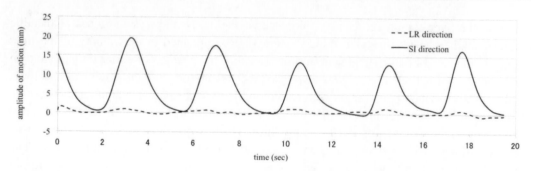

Figure 17. A typical respiratory motion pattern of the liver. The solid and dashed lines indicate liver motion in the SI and LR directions, respectively.

The liver motion with respiration can be estimated by the surface motion of the patient's abdomen near the diaphragm (Figure 18). This is because that there is a strong positive correlation between organ motion and surface motion of the abdomen near the diaphragm (Figure 19). This correlation differs for every patient and the correlation can change over prolonged observation. Previous studies have reported that the correlation ranges from 0.7-0.9 [41].

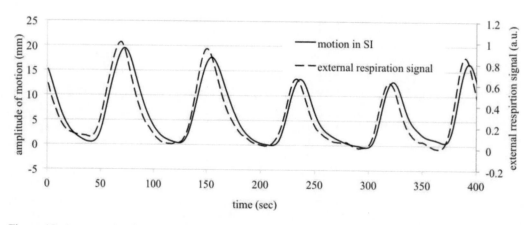

Figure 18. An example of the motion pattern of the liver and that of the respiration signal.

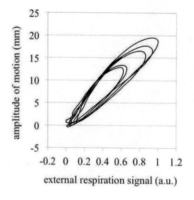

Figure 19. An example of the correlation with the motion pattern of the liver and that of the respiration signal.

5.2. Respiratory Control Method

The most effective and simple way to deal with respiratory motion is to limit timing of the CT scan or beam irradiation to a pre-defined phase: the Gating method. The respiratory exhalation phase is generally the most appropriate for this pre-defined phase because the organ motion is more stable during exhalation and the duration of exhalation is longer than inhalation, as noted previously. Figure 20 shows the timing structure for respiratory-gated beam extraction. From the perspective of CT imaging, selection of the exhalation phase is also suitable because, during the 0.5 s scan time required for the rotation of a general CT detector, organ motion should be minimized to reduce a motion artifact of the CT image.

Respiratory gating method for the treatment of liver tumor is categorized mainly as follows:

(1) Gating method using an external respiration signal
(2) Gating method using fluoroscopy

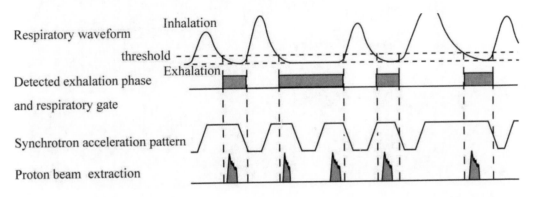

Figure 20. Timing structure of respiratory gated beam extraction. Detection of the exhalation phase gates the proton beam extraction.

(1) Gating method using an external respiration signal

The principle of this gating method using an external respiration signal was devised at the University of Tsukuba [29]. The motion of the skin surface of the patient's abdomen is generally used to monitor the external respiration waveform. From this waveform and adequate setting of thresholds, a gating signal for imaging or treatment is generated. There are mainly two types of detection methods.

The first method is direct measurement using a laser displacement sensor (Figure 21), which generates a waveform from a distance between the abdomen skin surface and the sensor in real-time. The AZ-733V (Anzai Medical Co.) is a system that is typically used for this method. An amplitude threshold can be set for the waveform to generate the gate for imaging or treatment.

The second method is indirect measurement using both an infrared reflective marker and an infrared tracking camera. The Real-time Position Management (RPM) system (Varian Medical System Co.) is a system that is typically used for this method. The infrared reflective marker is placed on the surface of the patient's abdomen and is captured as a video image by the infrared camera. The position of the marker for each frame is calculated automatically using a machine learning function. The gate for imaging or treatment is generated when the detected marker position is within a pre-defined range of amplitude or within a pre-defined phase.

An accuracy of the irradiation of these methods depends on the stability of the motion correlation between the tumor and the skin surface of patient.

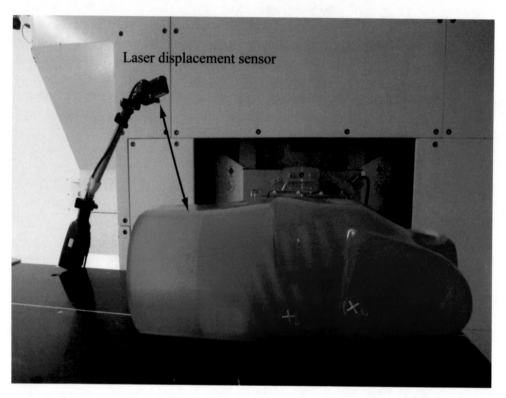

Figure 21. Laser displacement sensor for respiratory gating method at University of Tsukuba.

(2) Gating method using fluoroscopy

The first gating method using fluoroscopy, i.e., the Real-Time Tumor-Tracking (RTRT) system was developed at Hokkaido University (Figure 22) [42]. This system has a set of four kV X-ray fluoroscopic imaging units mounted around the MV X-ray Liniac system. This system can detect the position of 2 mm gold sphere markers implanted in the vicinity of the tumor with an accuracy of ±1 mm for each 33 ms during irradiation automatically by a machine learning function. The treatment beam is irradiated when the detected marker position is within the prescribed permissible range. With the exception of the case of marker migration, the RTRT system has sufficient accuracy and the reliability is higher than that of the gating system using an external respiratory signal. The disadvantage of this method is to increase the additional dose by the fluoroscopy to the patient during treatment. However, it has been reported that the amount of the additional dose is approximately 1% of the treatment beam and is within the clinical tolerance level. Hokkaido University plans to combine this RTRT system with a scanning irradiation system for proton therapy.

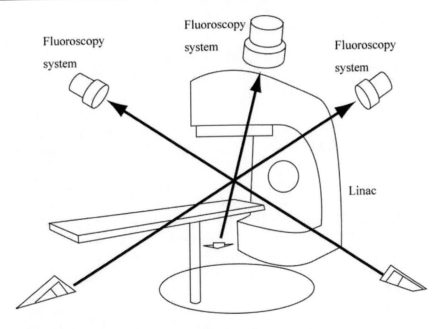

Figure 22. Illustration of RTRT system at Hokkaido University.

6. Principle of Radiation Therapy for Hepatocellular Carcinoma

6.1. Background

Historically, whole-liver irradiation was employed for the treatment of tumors in the liver, until the mid-1980s. This was because of the immaturity of both diagnostic imaging of the liver and the precision of radiotherapeutic technologies for moving targets. Ingold reported a dose-complication relationship for whole-liver irradiation in 1965 [43]. Radiation-induced liver disease (RILD) was observed in 1/8 patients who received 30-35 Gy over 3-4 weeks, and in 12/27 patients who received > 35 Gy over the same time-span. Hence, whole-liver irradiation has been performed for the palliative treatment of liver tumors.

In the 1990s, computer-assisted diagnosis and treatment planning led to partial liver radiation therapy, and dose escalation studies could be conducted. CT has allowed the local diagnosis of tumors, which has facilitated the application of partial liver irradiation for cases with a small number of lesions and tumor sizes within an acceptable range. With advances in treatment planning, it has become recognized that the tolerance dose for the liver with partial irradiation is completely different from that with whole liver irradiation, and now, treatment of intrahepatic localized lesions aims to achieve local control by irradiation. Localized intrahepatic tumors can now be irradiated with curative intent.

In this part, tolerance of the liver to ionizing radiation, and the clinical outcome of radiation therapy of hepatocellular carcinoma with photons and protons will be described.

6.2. Tolerance of the Liver to Ionizing Radiation

Radiation-induced liver disease (RILD) has long been reported as one of the most important treatment-related complications contributing to the difficulty of hepatic radiation therapy. Whole-liver radiation therapy has been found to be limited and unsatisfactory for patients with HCC, mainly due to the poor hepatic tolerance to ionizing radiation. Knowledge regarding tolerance of the liver to radiation therapy, however, has continued to accumulate over the past 30 years. RILD is now distinguished as either "classic" or "nonclassic" RILD [44].

Classic RILD is characterized by anicteric hepatomegaly, ascites and elevation of alkaline phosphatase levels at least two-fold greater than the upper normal limit. Classic RILD typically occurs between 2 weeks and 3 months after therapy. Pathologically, occlusion and obliteration of the central vein of the hepatic lobules, retrograde coagulation, and secondary hepatocyte necrosis are observed [45]. Classic RILD can occur in patients who have otherwise fairly well functioning pretreatment livers. Thus, the treatment options for this disease entity are very limited, and liver failure and death can result.

Emami reported that the dose leading to classical RILD, 5 years after whole liver irradiation, was 30 Gy / 15 times, at a probability of 5% [46]. RTOG 84-05 reported that the incidence of RILD caused by whole liver irradiation at a single dose of 1.5 Gy twice a day was 0/122 when the total dose was 27-30 Gy compared with 5/51 (9.8%) when the total dose was 33 Gy. In either case, it was impossible to control tumors for a sustained period of time at these doses.

Nonclassic RILD is characterized by elevated liver transaminase at least five-fold greater than the upper normal limit, or a decline in liver function (a worsening of the Child-Pugh score by 2 or more) in the absence of classic RILD, and can occur between 1 week and 3 months after therapy. The pathological background of nonclassic RILD remains unclear. These clinical manifestations have been described in HCC patients [44, 47, 48].

Advances in imaging, radiation planning, motion management and image guidance at the time of radiation delivery have made the delivery of ablative doses irradiation to focal liver tumors possible. However, it has been shown that only limited cases can be safely irradiated at a high dose, due to this nonclassic RILD. The incidence of nonclassic RILD after partial liver irradiation are reported in the literature [44, 49-51]. The significant parameters, to which greater importance have been attached, are the mean liver dose and V 30 (volume receiving > 30 Gy).

Among the factors increasing the risk of RILD, Child B,C poor liver function [44, 51-54], hepatitis B virus carrier, involvement of transcatheter chemoembolization, TACE [54] and portal vein tumor thrombosis, PVTT [48, 54-56] have been reported. There have also been reports of the analyses of cases treated with proton beam therapy. Kawashima reported the importance of V_{30} and ICG R15, in which proton-induced hepatic insufficiency (PHI) did not develop in patients with an ICG R15 lower than 20%, but V30 < 25% was recommended for patients with an ICG R15 of 20-50% [57]. In patients who have an ICG R15 ≥ 50%, the indication for proton beam therapy should be considered with extreme caution, in order to prevent life-threatening PHI. Mizumoto reported that liver function after proton beam therapy is significantly related to the percentage volume of the normal liver, i.e., not irradiated [58]. Four out of 7 patients who died of liver failure without tumor progression after proton beam therapy had an ICG R15 > 40%. It is obvious that the avoidance of additional doses to the surrounding normal liver tissue is important to maintain liver function after proton beam therapy.

There have been several reports on the changes in images after partial liver irradiation. In regions exposed to high-dose proton beam therapy, typical RILD has been visualized as low attenuation area on CT before contrast enhancement and as high attenuation area on contrast CT, 3-4 months after irradiation in 95.3% of cases [59-61]. On MRI, regions with low intensity on T1-weighted imaging and high intensity on T2-weighted imaging have been reported, and their intense and prolonged enhancement during dynamic study became significant after 13 months compared to those within 3 months after irradiation. These were histologically confirmed to be composed of collapsed lobules with hepatic small vein occlusions and rich extracellular matrices which retained extracellular fluid [62].

6.3. Conventional Radiotherapy for HCC

In the era of whole liver irradiation, a response rate of 20% was unachieveable [63-65]. Thus, neither the local effects nor the long-term follow-up results reached satisfactory levels.

However, partial liver irradiation has become possible, and consequently the therapeutic outcomes have gradually improved. In recent reports, the dose has increased to 50-60 Gy, and the local response rate in combination with TACE [54, 56, 66-68] or arterial injection [69] or irradiation alone [70, 71] has been 57-67%, and the median survival time (MST) was reported to be 10-35 months (Table 3). Thus, on meta-analysis, improvements of both the survival and response rates have been reported as a result of TACE + radiation therapy [72]. However, the 2-year survival rate continues to be about 40% in many reports, and long-term survival cannot be easily expected.

Intrahepatic metastasis and recurrence in other regions distant from the irradiated field have emerged as a recent issue. Zhao et al. are currently performing a phase I/II study in which sorafenib administration is continued as maintenance therapy following radiation therapy after TACE in patients with a 5 cm or larger solitary HCC, and the results are anticipated [73].

6.4. Proton Beam Therapy for HCC

Utilizing the characteristic of the dose distribution of proton beams, i.e., the capacity to markedly reduce the dose for regions deeper than the target, the dose for tumors can be set at a higher level in proton beam therapy. At the same time, the non-exposed non-cancerous regions can be secured in a large volume, which may increase the safety in liver cirrhosis patients with low hepatic function. These properties have facilitated the establishment of high single and total doses in proton beam therapy compared with those in conventional fractionated X-ray radiotherapy. As a result, outcomes of HCC treatment have been reported to markedly supercede those achieved by X-ray radiotherapy [57, 58, 74-79].

Table 3. Clinical results of photon therapy for HCC with or without transcatheter treatment

Author	year	Pt	treatment	dose (Gy)	response rate (%)	MST (M)	OS (%)	comment
Park W	2005	59	RT alone	30 - 55	66.1	10	27.4/ 2Y	
Kim DY	2005	59	RT alone	30 – 54	45.8	responder 10.7	40.7/ 1Y	PVTT
						non responder 5.3	25.0/ 1Y	PVTT
Ben-Josef E	2005	128	RT + i.a.	60.75		15.8	17 / 3Y	
Seong J	2003	158	RT: 51 RT+TACE :107	48.2	67.1	16	30.5/ 2Y 9/ 5Y	
Liang SX	2005	128	RT±TACE	53.6	55	20	65/ 1Y 43/ 2Y 33/ 3Y	
Yamada K	2005	19	RT + TACE	60	57.9	7	10.2/ 2Y	PVTT
Seo YS	2008	65	RT±TACE	61	56.9	responder 346D non responder 212D	34.7/ 12M 27.0/18M	
Koom WS	2010	107	RT + TACE	50.4	35	single nodular 35 M	82/ 1Y 48/ 3Y	
Oh D	2010	40	RT + TACE	54	62.8		72.0/ 1Y 45.6/ 2Y	

In many previous reports, proton beam therapy has been indicted for nodular-type HCC cases in which all lesions can be included in the irradiation field. Essentially, the indication is nodule-forming HCC, as described above, but favorable responses of cases with vascular invasion in the portal vein or inferior vena cava have also been reported [80, 81].

It has also been reported that proton beam therapy is safely applied to patients for whom other therapies are not suitable, due to complications [53] and elderly patients [82], and that irradiation may be possible for patients with serious liver dysfunction if certain conditions are met [52].

Determination of local tumor control after proton beam therapy should be based on the expression of tumor markers and radiographic evaluation. Alpha-fetoprotein (AFP) levels are expected to decrease when the treatment is successful [77, 83]. The AFP nadir is observed between 3 and 6 months after completion of treatment [83].

On radiographic evaluation, it is important to emphasize not only the changes of the tumor itself, but also changes of the surrounding liver parenchyma. The irradiated tumor is recognized as a nodule in the hepatic parenchyma suffering from radiation-induced liver injury on both CT and MRI [59, 60]. The importance of dynamic study for the differentiation between HCC and RILD has been reported [84]. Recurrent tumors and the irradiated area tend to exhibit similar image characteristics: low intensity in T(1)-WI and high intensity in T(2)-WI. In a gadolinium-enhanced dynamic study, recurrent HCC showed early enhancement, followed by a rapid washout. However, the irradiated liver parenchyma exhibited high intensity from the early phase, and contrast enhancement tended to be more prominent and prolonged at the end of the dynamic studies. However, long-term persistence of hypervascularity of HCC has been reported after irradiation [59, 60, 85]. Therefore, observation of the course of changes in the size is necessary to judge local control.

There have been a few reports on the histological changes that occur in tumors after proton beam therapy. Saito compared MIB-1 labeling index (LI) before and after proton beam therapy, and reported a significant reduction of LI from $13.0 \pm 8.5\%$ to $3.2 \pm 2.4\%$. All lesions that exhibited a reduction of MIB-1 LI at 3 weeks post-proton beam therapy were ultimately diagnosed as completely responsive at 1 year after treatment [86]. Many issues still remain to be investigated, including the assessment of therapeutic efficacy using the latest imaging and histological examination.

7. Treatment Results

Clinical data on the use of proton beam therapy for the treatment of hepatocellular carcinoma (HCC) has been published since 2000. Most of the studies reported are from Japan and the USA. In most of the previous studies, usually one or a few lesions could be included into a single irradiation field, the diameter of the tumor was less than 10 cm, and hepatic function was Child-Pugh class A or B.

7.1. Local Control

Bush et al. reported 34 cases of HCC in 2004 [83]. Their protocol used 63 GyE / 15fr and they reported that AFP levels decreased post treatment and achieved the lowest levels between 3 and 6 months after completion of treatment. In this report, 1 case with non-responsive AFP levels had gross residual disease, and 3 cases showed local recurrence in the treated area. They concluded that the 2-year local control rate (LC) was 75%. In their updated study in 2011, they also reported that 15 of 76 cases showed local failure between 2 and 60 months after treatment [78]. Only 3 of 15 cases experienced local treatment failure without having new lesions develop in other parts of the liver. In this report, a total of 7 cases showed increasing AFP levels, indicating local control failure.

Kawashima et al. reported 30 cases of HCC in 2005 [87]. Their protocol used 72.6 GyE / 16fr and they reported that a total of 24 cases achieved complete disappearance of the primary tumor for 5 to 20 months, 5 cases had residual tumor until death or at last follow up, and only 1 case having a single nodular tumor of 4.2 cm in diameter experienced local recurrence at 5 months after treatment. They reported that 29 of 30 patients were free from local progression until death or at last follow-up, and that the 2-year LC rates were 96%.

Chiba et al. retrospectively reviewed 162 cases of HCC in 2005 [88]. They used various treatment schedules from 55 GyE / 10fr to 92.4 GyE / 24fr and reported that 13 cases showed local recurrence between 7 and 43 months after treatment. The diameter of the tumors that had recurred was from 2.0 to 7.0 cm. However, since the tumor diameter did not show significant relation to the LC rate, they suggested that proton beam therapy could be used to treat patients with relatively large tumors on which conventional local treatments, such as percutaneous ethanol injection, microwave coagulation therapy, and radiofrequently ablation, were not the successful. They reported that the 5-year LC rate was 86.9%.

Hata et al. retrospectively reviewed 19 cases of HCC whose hepatic function was Child-Pugh C class [89]. They tested various treatment schedules between 55-92.4 GyE / 10-24fr and reported that the objective response (complete or partial response) was 63%, and all but one of the irradiated tumors was controlled at the median follow-up period of 17 months.

Fukumitsu et al. reported on 51cases of HCC in which the tumors were not adjacent to either the porta hepatis or the digestive organs in 2009 [90]. Their protocol used 66 GyE / 10fr and they reported that 3 cases showed local recurrence at 16, 18, and 41 months after treatment. They also found that the LC rate had no relationship among the prior treatments, number of tumors, tumor diameter, and AFP level. They reported that the 5-year LC rate was 87.8% (Figure 23).

Mizumoto et al. reported in 2008 on 53 cases of HCC in which the tumors were located adjacent to the porta hepatis [91]. Their protocol used 72.6 GyE / 22fr and they reported that 3 cases of HCC which were adjacent to the porta hepatis developed a local recurrence at 7, 14, and 30 months after treatment and simultaneously developed new liver tumors outside the irradiated area. They reported that the 3-years LC rate was 86%. They also retrospectively reviewed a total of 266 cases treated by 3 different treatment protocols (66 GyE / 10fr, 72.6 GyE / 22fr, and 77 GyE / 35fr) in 2011 [92]. They reported that the LC rate was 98, 87, and 81% at 1, 3, and 5 years, respectively. They concluded that no significant difference of LC rate was found among the 3 different protocols, and no prognostic factor for the response rate was also found in their review of 266 cases.

Komatsu et al. reported 242 cases of HCC in 2011 [55]. They used various treatment schedules between 52.8 GyE / 4fr to 84 GyE / 20fr and reported that the 5-year overall survival rate was 38%. They investigated whether the irradiation dose could affect the LC rate and found that the irradiation did not affect the LC rate.

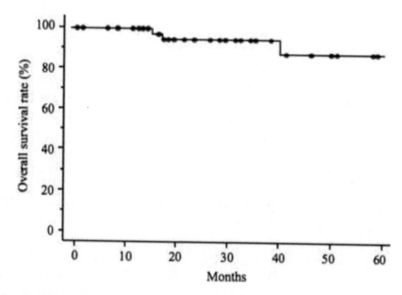

Figure 23. Local control rate at 66 GyE / 10 fractions reported by Fukumitsu N et al., University of Tsukuba. The 5-year local control rate is 87.8%.

Niizawa et al. investigated the change of blood flow after proton beam therapy using ultrasonography (US) [93]. They found a transient increase of blood flow in the tumor in more than half of the patients. At longer periods after irradiation, blood flow was gradually decreased and it was significantly reduced after 9 months. They also reported that this US finding was consistent with computed tomography (CT) and magnetic resonance imaging (MRI) findings. In our experience, several HCC cases showed no tumor size change and no tumor marker reduction during the treatment course, while a gradual reduction in both was observed several months later. Enhancement in a study of CT or MRI is sometimes found a few months after treatment. It is not unusual to find a necrotic mass in the liver long after treatment, especially in large HCC. Figure 24 shows a case of the change in HCC after proton beam therapy.

Taken together, the LC rate of HCC with single or multiple tumors that can be treated in a single irradiation field is about 85-90% at 3 years and 80-90% at 5 years. There are few differences among the tumor lesion types, and tumor shrinkage can be seen several months later. The definition of local control was not completely the same among the research groups. Japanese groups use similar evaluation criteria, that is, "no sign of regrowth and no new tumors in the treated volume". In contrast, groups from the USA include in addition to no new tumor growth "AFP elevation without any radiographic disease progression outside of the primary treatment area" which is more strict than the Japanese definition. The more strict definition of LC may be the main reason for the difference of LC rates between the USA and Japanese studies.

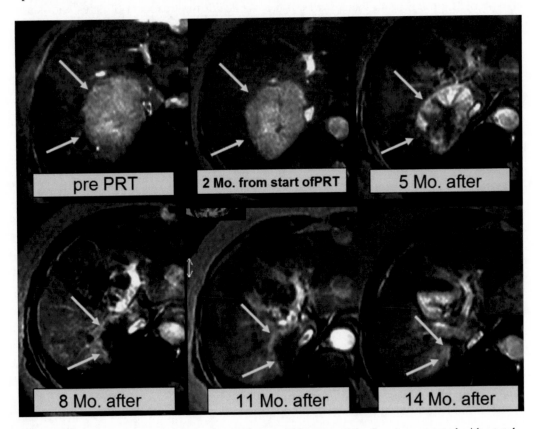

Figure 24. Change in HCC after proton beam therapy. This tumor (10 x 7 cm) was treated with a total of 81 GyE / 27 fractions. The tumor size was gradually decreased, then disappeared at 14 months after treatment.

7.2. Survival

Bush et al. reported that the 2-year overall survival (OS) rate of 34 cases was 55% [83]. Kawashima et al. reported that the OS rates of 30 cases were 77, 66, and 62% at 1, 2, and 3 years [87]. They also found that the 2-year OS rate of the cases where the indocyanine green clearance test employing a retention rate at 15 minutes (ICG R15) ≤ 40% was significantly higher than that of the cases with ICG R15 > 40% (80 and 30%, respectively).

Chiba et al. reported that the 5-year OS rate of 162 cases was 23.5% in their retrospective report [88]. They found that the 5-year OS rate of cases with chronic hepatitis and Child-Pugh class A were significantly better than for those with Child-Pugh class B and C cirrhosis. No significant difference was found between patients with Child-Pugh class B and C cirrhosis (Child-Pugh class A: 35.1%, B: 10.3%, C: 0%). With regard to the number of tumors, the OS rate of the 80 cases with solitary lesions was significantly higher than that of the 82 cases with multiple lesions. The causes of death were tumor progression (46.9%) and hepatic failure (37.9%).

Hata et al. reported that the 2-year OS rate of selected HCC patients whose hepatic function was Child-Pugh class C was 42% [89]. They found that even cases with Child-Pugh class C could survive longer than the reported OS of the patients treated only with supportive care. They concluded that although most of the previous studies selected cases of Child-Pugh class A or B, proton beam therapy was also a viable for the treatment of cases with severe hepatic function.

Fukumitsu et al. reported that the OS rate of 51cases in which the tumor location was not adjacent to either the porta hepatis or the digestive organs was 49.2% at 3 years and 38.7% at 5 years [90]. In this report, the causes of death were tumor progression (71%) and hepatic failure (10%).

Mizumoto et al. reported that the OS rate of 53 cases in which the tumor was located adjacent to the porta hepatis was 57 and 45% at 2 and 3 years [91]. In this report, the 2-year OS rate of 46 cases with Child-Pugh class A was 63.6%, which was significantly higher than 7 cases with either Child-Pugh class B or C (14.3%). With regard to the number of tumors, the 2-year OS rate of the 22 cases with a solitary lesion was 76.3%, which was significantly higher than that of the 31 cases with multiple lesions (43.4%). They reported that the 3-year OS rate of 14 cases who presented as Child-Pugh class A with a solitary HCC and an AFP level less than 100 ng/ml was 83.9% which was an excellent outcome.

The causes of death were intrahepatic recurrence (69.2%), distant metastasis (7.7%), and hepatic failure (11.5%), which were similar to the data in the Fukumitsu et al. report [90]. They also retrospectively reviewed a total of 266 cases treated by 3 different treatment protocols in 2011, and reported that the 5-year OS rate of 198 cases with Child-Pugh class A was 55.1%, which was significantly higher than that of the 61 patients with either Child-Pugh class B or C (11.4%) [92].

In this report, the OS rates of all cases was 61 % at 3-years and 48% at 5-years, and the OS rate of the cases, who were treated using either the 66 GyE / 10fr, 72.6 GyE / 22fr, or 77 GyE / 35fr protocol, were quite similar to each other (Figure 25).

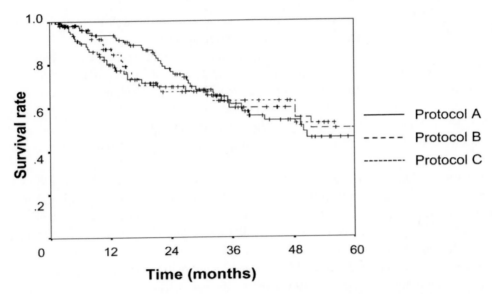

Figure 25. Overall survival rate. The 5-year OS rate is 48% with no significant differences among the 3 different protocols (A: 66 GyE / 10 fractions, B: 72.6 GyE / 22fr, C: 77 GyE / 35fr). The result was reported by M. Mizumoto et al., University of Tsukuba.

Komatsu et al. reported that the 5-year OS rate of 242 cases was 38% [55]. They found that the 5-year OS rate of the 184 cases with Child-Pugh class A was 46.6%, which was significantly higher than that of the 55 cases with Child-Pugh class B (8.7%) and that of the 3 cases with Child-Pugh class C (0%). The prognostic factors were performance status (PS), Child-Pugh class, and vascular invasion.

Taken together, the OS rate of HCC is about 55-65% at 2 years and 20-50% at 5 years. The causes of death are 50-70% due to tumor progression, followed by 10-40% due to hepatic dysfunction. The prognostic factors for survival are hepatic function, and number and size of tumors. Additionally AFP level, PS, and vascular invasion are also included as prognostic factors.

7.3. Adverse Effects

Bush et al. reported that acute adverse effects, such as fatigue, radiation dermatitis, and abdominal discomfort were found in approximately 60% of the patients [83]. None of the patients required hospitalization or interruption of treatment. They also reported small decrease in serum albumin levels and small increase in total serum bilirubin levels after treatment. The serum albumin levels returned to baseline at 6 months, and no patient was clinically jaundiced. They concluded that both the acute and adverse effects of proton beam therapy treatment in HCC were mild. They also found that severe adverse effects more than Grade 3 were not present in acute and in late stage treatment in their updated report in 2011 [78].

Kawashima et al. reported that 8 of 30 cases developed proton-induced hepatic insufficiency involving ascites and/or asterixis without a large elevation of either serum bilirubin or transaminase at 1 to 4 months after treatment [87]. They suggested that V30% in combination with ICG R15 might be a useful indicator for estimation of liver tolerance to proton beam therapy from their dose-volume histogram analysis.

Chiba et al. reported 5 of 162 cases with late adverse effects of Grade 2 or higher [88]. The late adverse effects in 5 cases included fibrotic stenosis of the common bile duct at 13 months, biloma at 29 and 36 months, and gastrointestinal tract bleeding at 4 and 6 months after treatment. No patients died due to the late adverse effects. Some acute adverse effects were noted but they subsided quickly without causing any problems. The acute adverse effects included elevation of aspartate transaminase and alanine transaminase levels in 18 cases.

Fukumitsu et al. reported that 4 of 51 cases showed late adverse effect more than Grade 3, such as 3 cases with a rib fracture at 3-27 months and 1 case of pneumonitis at 3 months [90]. However, no patients died of these late adverse effects. We conclude that patients whose tumor is located close to the body surface should be monitored more carefully with regard to the dose distribution to the skin and ribs.

Mizumoto et al. reported that all 53 cases in which the tumor was located adjacent to the porta hepatis did not show acute or late adverse effects more than Grade 3 [91]. They found that cases with severe late adverse effects, such as fibrotic stenosis of the common bile duct or biloma, had been treated with either 79.2 GyE / 16 fr or 91.3 GyE / 23fr in the Chiba et al. study [74]. Thus, their protocol was 72.6 GyE / 22fr which was a lower dose fractionation schedule and there was no difference in LC rate for tumors located adjacent to the porta hepatis. Consequently, only 5 cases showed Grade 2 acute adverse effects in the skin and in the gastrointestinal tract, and all 53 cases did not show acute and late adverse effects of more than Grade 3. They also retrospectively reviewed a total of 266 cases treated by 3 different treatment protocols in 2011, and reported that the adverse effects that were more than Grade 3 were acute dermatitis in 2, late rib fracture in 3, dermatitis in 1, and perforation, bleeding or inflammation of the digestive tract in 3 [92].

In the treatment of 242 cases, Komatsu et al. reported that all acute toxicities were transient, easily managed, and acceptable [55]. However, 4 cases had late adverse effects including refractory skin ulcers, and 1 case required skin transplantation. Moreover, a salvage drainage operation was required for 1 case of biloma at 10 months after treatment. In addition, although 8 cases showed late adverse effect on hepatic function of more than Grade 3, all of these cases with hematological disorders were asymptomatic and required no further treatment.

Taken together, acute adverse effects, such as dermatitis and hepatic dysfunction, are found in some cases. However they are generally transient, easily managed, and acceptable. With regard to the late adverse effects, bile duct damage, ulcer, dermatitis, and rib fracture potentially occur. However, these late adverse effects are quite rare, and could be avoided using recent fractionation schedules.

7.4. Conclusion

Most previous studies investigated HCC which consisted of a single tumor or a few tumors that were treated in one irradiation field, and hepatic function was Child-Pugh class A or B. The irradiation dose of the proton beam is variable. However, biologically effective doses of 75-100 GyE (α/β=10), and 80-130 GyE (α/β=3) have been used clinically resulting in an LC rate of about 85-90% at 3 years and 80-90% at 5 years. However, intrahepatic recurrence which is feature of HCC is observed in many patients. Consequently, the OS rate is about 55-65% at 2 years and 20-50% at 5 years. The cause of 50-70% of the deaths is tumor progression. The prognostic factors for survival are hepatic function, and number and size of tumors. Adverse effects are quite rare even in the acute and late phases. Table 4 summarized the reports of proton beam therapy for HCC in literature.

8. Treatment Factors for Proton Beam Therapy

8.1. Tumor Volume

There are various treatment options for patients with HCC. Tumor size is an important factor in determining the treatment modalities. For example, percutaneous ethanol injection is inappropriate for tumors larger than 3 cm [94]. Radiofrequency ablation is not usually indicated for tumors larger than 5 cm or for tumors adjacent to a large vessel, such as the portal vein or inferior vena cava [95-97]. Surgery seems the best choice for patients with large HCC, although only less than 20% of the patients are candidates for surgical resection.

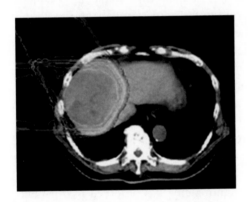 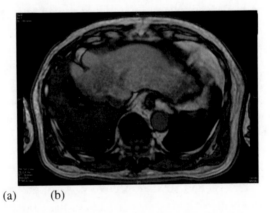

(a)   (b)

Figure 26. (a) Dose distributions for large HCC. Proton beam therapy of 72.6 GyE in 22 fractions was demonstrated. (b) MRI image taken 20 months after completion of proton beam therapy demonstrate tumor shrinkage.

Recently, radical photon radiotherapy has been used occasionally for HCC. The radiation tolerance of the liver is an important consideration and can be determined by the preserved functional capacity [98]. In photon radiotherapy, large tumors require a wide low dose area in normal liver. Therefore, when using photon radiotherapy, only stereotactic body radiotherapy (SBRT) is usually indicated for small tumors less than 5 cm, and large tumors are contraindicated for radical photon radiotherapy. In contrast, proton beams can focus more on the target area due to the Bragg-Peak, and a small number of ports (1-3 ports) can deliver sufficient doses to the tumor.

Therefore, proton beam therapy can offer radical treatment to larger HCC beyond the ability of photon radiotherapy. Sugahara et al. reported the results of 22 patients with large HCC of more than 10 cm in diameter [99]. In that study, the median dose of 72.6 GyE in 22 fractions was delivered (range: 47.3-89.1 GyE in 10-35 fractions). They reported a 2- year local tumor control and an overall survival of 87% (95% confidence interval (CI), 65-100) and 36% (15-56%), respectively. There were no severe toxicities due to the treatment. Figure 26 shows dose distribution of proton for large HCC [99].

The experience of proton beam therapy for large HCC has not been extensive enough to be accepted as a standard treatment modality. However, proton beam therapy seems well worth evaluation when other treatment modalities are not effective due to tumor size.

8.2. Tumor Location & Protocol

Tumors occur in various locations with some developing peripherally, and some developing centrally in the liver parenchyma. Also, some tumors grow in the hepatic portal region and sometimes invade the portal veins. Depending on the tumor location, different treatment protocols are necessary to protect certain tissues/organs. Some protocols have been suggested by the University of Tsukuba.

For the tumor that localizes in the hepatic portal regions, bile duct stenosis is a severe problem after high dose radiotherapy. Chiba et al. reported that 3 of the 162 patients experienced proton beam therapy-related bile duct stenosis with the dose of 79.2 GyE in 16 fractions and 92.4 GyE in 24 fractions [74]. Based on this finding, Mizumoto et al. conducted proton beam therapy in 55 patients with HCC adjacent to the porta hepatis with the dose of 72.6 GyE in 22 fractions [75]. They reported that the 3-year local control and overall survival were 86% and 50.0%, respectively, with no severe late toxicities, including bile duct stenosis.

Also, HCC is sometimes adjacent to the gastrointestinal tract. In this case, hemorrhage, ulceration, or perforation of the gastrointestinal tract should be prevented. Nakayama et al. used 72.6 GyE in 22 fractions and 77 GyE in 35 fractions for 47 patients with HCC which was located within 2 cm from the gastrointestinal tract [76]. They reduced the treatment margin to avoid excess radiation doses to the gastrointestinal tract at 33-39.6 GyE in 10-12 fractions with a total dose of either 72.6 GyE or 50.6-55 GyE in 10-21 fractions in a total dose of 77 GyE. They found that the 3-year local progression-free survival and overall survival were 88% and 50%, respectively. Also, gastrointestinal toxicity was observed in 4 patients; One with a Grade 2 hemorrhage of the stomach, 2 with Grade 2 and 3 colonic hemorrhages, and 1 with a Grade 2 hemorrhage in the hepatic flexure of the colon. The irradiated volume of 50 Gy or more was 5.4 ml, 5.1 ml, and 25.8 ml for the patients with stomach hemorrhages, Grade 3 colonic hemorrhage, and Grade 2 hemorrhage in the hepatic flexure of the colon, respectively.

On the other hand, dose escalation seems possible for the tumors located peripherally in the liver parenchyma. Fukumitsu et al. reported local control of 94.5% and 87.3% at 3 and at 5 years for HCC that was located more than 2 cm from either the porta hepatis or gastrointestinal tract with proton beam therapy of 66 GyE in 10 fractions [77]. The overall survival at 3- and 5-years was 49.2 and 38.7%, respectively. Three patients of the 51 developed rib fractures, but no patient suffered from liver failure secondary to proton beam therapy. In this protocol, a V60 (60 Gy equivalent dose at 2 Gy fractions [EQD2], when alpha beta ration = 3) of the rib ≥ 4.48 cm^3 is one of the useful indications to expect rib fractures [100].

A comparison of these 3 treatment protocols was performed, but there were not significant differences in the treatment results. The overall survival at 3- and at 5-years was

61% (95% CI: 53-68%) and 48% (38-57%), respectively, and the local control at 3- and at 5-years was 87% (81-97%) and 81% (68-94%), respectively [58].

Recently, Kawashima et al. and Bush et al. each reported a phase 2 study for HCC treated with proton beam therapy [57, 78]. The tumor location was not mentioned in these 2 reports. Kawashima et al. used 76 GyE in 3.8 GyE once-daily fractions at four fractions in a week, and the 2 year local progression-free survival and overall survival were reported as 96% (95% CI, 88-100%) and 66% (48-84%), respectively. Four of the 30 patients died of hepatic insufficiency without tumor recurrence during the 6-9 months after the proton beam therapy. Bush et al. used 63 Gy in 4.2 Gy-daily fractions in 15 fractions over 3 weeks. They reported the median survival time was 36 months (95% CI, 30- 42 M) and local treatment failure was observed in 15 of the 76 (20%) patients with a mild treatment toxicity of Grade 2: gastrointestinal ulceration or inflammation observed in 5 of the 76 patients.

The local control was excellent and the overall survival was favorable in all these reports (Table 5). Since the feasible dose fractionation varied, it is important that tumor location, especially doses for those near the gastrointestinal tract, should be taken into consideration in the selection of treatment fractionation.

8.3. Liver Function & Coexistence of Disease

HCCs often develop from cirrhotic liver. Liver cirrhosis is a progressive disease and the treatment modality for HCC is strictly limited for these patients because of the potential risk of liver failure.

Therefore, HCC patients with severe cirrhosis are usually treated with palliative care. The median survival time of these patients is 3-9 months, and all die within 3 years [101-103]. Radiotherapy is not suggested for these patients. The risk of radiation-induced liver disease (RILD) increases for patients with poor liver function. Chang et al. reported the results of stereotactic body radiotherapy (SBRT) for 16 patients [104]. In this report, there was no treatment-related toxicity for Child-Pugh score A patients, but severe liver failure was observed for 2 Child-Pugh score B patients.

Also, Cardenes et al. reported the results of a dose escalation study using SBRT [105]. They planned 48 Gy in 3 fractions for Child-Pugh A patients and 42 Gy in 3 fractions for Child-Pugh B patients. However, toxicity was observed in the Child-Pugh B patients' group, therefore, the treatment doses were decreased to 40 Gy in 5 fractions. Nevertheless, RILD was observed in 3 patients with a Child-Pugh score ≥ 7.

Liver function was not only a risk factor for RILD, but also an important determining factor for proton beam therapy. Mizumoto et al. found that a favorable Child-Pugh score was significantly associated with a good prognosis [58], and Kawashima et al. reported that that the level of indocyanine green retention at 15 minutes (ICG 15) was related to good overall survival [57].

Table 4. Summary of proton beam therapy for hepatocellular carcinoma

	N	Number of tumors (single/ multiple)	Size (<5/≧ 5mm)	Child- Pugh (A/B/C)	Dose	Survival	Local control	Prognostic factor	Adverse effect
Bush [83]	34	32/2		14/7/7	63GyE/15fr	55% (2Y)	75% (2Y)		
Kawashima [87]	30	30/0	19/11	20/10/0	72GyE/16fr	66% (2Y)	96% (2Y)	hepatic function	ascites/asterixis: 4
Chiba [88]	162	80/82	156/88	90/62/10	55-92.4GyE/10- 24fr	23.5% (5Y)	86.9% (5Y)	Child-pugh No of tumors	bile duct stenosis: 1 biloma: 2 digestive organ bleeding: 2
Mizumoto [91]	53	22/31	31/22	46/6/1	72.6GyE/22fr	45.1% (3Y)	86% (3Y)	No of tumors Child-Pugh AFP	
Fukumitsu [90]	51	31/20	45/6	41/10/0	66GyE/10fr	38.7% (5Y)	87.8% (5Y)		rib fracture:3 pneumonitis 1
Bush [78]	76	65/11	39/37	22/36/18	63GyE/15fr				
Mizumoto [92]	266	124/142	196/70	203/60/3	66-77GyE/10- 35fr	48% (5Y)	81% (5Y)	CTV Child-Pugh prior treatment	Intratumor hemorrhage: 1
Komatsu [55]	242	238/40	196/82	184/55/3	52.8-84 GyE/4- 38fr	38% (5Y)		PS Child-Pugh vascular invasion	skin ulcer: 5

Table 5. Tumor location and treatment protocols

Treatment protocol							
Author	**Year**	**Patients No**	**Tumor location**	**Total dose (GyE)**	**Fractionation**	**Local control**	**Overall survival**
Mizumoto	2008	55	adjacent to the porta hepatis	72.6	22	3y 86%	3y 50%
Nakayama	2011	47	2 cm from the gastrointestinal tract	72.6	22	3y 88%	3y 88%
				74	37		
Fukumitsu	2009	51	2 cm from the porta hepatis or gastrointestinal tract	66	10	3y 95%	3y 49%
Kawashima	2005	30	-	76	20	2y 96%	2y 66%
Bush	2011	76	-	63	15	Local failure 20%	MST 36 M

On the other hand, there was a report that proton beam therapy affected liver function. Hata et al. studied proton beam therapy use in 19 patients with Child-Pugh C cirrhosis [52], who received total doses of 50-84 GyE in 3-5 GyE fractions. The 2 year overall survival was 42% with a 63% objective response rate (complete response and partial response), and neither Grade 3 nor more severe treatment toxicity was observed. Also, there was no deterioration in the Child-Pugh score, but rather, it improved in 14 patients. These results suggested that proton beam therapy is less toxic for normal liver, and inhibition of the tumor progression improves liver function.

Also, patients with limited treatment options due to old age, unfavorable conditions, and comorbidities were analyzed. [53, 82] For patients older than 80 years, 66 GyE in 10 fractions, 72.6 GyE in 22 fractions, and 77 GyE in 35 fractions were delivered based on the tumor locations, as mentioned previously. Severe toxicity was not observed, and the 3-year cause-specific survival was 88% even though the overall survival at 3 years was 62%. These results were compared with the data from other patients. These reports were all from retrospective and small studies. Proton beam therapy seems applicable for variety of patients with HCC who are not suitable for other treatments.

8.4. Portal Vein Tumor Thrombosis (PVTT), Inferior Vena Cava Tumor Thrombosis (IVCTT)

The prognosis of advanced HCC remains poor, especially in patients with tumor thrombosis in either the portal vein or inferior vena cava (IVC). The incidence of portal vein tumor thrombosis (PVTT) and of IVC tumor thrombosis (IVCTT) is high in patients with HCC; 44-84% and 31-50% according to autopsy and to clinical data, respectively [106-108]. There are many treatment options for HCC, however, the effectiveness is strictly limited and controversial for these patients, and the prognosis for these patients if untreated remains extremely poor with a median survival of only 2-3 months [109-112].

Standalone photon radiotherapy is also sometimes used, but the objective of such treatment is often palliative care due to the low tolerance of the whole liver to radiation. Also, photon radiotherapy in combination with transarterial chemoembolization (TACE) has also been used [113-117]. In this type of treatment, radiotherapy is usually employed to treat the PVTT only with a median total dose of 45-50 Gy delivered to the PVTT in 1.8-2.0 Gy, then TACE is used to address the intrahepatic tumors. The objective response was 50-79%, and the overall survival at 1 year and 2 years was 25-45% and 10-25%, respectively with the median survival ranging from 5.3 to 8.0 months. Severe treatment toxicities including gastrointestinal ulcers and bleeding were reported in 2-26% of the patients.

Meanwhile, there are some reports of proton beam therapy use for PVTT and IVCTT therapy. The first report of proton beam therapy for PVTT was from the University of Tsukuba [118]. In this report, 12 patients with a tumor thrombus in the main trunk and in the major branches of the portal vein were treated with the total dose of 50-72 Gy in 10-22 fractions (The RBE was calculated as 1.0 at that time). All treated tumor thrombi were reported to be controlled in the follow up period which ranged from 0.3-7.3 years without ≥Grade 3 toxicities. Sugahara et al. reported the results of 35 patients with PVTT treated by proton beam therapy [81]. They delivered 72.6 GyE in 22 fractions (Figure 27). They reported that 29 of the 35 patients showed an objective response and that the overall survival at 2 and at 5 years was 48% and 21%, respectively and the median survival time was 22 months (range, 2-88 months). They reported that there were no severe toxicities.

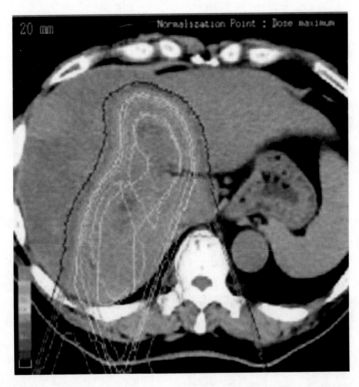

Figure 27. The isodose distributions of proton beam therapy for a patient having HCC with bilateral PVTT. 90% isodose curve (pink line), which is shaped by proton beams from posterior oblique ports, encompass the entire HCC and PVTT. Proton beam therapy of 72.6 GyE in 22 fractions was demonstrated.

The first results of proton beam therapy for IVCTT were reported by Mizumoto et al. [80]. In this report, proton beam therapy was used on 3 patients, and IVC was re-canalized in all patients after the treatment without severe toxicities. In 2011, Komatsu et al. reported the results of 16 patients with IVCTT treated with particle radiotherapy [79]. Thirteen of the 16 patients were treated by proton beams, with the dose of 56-76 GyE in 8 to 38 fractions (Figure 28). Three additional patients were treated with carbon ion. They showed an overall survival of 100% and 60%, respectively at 1 and 3 years for patients in the curative treatment group, and all irradiated tumors showed complete tumor shrinkage without severe toxicities.

The proton beam therapy treatment results for PVTT and for IVCTT were positive, and suggested that proton beam therapy may be effective and safe for patients who cannot be treated with other treatment modalities. However, these reports are all from retrospective studies from a single facility. Additional larger and prospective studies are required to establish the efficacy of proton beam therapy for both PVTT and IVCTT in the future.

8.5. Re-Irradiation

HCC generally is a multicentric disease, especially when it is associated with HCV, therefore, new tumors often develop sequentially, and repeated treatment is an unavoidable necessity.

When liver is irradiated widely with a high dose, radiation-induced liver disease will occur.

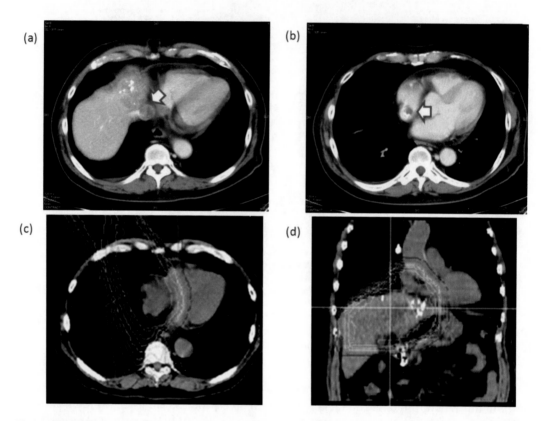

Figure 28. Pretreatment contrast-enhanced computed tomography scans demonstrate HCC with an inferior vena cava tumor thrombus (a: arrow) extending into right atrium (b; arrow). Ninety % isodose curve (pink line), which is shaped by proton beams could cover the entire HCC, IVCTT and right atrium (c and d). Proton beam therapy of 72.6 GyE in 22 fractions was demonstrated.

Emami et al. reported tolerance doses of 30, 35, and 50 Gy for the entire liver, two-thirds, and one-third of the liver, respectively [46]. Dawson et al. reported that the tolerance dose was more than 90 Gy when the irradiated volume was limited to one third of the liver [119].

Using photon beams, SBRT is commonly used for small liver tumors (mainly liver metastases). In SBRT, multiple beams are used, resulting in a large low dose area in the liver. Therefore, repeated radiotherapy for HCC is not common, because it is difficult to avoid overlap of the beams and the tissue functional capacity is decreased. In contrast, proton beam therapy can be performed with minimal ports. Generally, 1-3 ports are used for one tumor, therefore, the low dose area is small, and repeated proton beam therapy can be considered. Hashimoto et al. reported the results of repeated proton beam therapy for 68 lesions in 27 patients [120]. The local control response was 87.8%. Acute Hepatic failure was observed for only 2 patients with Child-Pugh classes B and C, and they concluded that the repeated proton beam therapy for HCC was safe when both the tumor was located in the peripheral region of the liver and the liver function was Child-Pugh class A.

However, there is little knowledge about repeated proton beam therapy related to the dose-volume relationship. Accurate analysis would be difficult, because the liver becomes atrophic and deformed over a long period due to either irradiation or liver cirrhosis. Also, effects from other treatment or effects on other treatment, such as TACE, tissue-ablating therapy, or drug therapy are not clarified. Repeated proton beam therapy for HCC seems possible and safe, and should be considered when other treatment modalities are not recommended.

9. Techniques and Results of New Radiotherapies for Hepatocellular Carcinoma

9.1. Stereotactic Radiotherapy

Stereotactic body radiotherapy (SBRT) is an external beam radiotherapy method used to very precisely deliver a high dose of therapeutic radiation to an extracranial target within the body using either a single fraction or a small number of fractions [121]. Hypofractionation defined as the delivery of a small number of large doses of radiation is very different from the standard radiotherapy. The typical fractionation of standard radiotherapy to epithelial tumors with curative intent, which is called conventional fractionation, involves the use of 30 or more fractions at 1.8 to 2.0 Gy per fraction delivered 5 days per week. The very large hypofractionated doses used in SBRT can be given safely because *(a)* the treated volumes are small with tight margins, and *(b)* the technique employs a large number of beams (eight or more), which individually contribute a small dose along their path but together result in a much larger dose where they intersect and are combined at the locus of the cancer [122]. In the 1990s, SBRT emerged in clinical use due to advances in both computer and imaging technologies. SBRT was commonly applied to treating both primary non-small cell lung cancer (NSCLC) and metastatic pulmonary tumors. SBRT achieved good local control and overall survival comparable to that of lobectomy in non-randomized and population-based comparisons in medically inoperable or older patients. Today, SBRT is an alternative treatment option for patients with early-stage NSCLC who are medically inoperable or who refuse surgery.

The role of external beam radiotherapy has been limited in the management of patients with hepatocellular carcinoma (HCC) because of concerns about radiation-induced liver disease (RILD) and the existence of more efficient, or less time-consuming, treatment options. The tolerance dose of the whole liver to radiotherapy is about 30 Gy in 2.0 Gy per fraction [46] in most patients but the dose is generally lower in patients with liver cirrhosis. This tolerance dose (30 Gy in 15 fractions) of normal liver tissue is far lower than that required to eradicate a tumor. In addition to liver toxicities, normal tissues adjacent to the liver, such as the stomach, the duodenum, and the kidneys, are also at risk of injury from radiotherapy. SBRT has made it possible to deliver precise, high-dose radiotherapy to liver tumors while sparing the uninvolved liver and other normal tissues (Figure 29).

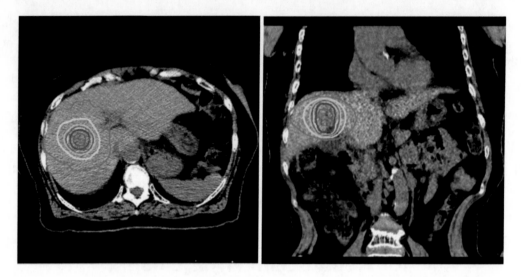

Figure 29. Stereotactic body radiation therapy with dynamic conformal multiple arc therapy. The prescribed dose is 40 Gy in 5 fractions. It is defined as 70% of the maximal dose to cover more than 95% of the PTV. Isodose lines from inner to outer represent 90% (brown), 70% (red), 60% (orange), 40% (yellow), and 20% (green), respectively. (Courtesy of Dr. A. Takeda, Ofuna Chuo Hospital).

There have been no randomized clinical trials that have studied the efficacy of SBRT for patients with HCC. Retrospective studies and Phase I/II prospective studies have suggested that SBRT can be an effective and safe treatment option for patients with HCC. Those studies included patients with Child-Pugh A or B scores for liver function, who are unsuitable for other treatment options, such as surgery, trans-arterial chemoembolization (TACE), and radiofrequency ablation (RFA).

In a Phase I study of 102 patients with locally advanced HCC or intrahepatic cholangiocarcinoma (IHC), Tse et al. reported that individualized six-fraction SBRT with doses ranging from 24 Gy to 54 Gy did not induce RILD or treatment-related grade 4/5 toxicities and the patients had a better outcome than those of historical controls [123]. They concluded that six-fraction SBRT was a safe treatment for HCC and IHC. In a retrospective study that evaluated the safety and efficacy of SBRT for HCC, Andolino et al. reported that the 2-year local control response, progression-free survival, and overall survival were 90%, 48%, and 67%, respectively [124]. In another study that evaluated the outcomes of SBRT for HCC, Sanuki et al. reported that the 3-year local control response and overall survival were 91% and 70%, respectively [125]. Similarly, Choi et al. reported an overall response of 80%, with a 1- and 2-year overall survival of 70.0% and 43.1%, respectively [126]. In recent sequential Phase I and II trials using SBRT for treating locally advanced HCC, Bujold et al. reported that the 1-year local control response was 87% with a median survival of 17 months [127]. Overall, the responses reported ranged from 49% to 86%. The 1-year local responses were from 65% to 100%, and the 1-year overall survivals were from 51% to 92.2% [68, 123-133].

SBRT for HCC is generally used to treat patients with 1 to 3 tumors without extrahepatic disease. Although there is no established size limitation, SBRT is given to patients with relatively small tumors. In Japan, SBRT for one tumor less than 5 cm in diameter without any extrahepatic disease is permitted by our health insurance for medical treatment. The optimal radiation dose and schedules have not been established, but recent reports with SBRT for

HCC have resulted in the use of 20 to 50 Gy at one to six fractions. Patients with Child-Pugh A liver function receive SBRT with acceptable liver toxicities. Treatment for those patients with Child-Pugh C is contraindicated. Patients with Child-Pugh B are treated with caution with SBRT, because they tend to develop RILD more frequently than those with Child-Pugh A [134]. Dose modifications and strict dose constraints may be needed in treating patients with Child-Pugh B.

There has been no evidence supporting prolonged survival of patients with HCC so far with conventional treatments. However, promising results using SBRT for relatively small HCC unsuitable for other local therapies have been reported. SBRT can be considered as an alternative therapy when other local therapies are contraindicated or have been failed.

9.2. Carbon Beam Therapy

The clinical application of helium ion beams began in the early 1950s at the Lawrence Berkeley National Laboratory in the United States, and clinical trials using heavy ion beams were later initiated in 1970s [14, 135, 136]. The National Institute of Radiological Sciences (NIRS) in Japan, which is the world's first facility dedicated to cancer therapy using heavy ion beams, constructed the Heavy Ion Medical Accelerator in Chiba (HIMAC) in 1993 [137]. A year later, in 1994, clinical studies using carbon ions generated from the HIMAC were initiated for cancer treatment. Based on a substantial amount of biological evidence that carbon ion radiation therapy (C-ion RT) is effective even for tumors, which are biologically and/or histopathologically radioresistant, with minimum morbidity, there are now 7 facilities using C-ion RT for cancer treatment.

Carbon ion beams offer advantageous physical and biological properties in RT [137, 138]. They exhibit a Bragg peak which is also seen with protons, and can create a better dose distribution for the target volume by specified beam modulations, such as utilizing a spread-out Bragg peak (SOBP) [139]. When comparing dose distributions of carbon ion beams with those of proton beams, almost no dose is deposited in protons but a small dose in carbon ions in the region beyond the distal end of the peak is deposited. This is because the primary carbon ions undergo nuclear interactions and fragment into particles with a lower atomic number, producing a fragmentation tail beyond the peak. However, the biological effect of this fragmentation tail seems to be very small, because the tail contains only fragments with a low atomic number [137]. Furthermore, the lateral fall-off around the target volume is more rapid with carbon ion beams than that with proton beams. A typical dose distribution of carbon beam therapy for HCC is shown in Figure 30.

Carbon ion beams have a relatively powerful biological effectiveness (RBE) resulting from high linear energy transfer (LET), similarly to neutron beams. The rate at which particle beams lose energy when penetrating into the tissue increases with the mass of the particles is known as LET. Photons and protons are sparsely ionizing radiations and are regarded as low-LET radiations, whereas fast neutrons and carbon ions are densely ionizing and are referred to as high-LET radiations. There is a close relationship between LET and the biological effects of radiations; it is known that the RBE increases if the LET increases [140]. Previous studies revealed that the cytocidal effect of carbon ions is estimated to be about 3 times that of photons and protons, since carbon ions directly cleave double-stranded DNA at multiple sites even at low oxygen content. This damage allows access to hypoxic parts of the tumors that would be resistant to low LET radiotherapy [141]. In contrast to neutron beams whose LET remains uniform at any depth in the body, the LET of carbon ion beams increases steadily from the point of entrance in the body with increasing depth to reach a maximum in the target region [142]. In addition, experiments with both neutrons and carbon ions have demonstrated that a larger fraction dose tends to lower RBE for both tumor and normal tissues, but the RBE for the tumor does not decrease as rapidly as that for the normal tissues [143]. These results may indicate that the therapeutic ratio increases when the fraction dose is increased. Based on these unique physical and biological properties of carbon ion beams, it is theoretically possible to deliver hypofractionated radiotherapy using significantly smaller number of fractions than those used in conventional RT.

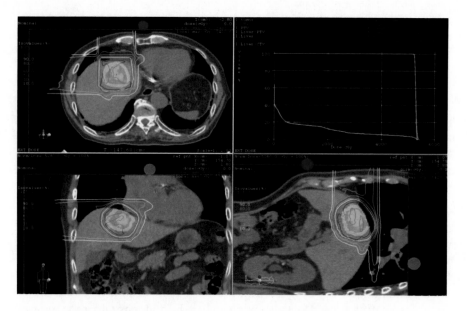

Figure 30. A typical dose distribution of carbon beam therapy for HCC.

The eligibility criteria for enrollment for carbon ion RT at NIRS was that other therapies appeared to offer less potential for sufficient efficacy or other treatments had proved ineffective in local HCC tumor control [142]. Kato et al. [144] reported the first prospective phase I/II study of C-ion RT using a 15 fraction regimen for HCC. Between June 1995 and February 1997, 24 patients with histopathologically proven HCC were treated. A dose escalation was performed to determine the optimal dose fractionation schedule by stepping up the fraction dose in increments of 10 % from 3.3 to 5.3 GyE, and a total dose ranging from 49.5 to 79.5 Gray equivalents (GyE) was delivered over 5 weeks. No severe liver injury occurred, and the Child-Pugh score did not increase by >2 points at any time. Within 3 months and 4-12 months after the start of therapy, no change or only a 1-point increase in the Child-Pugh score was observed in 18 (78%) of 23 patients and in 15 (75%) of 20 patients, respectively. The number of patients included in the minor or major change groups did not depend on the initial Child-Pugh grade, tumor size, or disease stage. During a median follow-up of 71 months (range, 63-83 months), 4 local recurrences (17%), 14 regional recurrences in the liver (58%), and 6 distant metastases (25%) developed. Five of the 6 patients with distant metastases had Stage IVA disease before the start of C-ion RT. The tumor response was complete in 10 patients, partial in 7, stable in 3, and progressive in 4. The 3-year level of local tumor control and overall survival was 81% (95% CI 60–100%) and 50% (95% CI, 30–70%), respectively, and the median survival time was 37 months. The treatment outcome of a phase II clinical trial using more hypofractioned C-ion RT for 44 patients with histologically proven HCC was also reported [145]. This study was carried out between April 2001 and February 2003, and a total dose of 52.8 GyE was delivered in 4 fractions over 1 week. No treatment-related deaths occurred. Within 3 months after the start of therapy, grade 3 morbidity in the liver was observed in 3% of the subjects, but no grade 3 or severe hepatic reaction was observed thereafter. The 2-year rates of local control and overall survival were 89% and 85%, respectively. None of the subjects died of hepatic failure within 1 year after the start of therapy. This fractionation schedule for HCC has been also used at Gunma University which started C-ion RT for HCC in 2010 [146].

NIRS has also used C-ion RT for centrally located HCC. Imaeda et al. compared the efficacy and toxicity after C-ion RT at a total dose of 52.8 GyE in 4 fractions for HCC based on tumor location [147]. The 5-year overall survival and local control were 22.2% and 87.8%, respectively, in 18 patients with HCC located within 2 cm of the main portal vein. The corresponding responses for survival and local control were 34.8% and 95.7%, respectively, in 46 patients with HCC located far from the porta hepatis. There were no significant differences in the responses between both groups. In Germany, the first clinical phase I dose-escalation study of C-ion RT delivered by intensity-modulated rasterscanning for advanced HCC (PROMETHEUS-01 trial) is ongoing to determine the optimal dose [148]. Recently, they reported the findings of the first 6 patients who received C-ion RT at a total dose of 40 GyE in 4 fractions [149]. Fortunately, all patients had HCC that was locally controlled and experienced no toxicities at the median follow up time of 11.0 months (range, 3.4-12.7 months). They concluded therefore that additional patients will be included in the clinical study. In conclusions, theoretically, C-ion RT is a promising treatment method for advanced HCC, since the tumors likely have radioresistance because of their large size in addition to their pathological characteristics. However, there is still little evidence showing the effectiveness of C-ion RT for HCC. Although proton beam therapy has been widely applied for HCC, the clinical outcomes of C-ion RT for HCC have been reported only from NIRS in the last decade. Furthermore, 2 facilities recently started C-ion RT in Japan. A new C-ion RT facility is under construction in the Kanagawa Cancer Center, and it will become the fifth C-ion RT center in Japan in 2016. Thus, it will be possible to carry out a multicenter prospective trial to validate the feasibility and effectiveness of C-ion RT for HCC. Accumulation of the collected data may more clearly determine the differences in the outcomes and the appropriate eligibility criteria between proton beam therapy and C-ion RT in the future.

10. Application for Proton Beam Therapy for Other Liver Tumors

10.1. Intrahepatic Cholangiocellular Carinoma (CCC)

Among the primary liver tumors, the incidence of hepatocellular carcinoma (HCC) is the highest, followed by intrahepatic cholangiocarcinoma (CCC). In Japan, 94.2 and 4.1% of primary liver tumors are registered as HCC and ICC, respectively [150]. CCC frequently metastasizes to other organs and lymph nodes, compared with HCC. Jaundice is likely to occur due to tumor progression in the liver, and the prognosis is poor in many cases. Park et al. reported the natural history of untreated unresectable cholangiocarcinoma, in which the overall median survival time of 203 patients with CCC plus 127 patients with hilar cholangiocarcinoma was 3.9 months. The prognosis of CCC patients was worse than that of hilar cholangiocarcinoma patients, and the median survival time was 3.0 months in CCC compared with 5.9 months in hilar cholangiocarcinoma [70]. CCC may be very aggressive tumor among the liver tumors.

Tumor resection is the most radical treatment for CCC, but radical resection is only applicable to about 30% of patients [151]. Sulpice et al. reported that the median survival of 87 CCC patients who could be treated with radical partial liver resection was 33 months, and that the 3-year and 5-year survival rates were 47 and 31%, respectively [152]. Wang et al. investigated 367 patients treated with partial liver resection, and observed that the median survival time was 21 months, and the 3-year and 5-year survival rates were 40.8 and 35.2%, respectively [153]. In these reports, important prognostic factors included serum CEA, CA 19-9, tumor diameter and number, vascular invasion, lymph node metastasis, direct invasion, and local extrahepatic metastasis. It has also been reported that the tumor location influences the prognosis based on surgical cases of perihilar cholangiocarcinoma, which arises in the liver hilar region. Ebata et al. reported that the 3-year survival rate of patients with extrahepatic cholangiocarcinoma (EHC) was 43%, whereas that of CCC was 29% [154]. Based on the above reports, the prognosis of CCC remains poor, even though radical resection is performed. From a surgical viewport, the wider resection may improve the prognosis. Ohtsuka et al. reported the results of many cases of hemi- or more extensive hepatectomy, in which the median survival time was 26 months and the 3-year and 5-year survival rates were 38 and 23%, respectively [155]. Based on these reports, surgery should be firstly considered for this difficult tumor, but local recurrence and distant metastasis frequently occur even though extensive hepatectomy is performed, and the improvement of the prognosis of CCC is insufficient.

Unresectable CCC accounts for about 70% of cases, for which chemotherapy is performed, but cure is not achieved by chemotherapy alone [70]. In general, gemcitabine is the most effective drug for unresectable biliary duct cancer. In addition, cisplatin, oxaliplatin, and capecitabine are used as effective agents in combination. In clinical trials verifying chemotherapy including gemcitabine, the median survival time was mostly 8.8-12.7 months [156-158]. The effect of systemic standard chemotherapy for unresectable CCC is limited, and meta-analysis has shown that chemotherapy-based transarterial therapy prolonged the survival time by only several months [159].

Radiofrequency ablation (RFA) is another treatment method. Fu et al. reported a median survival time of 30 months after RFA; although the number of patients was small [160]. However, RFA is basically indicated only for tumors that are 3-cm or smaller, and it may not be applied to most CCC cases.

The usefulness of radiation therapy for CCC has not yet been clarified. Palliative radiation therapy for unresectable CCC has been reported. Shinohara et al. investigated patients treated with radiation therapy using the Surveillance, Epidemiology, and End Results (SEER) database, in which the prognosis was significantly more favorable in patients treated with radiation therapy in addition to surgery compared with those undergoing surgery alone, and in patients treated with radiation therapy compared with untreated patients [161]. Chen et al. reported that, when conventional fractionated radiation therapy at about 50 Gy was performed with palliative intent, the survival time of irradiated patients was significantly prolonged compared with non-irradiated patients [162]. These reports on CCC suggest that not only the symptoms but also the prognosis may be improved by a radiation therapy, even though it is palliative.

Radiation therapy has recently advanced markedly, and improvement of the dose distribution has facilitated elevation of the treatment intensity for tumors while maintaining the safety for normal tissue. Stereotactic body radiation therapy (SBRT) is one such approach. SBRT is useful for small tumors with a size of about 3 cm, but it may be rarely applied to tumors that are not discovered until the size exceeds 5 cm, such as CCC.

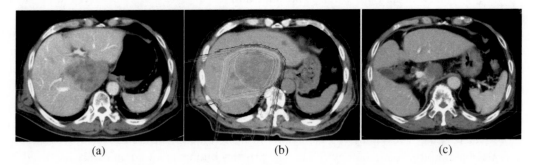

(a)   (b)   (c)

Figure 31. A treatment course of CCC patient using proton beam therapy. (a) CT image before proton beam therapy. (b) Dose-distribution of administration of a total proton dose of 72.6 GyE in 22 fractions. Isodose curves representing 100% to 10% of the prescribed dose are shown at 10% intervals. (c) CT images showing the treatment course at and 41 months after proton beam therapy.

Proton beam therapy is another technique capable of concentrating the dose to liver tumors regardless of the size while maintaining the safety for normal tissue. Proton beam therapy achieved efficacy for HCC, but it has not yet been shown whether it exhibits a similar effect on CCC. Proton beam therapy has been performed in 20 patients with 15-140 mm (median: 50 mm) unresectable CCC by 2010 at the University of Tsukuba. The dose was 72.6 GyE in 22 fractions. Chemotherapy was simultaneously administered during proton beam therapy in 4 patients. Proton beam therapy was performed with curative intent in 12 patients and as a palliative therapy in the other 8 patients. No recurrence in the irradiated field over the observation course for 8.6-62.6 months (median: 20.8 months) in 9 of the 12 patients treated with curative intent. The median survival time of the 12 patients was 27.5 months, the 1-year and 3-year survival rates were 82 and 38%, respectively; some patients survived 5 years. The prognosis was poor in patients with symptoms of jaundice at the time of treatment initiation. Patients treated with proton beam therapy for CCC are shown in Figure 31. Grade-2 gastric ulcer developed in one of the 20 patients, but no grade-2 or more severe complications were noted in any other patients.

Although our experience is still insufficient, proton beam therapy is a safe treatment for unresectable CCC with no distant metastasis, and the therapeutic effect may be high. Since some treated patients survived for a prolonged time, it is necessary to investigate combination with chemotherapy, and develop the optimum therapeutic method for unresectable CCC.

10.2. Metastatic Liver Tumors

Although many reports have been published on the treatment of hepatocellular carcinoma (HCC) using proton beam therapy, reports on the treatment of metastatic liver tumors with this approach are rare. Gohongi et al. reported on one patient with a metastatic liver tumor originating from gastric cancer who received proton beam therapy combined with concurrent chemotherapy and survived more than 2 years without severe adverse effects [163]. Kanemoto et al. reported on five cases of metastatic liver tumors originating from breast cancer who received proton beam therapy combined with adjuvant chemotherapy and/or hormone therapy and survived longer than that expected with standard systemic therapy alone [164].

Only a few case reports found that proton beam therapy was safe and effective in cases with metastatic liver tumors. In those studies, all patients received systemic treatments, such as chemotherapy or hormone therapy, combined with proton beam therapy. Proton beam therapy provides excellent dose localization, and its usefulness has been reported not only for HCC but also for many kinds of malignant tumors. If proton beam therapy is effective in local control and the irradiation of the lesions prolongs survival or improves the quality of life (QOL) of the patients, proton beam therapy would be a possible treatment for metastatic liver tumors.

In our institute, University of Tsukuba, more than 150 cases with metastatic liver tumors have received proton beam therapy so far. The primary tumors are predominantly localized in the colon and rectum, followed by pancreas and breast. The therapeutic purpose is mostly palliative, followed by local control, and then curative. The irradiation dose is generally similar to that of HCC. However, reduction of the total irradiation dose or fractionation is sometimes necessary for cases that present with poor status to avoid any adverse effects.

Proton beam therapy is sometimes used in cases of liver metastasis as below.

1. Solitary liver metastasis without any tumor lesion outside the liver.
2. Multiple liver metastases, with one large tumor that can be controlled by proton beam therapy, to prolong survival when combined with other systemic treatments or surgery.
3. Tumor thrombosis in either the portal vein or hepatic vein, where growth control of the tumor is expected to avoid a sudden decline in the patients' status.
4. Metastasis which would likely cause bile duct stenosis and jaundice, and tumor growth control can contribute to the patients' QOL.

However, there are not many clinical studies to prove the utility of proton beam therapy. Defining the benefit for the patients and type of proton beam theapy that can contribute to the whole treatment should be evaluated carefully on a patient by patient basis with physicians who specialize in either surgery or chemotherapy.

There are few previous studies on the use of proton beam therapy for treating metastatic liver tumors, and the clinical usefulness has not been previously demonstrated. There are cases in which high dose localization of proton beam therapy to the tumor has provided a positive benefit. Proton beam therapy has potential as one possible treatment when combined with other treatments in cases where proton beam therapy can contribute to survival and to the QOL of the patients.

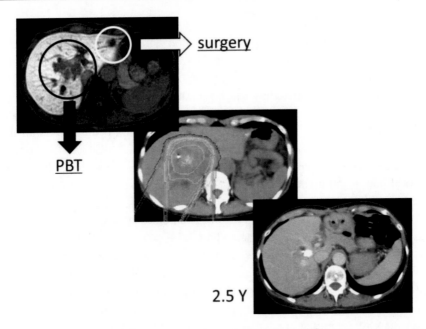

Figure 32. A 65-year-old woman with post-operative colon carcinoma. The metastatic liver tumor in the porta hepatis was treated with proton beam therapy, and the tumor in the left lobe was treated by surgery. Oral intake of TS-1 (tegafur, gimeracil, oteracil potassium) was continued after that. No recurrence was observed in the follow-up CT (2.5 years later) and the patient has now survived more than 4 years.

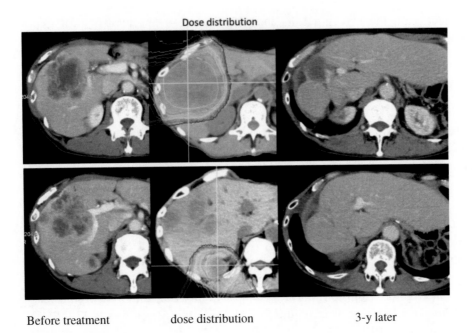

Figure 33. A 61-year-old man with post-operative gastric carcinoma. Metastatic liver tumors were treated with proton beam therapy alone. No recurrence was observed in the follow-up CT (3 years later) and the patient is still alive.

10.2.1. Case presentation

A 65-year-old woman with post-operative colon carcinoma (Figure 32). A metastatic liver tumor was found 7 years after she received a right hemicolectomy. The 2 cm diameter tumor was located in the left lobe, and another 5 cm diameter tumor was located in the porta hepatis. Several types of chemotherapy had been administered, but an effective response was not observed. Surgery was considered risky, especially for the tumor in the porta hepatis. Because the tumor size was too large to be irradiated by photon beam, the tumor in the porta hepatis was treated with proton beam therapy at the dose of 72.6 GyE/22fr, and tumor in the left lobe was removed by surgery. Oral intake of TS-1 (tegafur, gimeracil, oteracil potassium) was continued and at the present time the patient has survived without recurrence for more than 4 years.

A 61-year-old man with post-operative gastric carcinoma (Figure 33). A metastatic liver tumor was found 1 year after he had received a total gastrectomy. Although several kinds of chemotherapy were continued for more than 2 years, the size and number of the tumors increased. Multiple tumor lesions were found in the right lobe of the liver when he came to our hospital. Because most of the lesions were located in S5/8, those lesions were included into a single field and treated with proton beam therapy at the dose of 72.6 GyE/22fr (upper). A small tumor in S6/7 was also treated with proton beam therapy at the dose of 66 GyE/10fr (lower). After more than 3 years, this patient is alive and has no metastatic lesions.

Conclusion

Proton beam therapy is a safe and effective treatment modality for hepatocellular carcinoma in many conditions.

Acknowledgments

The authors express special thanks to all of the staffs who have been involved in proton beam therapy at University of Tsukuba. This work was supported by Grant-in-Aid from the Ministry of Education, Science, Sports and Culture of Japan.

References

[1]   Rutherford, E. Collisions of alpha particles with light atoms. II. Nitrogen and oxygen atoms. *Philos Mag*, 1919, 37(222), 571-80.

[2]   Rutherford, E. Collision of Particles with Light Atoms. IV. An Anomalous Effect in Nitrogen (Reprinted from Philosophical Magazine Series 6, vol 37, 581-587, 1919). *Philos Mag*, 2010, 90, 31-7.

[3]   Wilson, RR. Radiological use of fast protons. *Radiology*, 1946, 47(5), 487-91. Epub 1946/11/01.

[4] Koehler, AM; Preston, WM. Protons in radiation therapy. Comparative dose distributions for protons, photons, and electrons. *Radiology*, 1972, 104(1), 191-5. Epub 1972/07/01.

[5] Tobias, CA; Anger, HO; Lawrence, JH. Radiological use of high energy deuterons and alpha particles. *The American journal of roentgenology, radium therapy, and nuclear medicine*, 1952, 67(1), 1-27. Epub 1952/01/01.

[6] Falkmer, S; Larsson, B; Stenson, S. Effects of single dose proton irradiation of normal skin and Vx2 carcinoma in rabbit ears: a comparative investigation with protons and roentgen rays. *Acta radiologica*, 1959, 52, 217-34. Epub 1959/09/01.

[7] Larsson, B; Kihlman, BA. Chromosome aberrations following irradiation with high-energy protons and their secondary radiation: a study of dose distribution and biological efficiency using root-tips of Vicia faba and Allium cepa. *International journal of radiation biology*, 1960, 2, 8-19. Epub 1960/01/01.

[8] Robertson, JB; Williams, JR; Schmidt, RA; Little, JB; Flynn, DF; Suit, HD. Radiobiological studies of a high-energy modulated proton beam utilizing cultured mammalian cells. *Cancer*, 1975, 35(6), 1664-77. Epub 1975/06/01.

[9] Wainson, AA; Lomanov, MF; Shmakova, NL; Blokhin, SI; Jarmonenko, SP. The RBE of accelerated protons in different parts of the Bragg curve. *The British journal of radiology*, 1972, 45(535), 525-9. Epub 1972/07/01.

[10] Luft, R; Olivecrona, H. Experiences with hypophysectomy in man. *Journal of neurosurgery*, 1953, 10(3), 301-16. Epub 1953/05/01.

[11] Luft, R; Olivecrona, H. Hypophysectomy in man; experiences in metastatic cancer of the breast. Cancer. 1955, 8(2), 261-70. Epub 1955/03/01.

[12] Lawrence, JH. Proton irradiation of the pituitary. *Cancer*, 1957, 10(4), 795-8. Epub 1957/07/01.

[13] Lawrence, JH; Tobias, CA; Linfoot, JA; Born, JL; Lyman, JT; Chong, CY; et al. Successful treatment of acromegaly: metabolic and clinical studies in 145 patients. *The Journal of clinical endocrinology and metabolism*, 1970, 31(2), 180-98. Epub 1970/08/01.

[14] Castro, JR. *Future researth strategy for heavy ion radiothreaoy*. Kogelnik HD, editor1995.

[15] Falkmer, S; Fors, B; Larsson, B; Lindell, A; Naeslund, J; Stenson, S. Pilot study on proton irradiation of human carcinoma. *Acta radiologica*, 1962, 58, 33-51. Epub 1962/02/01.

[16] Kjellberg, RN; Hanamura, T; Davis, KR; Lyons, SL; Adams, RD. Bragg-peak proton-beam therapy for arteriovenous malformations of the brain. *The New England journal of medicine*, 1983, 309(5), 269-74. Epub 1983/08/04.

[17] Kjellberg, RN; Shintani, A; Frantz, AG; Kliman, B. Proton-beam therapy in acromegaly. *The New England journal of medicine*, 1968, 278(13), 689-95. Epub 1968/03/28.

[18] Suit, H; Goitein, M; Munzenrider, J; Verhey, L; Blitzer, P; Gragoudas, E; et al. Evaluation of the clinical applicability of proton beams in definitive fractionated radiation therapy. *International journal of radiation oncology, biology, physics*, 1982, 8(12), 2199-205. Epub 1982/12/01.

[19] Gragoudas, ES; Goitein, M; Koehler, AM; Verhey, L; Tepper, J; Suit, HD; et al. Proton irradiation of small choroidal malignant melanomas. *American journal of ophthalmology*, 1977, 83(5), 665-73. Epub 1977/05/01.

[20] Constable, IJ; Goitein, M; Koehler, AM; Schmidt, RA. Small-field irradiation of monkey eyes with protons and photons. *Radiation research*, 1976, 65(2), 304-14. Epub 1976/02/01.

[21] Goitein, M; Miller, T. Planning proton therapy of the eye. *Medical physics*, 1983, 10(3), 275-83. Epub 1983/05/01.

[22] Gragoudas, ES; Lane, AM; Munzenrider, J; Egan, KM; Li, W. Long-term risk of local failure after proton therapy for choroidal/ciliary body melanoma. *Transactions of the American Ophthalmological Society*, 2002, 100, 43-8, discussion 8-9. Epub 2003/01/28.

[23] Drzymala, RE; Mohan, R; Brewster, L; Chu, J; Goitein, M; Harms, W; et al. Dose-volume histograms. *International journal of radiation oncology, biology, physics*, 1991, 21(1), 71-8. Epub 1991/05/15.

[24] Goitein, M; Abrams, M; Rowell, D; Pollari, H; Wiles, J. Multi-dimensional treatment planning: II. Beam's eye-view, back projection, and projection through CT sections. *International journal of radiation oncology, biology, physics*, 1983, 9(6), 789-97. Epub 1983/06/01.

[25] Matsuzaki, Y; Osuga, T; Saito, Y; Chuganji, Y; Tanaka, N; Shoda, J; et al. A new, effective, and safe therapeutic option using proton irradiation for hepatocellular carcinoma. *Gastroenterology*, 1994, 106(4), 1032-41. Epub 1994/04/01.

[26] Tsujii H; Tsuji H; Inada T; Maruhashi A; Hayakawa Y; Takada Y; et al. Clinical-Results of Fractionated Proton Therapy. *Int J Radiat Oncol*, 1993, 25(1), 49-60.

[27] Tsujii, H; Inada, T; Maruhashi, A; Hayakawa, Y; Tsuji, H; Ohara, K; et al. [Field localization and verification system for proton beam radiotherapy in deep-seated tumors]. *Nihon Igaku Hoshasen Gakkai zasshi Nippon acta radiologica*, 1989, 49(5), 622-9. Epub 1989/05/25.

[28] Arimoto, T; Takase, Y; Ishikawa, N; Yoshii, Y; Ishikawa, S; Otani, M; et al. [Investigation of marking procedure for markers in deep-seated organs by proton beam therapy]. *Gan no rinsho Japan journal of cancer clinics*, 1988, 34(4), 395-403. Epub 1988/04/01.

[29] Ohara, K; Okumura, T; Akisada, M; Inada, T; Mori, T; Yokota, H; et al. Irradiation Synchronized with Respiration Gate. *Int J Radiat Oncol*, 1989, 17(4), 853-7.

[30] Beeckman, W; Jongen, Y; Laisne, A; Lannoye, G. Preliminary Design of a Reduced Cost Proton Therapy Facility Using a Compact, High-Field Isochronous Cyclotron. *Nucl Instrum Meth B*, 1991, 56-7, 1201-4.

[31] Bethesda, MD. Clinical Proton Dosimetry Part1: Beam Production, Beam Delivery and Measurement of Absorbed Dose. *ICRU Report*, 59. 1998.

[32] Blosser, HG; Gelbke, GK; Lawton, D; Marti, E; Vincent, J; York, RC; et al. Proposal to construct a 250 MeV Superconducting Isochronous Cyclotron to Serve as an Advanced Cancer Treatment Facility and as a Manufacturing Prototype for Commercial Productions of such Cyclotron. National Superconducting Cyclotron Laboratory, Michigan State University, East Lansing, MI, 1998.

[33] Hiramoto, K; Umezawa, M; Saito, K; Tootake, S; Nishiuchi, H; Hara, S; et al. The synchrotron and its related technology for ion beam therapy. *Nucl Instrum Meth B*, 2007, 261(1-2), 786-90.

[34] Cole, F; Livdahl, PV; Mills, F; Teng, L. editors. Design and application of a proton therapy accelerator. 1987 IEEE Particle Accelerator Conference, 1987, IEEE.

[35] Fukumoto, S; Endo, K; Muto, K; Akisada, M; Kitagawa, T; Inada, T; et al. Tsukuba Medical Proton Synchrotron. *PSI Report*, 1989, 69, 70.

[36] Koehler, AM. Preliminary design study for a corkscrew gantry. *Proceedings of Fifth Proton Therapy Co-Operative Group Meeting*, 1987, 147-58.

[37] Pedroni, E; Bearpark, R; Bohringer, T; Coray, A; Duppich, J; Forss, S; et al. The PSI Gantry 2: a second generation proton scanning gantry. *Zeitschrift fur medizinische Physik*, 2004, 14(1), 25-34. Epub 2004/04/24.

[38] Takada, Y. Optimum solution of dual-ring double-scattering system for an incident beam with given phase space for proton beam spreading. *Nucl Instrum Meth A*, 2002, 485(3), 255-76.

[39] Chu, WT; Ludewigt, BA; Renner, TR. Instrumentation for Treatment of Cancer Using Proton and Light-Ion Beams. Rev Sci Instrum, 1993, 64(8), 2055-122.

[40] Kraft, G. Tumor therapy with heavy charged particles. *Prog Part Nucl Phys*, 2000, 45, S473-S544.

[41] Keall, PJ; Mageras, GS; Balter, JM; Emery, RS; Forster, KM; Jiang, SB; et al. The management of respiratory motion in radiation oncology report of AAPM Task Group 76. *Medical physics*, 2006, 33(10), 3874-900.

[42] Shirato, H; Shimizu, S; Kitamura, K; Nishioka, T; Kagei, K; Hashimoto, S; et al. Four-dimensional treatment planning and fluoroscopic real-time tumor tracking radiotherapy for moving tumor. *Int J Radiat Oncol*. 2000, 48(2), 435-42.

[43] Ingold, JA; Reed, GB; Kaplan, HS; Bagshaw, MA. Radiation Hepatitis. *The American journal of roentgenology, radium therapy, and nuclear medicine*, 1965, 93, 200-8. Epub 1965/01/01.

[44] Xu, ZY; Liang, SX; Zhu, J; Zhu, XD; Zhao, JD; Lu, HJ; et al. Prediction of radiation-induced liver disease by Lyman normal-tissue complication probability model in three-dimensional conformal radiation therapy for primary liver carcinoma. *International journal of radiation oncology, biology, physics*, 2006, 65(1), 189-95. Epub 2006/03/18.

[45] Lawrence, TS; Robertson, JM; Anscher, MS; Jirtle, RL; Ensminger, WD; Fajardo, LF. Hepatic Toxicity Resulting from Cancer-Treatment. *Int J Radiat Oncol*, 1995, 31(5), 1237-48.

[46] Emami, B; Lyman, J; Brown, A; Coia, L; Goitein, M; Munzenrider, JE; et al. Tolerance of normal tissue to therapeutic irradiation. *International journal of radiation oncology, biology, physics*, 1991, 21(1), 109-22. Epub 1991/05/15.

[47] Cheng, JC; Wu, JK; Huang, CM; Liu, HS; Huang, DY; Cheng, SH; et al. Radiation-induced liver disease after three-dimensional conformal radiotherapy for patients with hepatocellular carcinoma: dosimetric analysis and implication. *International journal of radiation oncology, biology, physics*, 2002, 54(1), 156-62. Epub 2002/08/17.

[48] Kim, TH; Kim, DY; Park, JW; Kim, SH; Choi, JI; Kim, HB; et al. Dose-volumetric parameters predicting radiation-induced hepatic toxicity in unresectable hepatocellular carcinoma patients treated with three-dimensional conformal radiotherapy.

International journal of radiation oncology, biology, physics, 2007, 67(1), 225-31. Epub 2006/10/24.

[49] Dawson, LA; Normolle, D; Balter, JM; McGinn, CJ; Lawrence, TS; Ten Haken, RK. Analysis of radiation-induced liver disease using the Lyman NTCP model. *Int J Radiat Oncol*, 2002, 53(4), 810-21.

[50] Jackson, A; Ten Haken, RK; Robertson, JM; Kessler, ML; Kutcher, GJ; Lawrence, TS. Analysis of clinical complication data for radiation hepatitis using a parallel architecture model. *International journal of radiation oncology, biology, physics*, 1995, 31(4), 883-91. Epub 1995/02/15.

[51] Wu, DH; Liu, L; Chen, LH. Therapeutic effects and prognostic factors in three-dimensional conformal radiotherapy combined with transcatheter arterial chemoembolization for hepatocellular carcinoma. *World journal of gastroenterology: WJG*, 2004, 10(15), 2184-9. Epub 2004/07/20.

[52] Hata, M; Tokuuye, K; Sugahara, S; Fukumitsu, N; Hashimoto, T; Ohnishi, K; et al. Proton beam therapy for hepatocellular carcinoma patients with severe cirrhosis. Strahlentherapie und Onkologie: Organ der Deutschen Rontgengesellschaft [et al.]. 2006, 182(12), 713-20. Epub 2006/12/07.

[53] Hata, M; Tokuuye, K; Sugahara, S; Fukumitsu, N; Hashimoto, T; Ohnishi, K; et al. Proton beam therapy for hepatocellular carcinoma with limited treatment options. *Cancer*, 2006, 107(3), 591-8. Epub 2006/06/29.

[54] Liang, SX; Zhu, XD; Lu, HJ; Pan, CY; Li, FX; Huang, QF; et al. Hypofractionated three-dimensional conformal radiation therapy for primary liver carcinoma. *Cancer*, 2005, 103(10), 2181-8.

[55] Komatsu, S; Fukumoto, T; Demizu, Y; Miyawaki, D; Terashima, K; Sasaki, R; et al. Clinical results and risk factors of proton and carbon ion therapy for hepatocellular carcinoma. *Cancer*, 2011, 117(21), 4890-904. Epub 2011/04/16.

[56] Seong, J; Park, HC; Han, KH; Chon, CY. Clinical results and prognostic factors in radiotherapy for unresectable hepatocellular carcinoma: a retrospective study of 158 patients. *International journal of radiation oncology, biology, physics*, 2003, 55(2), 329-36. Epub 2003/01/16.

[57] Kawashima, M; Furuse, J; Nishio, T; Konishi, M; Ishii, H; Kinoshita, T; et al. Phase II study of radiotherapy employing proton beam for hepatocellular carcinoma. *Journal of clinical oncology: official journal of the American Society of Clinical Oncology*, 2005, 23(9), 1839-46. Epub 2005/03/19.

[58] Mizumoto, M; Okumura, T; Hashimoto, T; Fukuda, K; Oshiro, Y; Fukumitsu, N; et al. Proton beam therapy for hepatocellular carcinoma: a comparison of three treatment protocols. *International journal of radiation oncology, biology, physics*, 2011, 81(4), 1039-45. Epub 2010/10/05.

[59] Ahmadi, T; Itai, Y; Onaya, H; Yoshioka, H; Okumura, T; Akine, Y. CT evaluation of hepatic injury following proton beam irradiation: appearance, enhancement, and 3D size reduction pattern. *Journal of computer assisted tomography*, 1999, 23(5), 655-63. Epub 1999/10/19.

[60] Ahmadi, T; Okumura, T; Onaya, H; Akine, Y; Itai, Y. Preservation of hypervascularity in hepatocellular carcinoma after effective proton-beam radiotherapy - CT observation. *Clin Radiol*, 1999, 54(4), 253-6.

[61] Okumura, T; Itai, Y; Tsuji, H; Matsueda, K; Matsuzaki, Y; Tsujii, H. Focused Radiation Hepatitis after Bragg-Peak Proton Therapy for Hepatocellular-Carcinoma - Ct Findings. *Journal of computer assisted tomography*, 1994, 18(5), 821-3.

[62] Onaya, H; Itai, Y; Yoshioka, H; Ahmadi, T; Niitsu, M; Okumura, T; et al. Changes in the liver parenchyma after proton beam radiotherapy: evaluation with MR imaging. *Magn Reson Imaging*, 2000, 18(6), 707-14. Epub 2000/08/10.

[63] Cochrane, AM; Murray-Lyon, IM; Brinkley, DM; Williams, R. Quadruple chemotherapy versus radiotherapy in treatment of primary hepatocellular carcinoma. *Cancer*, 1977, 40(2), 609-14. Epub 1977/08/01.

[64] Friedman, MA; Volberding, PA; Cassidy, MJ; Resser, KJ; Wasserman, TH; Phillips, TL. Therapy for hepatocellular cancer with intrahepatic arterial adriamycin and 5-fluorouracil combined with whole-liver irradiation: a Northern California Oncology Group Study. *Cancer treatment reports*, 1979, 63(11-12), 1885-8. Epub 1979/11/01.

[65] Stillwagon, GB; Order, SE; Guse, C; Klein, JL; Leichner, PK; Leibel, SA; et al. 194 hepatocellular cancers treated by radiation and chemotherapy combinations: toxicity and response: a Radiation Therapy Oncology Group Study. *International journal of radiation oncology, biology, physics*, 1989, 17(6), 1223-9. Epub 1989/12/01.

[66] Koom, WS; Seong, J; Han, KH; Lee, DY; Lee, JT. Is Local Radiotherapy Still Valuable for Patients with Multiple Intrahepatic Hepatocellular Carcinomas? *Int J Radiat Oncol*, 2010, 77(5), 1433-40.

[67] Oh, D; Lim do, H; Park, HC; Paik, SW; Koh, KC; Lee, JH; et al. Early three-dimensional conformal radiotherapy for patients with unresectable hepatocellular carcinoma after incomplete transcatheter arterial chemoembolization: a prospective evaluation of efficacy and toxicity. *American journal of clinical oncology*, 2010, 33(4), 370-5. Epub 2010/02/10.

[68] Seong, J; Lee, IJ; Shim, SJ; Lim do, H; Kim, TH; Kim, JH; et al. A multicenter retrospective cohort study of practice patterns and clinical outcome on radiotherapy for hepatocellular carcinoma in Korea. *Liver international: official journal of the International Association for the Study of the Liver*, 2009, 29(2), 147-52. Epub 2008/09/18.

[69] Ben-Josef, E; Normalle, D; Ensminger, WD; Walker, S; Tatro, D; Ten Haken, RK; et al. Phase II trial of high-dose conformal radiation therapy with concurrent hepatic artery floxuridine for unresectable intrahepatic malignancies. *Journal of Clinical Oncology*, 2005, 23(34), 8739-47.

[70] Park, J; Kim, MH; Kim, KP; Park, DH; Moon, SH; Song, TJ; et al. Natural History and Prognostic Factors of Advanced Cholangiocarcinoma without Surgery, Chemotherapy, or Radiotherapy: A Large-Scale Observational Study. *Gut Liver*. 2009, 3(4), 298-305.

[71] Kim, DY; Park, W; Lim, DH; Lee, JH; Yoo, BC; Paik, SW; et al. Three-dimensional conformal radiotherapy for portal vein thrombosis of hepatocellular carcinoma. *Cancer*, 2005, 103(11), 2419-26. Epub 2005/04/12.

[72] Meng, MB; Cui, YL; Lu, Y; She, B; Chen, Y; Guan, YS; et al. Transcatheter arterial chemoembolization in combination with radiotherapy for unresectable hepatocellular carcinoma, a systematic review and meta-analysis. *Radiotherapy and oncology: journal of the European Society for Therapeutic Radiology and Oncology*, 2009, 92(2), 184-94. Epub 2008/12/02.

[73] Zhao, JD; Liu, J; Ren, ZG; Gu, K; Zhou, ZH; Li, WT; et al. Maintenance of Sorafenib following combined therapy of three-dimensional conformal radiation therapy/intensity-modulated radiation therapy and transcatheter arterial chemoembolization in patients with locally advanced hepatocellular carcinoma: a phase I/II study. *Radiat Oncol*, 2010, 5, 12. Epub 2010/02/13.

[74] Chiba, T; Tokuuye, K; Matsuzaki, Y; Sugahara, S; Chuganji, Y; Kagei, K; et al. Proton beam therapy for hepatocellular carcinoma: a retrospective review of 162 patients. *Clinical cancer research: an official journal of the American Association for Cancer Research*, 2005, 11(10), 3799-805. Epub 2005/05/18.

[75] Mizumoto, M; Tokuuye, K; Sugahara, S; Nakayama, H; Fukumitsu, N; Ohara, K; et al. Proton beam therapy for hepatocellular carcinoma adjacent to the porta hepatis. *International journal of radiation oncology, biology, physics*, 2008, 71(2), 462-7. Epub 2008/02/05.

[76] Nakayama, H; Sugahara, S; Fukuda, K; Abei, M; Shoda, J; Sakurai, H; et al. Proton beam therapy for hepatocellular carcinoma located adjacent to the alimentary tract. *International journal of radiation oncology, biology, physics*, 2011, 80(4), 992-5. Epub 2011/05/06.

[77] Fukumitsu, N; Sugahara, S; Nakayama, H; Fukuda, K; Mizumoto, M; Abei, M; et al. A prospective study of hypofractionated proton beam therapy for patients with hepatocellular carcinoma. *International journal of radiation oncology, biology, physics*, 2009, 74(3), 831-6. Epub 2009/03/24.

[78] Bush, DA; Kayali, Z; Grove, R; Slater, JD. The safety and efficacy of high-dose proton beam radiotherapy for hepatocellular carcinoma: a phase 2 prospective trial. *Cancer*, 2011, 117(13), 3053-9. Epub 2011/01/26.

[79] Komatsu, S; Fukumoto, T; Demizu, Y; Miyawaki, D; Terashima, K; Niwa ,Y; et al. The effectiveness of particle radiotherapy for hepatocellular carcinoma associated with inferior vena cava tumor thrombus. *Journal of gastroenterology*, 2011, 46(7), 913-20. Epub 2011/04/26.

[80] Mizumoto, M; Tokuuye, K; Sugahara, S; Hata, M; Fukumitsu, N; Hashimoto, T; et al. Proton beam therapy for hepatocellular carcinoma with inferior vena cava tumor thrombus: report of three cases. *Japanese journal of clinical oncology*, 2007, 37(6), 459-62. Epub 2007/06/08.

[81] Sugahara, S; Nakayama, H; Fukuda, K; Mizumoto, M; Tokita, M; Abei, M; et al. Proton-beam therapy for hepatocellular carcinoma associated with portal vein tumor thrombosis. Strahlentherapie und Onkologie: Organ der Deutschen Rontgengesellschaft [et al.]. 2009, 185(12), 782-8. Epub 2009/12/17.

[82] Hata, M; Tokuuye, K; Sugahara, S; Tohno, E; Nakayama, H; Fukumitsu, N; et al. Proton beam therapy for aged patients with hepatocellular carcinoma. *International journal of radiation oncology, biology, physics*, 2007, 69(3), 805-12. Epub 2007/05/26.

[83] Bush, DA; Hillebrand, DJ; Slater, JM; Slater, JD. High-dose proton beam radiotherapy of hepatocellular carcinoma: preliminary results of a phase II trial. *Gastroenterology*, 2004, 127(5 Suppl 1), S189-93. Epub 2004/10/28.

[84] Onaya, H; Itai, Y; Ahmadi, T; Yoshioka, H; Okumura, T; Akine, Y; et al. Recurrent hepatocellular carcinoma versus radiation-induced hepatic injury: differential diagnosis with MR imaging. *Magn Reson Imaging*, 2001, 19(1), 41-6.

[85] Niizawa, G; Ikegami, T; Matsuzaki, Y; Saida, Y; Tohno, E; Kurosawa, T; et al. Monitoring of hepatocellular carcinoma, following proton radiotherapy, with contrast-enhanced color Doppler ultrasonography. *Journal of gastroenterology*, 2005, 40(3), 283-90. Epub 2005/04/15.

[86] Saito, Y; Matsuzaki, Y; Honda, A; Iwamoto, J; Ikegami, T; Chiba, T; et al. Post-therapeutic needle biopsy in patients with hepatocellular carcinoma is a useful tool to evaluate response to proton irradiation. *Hepatology research: the official journal of the Japan Society of Hepatology*, 2013. Epub 2013/04/24.

[87] Kawashima, M; Furuse, J; Nishio, T; Konishi, M; Ishii, H; Kinoshita, T; et al. Phase II study of radiotherapy employing proton beam for hepatocellular carcinoma. *J Clin Oncol*, 2005, 23(9), 1839-46. Epub 2005/03/19.

[88] Chiba, T; Tokuuye, K; Matsuzaki, Y; Sugahara, S; Chuganji, Y; Kagei, K; et al. Proton beam therapy for hepatocellular carcinoma: a retrospective review of 162 patients. *Clin Cancer Res*, 2005, 11(10), 3799-805. Epub 2005/05/18.

[89] Hata, M; Tokuuye, K; Sugahara, S; Fukumitsu, N; Hashimoto, T; Ohnishi, K; et al. Proton beam therapy for hepatocellular carcinoma patients with severe cirrhosis. *Strahlenther Onkol*, 2006, 182(12), 713-20. Epub 2006/12/07.

[90] Fukumitsu, N; Sugahara, S; Nakayama, H; Fukuda, K; Mizumoto, M; Abei, M; et al. A prospective study of hypofractionated proton beam therapy for patients with hepatocellular carcinoma. *Int J Radiat Oncol Biol Phys*, 2009, 74(3), 831-6. Epub 2009/03/24.

[91] Mizumoto, M; Tokuuye, K; Sugahara, S; Nakayama, H; Fukumitsu, N; Ohara, K; et al. Proton beam therapy for hepatocellular carcinoma adjacent to the porta hepatis. *Int J Radiat Oncol Biol Phys*, 2008, 71(2), 462-7. Epub 2008/02/05.

[92] Mizumoto, M; Okumura, T; Hashimoto, T; Fukuda, K; Oshiro, Y; Fukumitsu, N; et al. Proton beam therapy for hepatocellular carcinoma: a comparison of three treatment protocols. *Int J Radiat Oncol Biol Phys*, 2011, 81(4), 1039-45. Epub 2010/10/05.

[93] Niizawa, G; Ikegami, T; Matsuzaki, Y; Saida, Y; Tohno, E; Kurosawa, T; et al. Monitoring of hepatocellular carcinoma, following proton radiotherapy, with contrast-enhanced color Doppler ultrasonography. *J Gastroenterol*, 2005, 40(3), 283-90. Epub 2005/04/15.

[94] Sitruk, V; Seror, O; Grando-Lemaire, V; Mohand, D; N'Kontchou, G; Ganne-Carrie, N; et al. [Percutaneous ablation of hepatocellular carcinoma]. *Gastroenterologie clinique et biologique*, 2003, 27(4), 381-90. Epub 2003/05/22. Traitement percutane du carcinome hepatocellulaire.

[95] Lencioni, RA; Allgaier, HP; Cioni, D; Olschewski, M; Deibert, P; Crocetti, L; et al. Small hepatocellular carcinoma in cirrhosis: randomized comparison of radio-frequency thermal ablation versus percutaneous ethanol injection. *Radiology*, 2003, 228(1), 235-40. Epub 2003/05/22.

[96] Lin, SM; Lin, CJ; Lin, CC; Hsu, CW; Chen, YC. Radiofrequency ablation improves prognosis compared with ethanol injection for hepatocellular carcinoma < or =4 cm. *Gastroenterology*, 2004, 127(6), 1714-23.

[97] Shiina, S; Teratani, T; Obi, S; Sato, S; Tateishi, R; Fujishima, T; et al. A randomized controlled trial of radiofrequency ablation with ethanol injection for small hepatocellular carcinoma. *Gastroenterology*, 2005, 129(1), 122-30. Epub 2005/07/14.

[98] Ohara, K; Okumura, T; Tsuji, H; Chiba, T; Min, M; Tatsuzaki, H; et al. Radiation tolerance of cirrhotic livers in relation to the preserved functional capacity: analysis of patients with hepatocellular carcinoma treated by focused proton beam radiotherapy. *International journal of radiation oncology, biology, physics*, 1997, 38(2), 367-72. Epub 1997/05/01.

[99] Sugahara, S; Oshiro, Y; Nakayama, H; Fukuda, K; Mizumoto, M; Abei, M; et al. Proton beam therapy for large hepatocellular carcinoma. *International journal of radiation oncology, biology, physics*, 2010, 76(2), 460-6. Epub 2009/05/12.

[100] Kanemoto, A; Mizumoto, M; Okumura, T; Takahashi, H; Hashimoto, T; Oshiro, Y; et al. Dose-volume histogram analysis for risk factors of radiation-induced rib fracture after hypofractionated proton beam therapy for hepatocellular carcinoma. *Acta Oncol*, 2013, 52(3), 538-44. Epub 2012/09/07.

[101] Blum, HE. Treatment of hepatocellular carcinoma. *Best practice & research Clinical gastroenterology*, 2005, 19(1), 129-45. Epub 2005/03/11.

[102] Llovet, JM; Bustamante, J; Castells, A; Vilana, R; Ayuso Mdel, C; Sala, M; et al. Natural history of untreated nonsurgical hepatocellular carcinoma: rationale for the design and evaluation of therapeutic trials. *Hepatology*, 1999, 29(1), 62-7. Epub 1998/12/24.

[103] Markovic, S; Gadzijev, E; Stabuc, B; Croce, LS; Masutti, F; Surlan, M; et al. Treatment options in Western hepatocellular carcinoma: a prospective study of 224 patients. *Journal of hepatology*, 1998, 29(4), 650-9. Epub 1998/11/21.

[104] Chan, LC; Chiu, SK; Chan, SL. Stereotactic radiotherapy for hepatocellular carcinoma: report of a local single-centre experience. *Hong Kong medical journal = Xianggang yi xue za zhi / Hong Kong Academy of Medicine*, 2011, 17(2), 112-8. Epub 2011/04/08.

[105] Cardenes, HR; Price, TR; Perkins, SM; Maluccio, M; Kwo, P; Breen, TE; et al. Phase I feasibility trial of stereotactic body radiation therapy for primary hepatocellular carcinoma. *Clinical & translational oncology: official publication of the Federation of Spanish Oncology Societies and of the National Cancer Institute of Mexico*, 2010, 12(3), 218-25. Epub 2010/03/17.

[106] Pirisi, M; Avellini, C; Fabris, C; Scott, C; Bardus, P; Soardo, G; et al. Portal vein thrombosis in hepatocellular carcinoma: age and sex distribution in an autopsy study. *Journal of cancer research and clinical oncology*, 1998, 124(7), 397-400. Epub 1998/08/27.

[107] Stuart, KE; Anand, AJ; Jenkins, RL. Hepatocellular carcinoma in the United States. Prognostic features, treatment outcome, and survival. *Cancer*, 1996, 77(11), 2217-22. Epub 1996/06/01.

[108] Fong, Y; Sun, RL; Jarnagin, W; Blumgart, LH. An analysis of 412 cases of hepatocellular carcinoma at a Western center. *Ann Surg*, 1999, 229(6), 790-9; discussion 9-800. Epub 1999/06/11.

[109] Lee, HS; Kim, JS; Choi, IJ; Chung, JW; Park, JH; Kim, CY. The safety and efficacy of transcatheter arterial chemoembolization in the treatment of patients with hepatocellular carcinoma and main portal vein obstruction. A prospective controlled study. *Cancer*, 1997, 79(11), 2087-94. Epub 1997/06/01.

[110] Okuda, K; Ohtsuki, T; Obata, H; Tomimatsu, M; Okazaki, N; Hasegawa, H; et al. Natural history of hepatocellular carcinoma and prognosis in relation to treatment. Study of 850 patients. *Cancer*, 1985, 56(4), 918-28. Epub 1985/08/15.

[111] Pawarode, A; Voravud, N; Sriuranpong, V; Kullavanijaya, P; Patt, YZ. Natural history of untreated primary hepatocellular carcinoma: a retrospective study of 157 patients. *American journal of clinical oncology*, 1998, 21(4), 386-91. Epub 1998/08/26.

[112] Nagasue, N; Yukaya, H; Hamada, T; Hirose, S; Kanashima, R; Inokuchi, K. The natural history of hepatocellular carcinoma. A study of 100 untreated cases. *Cancer*, 1984, 54(7), 1461-5. Epub 1984/10/01.

[113] Obi, S; Yoshida, H; Toune, R; Unuma, T; Kanda, M; Sato, S; et al. Combination therapy of intraarterial 5-fluorouracil and systemic interferon-alpha for advanced hepatocellular carcinoma with portal venous invasion. *Cancer*, 2006, 106(9), 1990-7. Epub 2006/03/28.

[114] Hsu, WC; Chan, SC; Ting, LL; Chung, NN; Wang, PM; Ying, KS; et al. Results of three-dimensional conformal radiotherapy and thalidomide for advanced hepatocellular carcinoma. *Japanese journal of clinical oncology*, 2006, 36(2), 93-9. Epub 2006/03/07.

[115] Ishikura, S; Ogino, T; Furuse, J; Satake, M; Baba, S; Kawashima, M; et al. Radiotherapy after transcatheter arterial chemoembolization for patients with hepatocellular carcinoma and portal vein tumor thrombus. *American journal of clinical oncology*, 2002, 25(2), 189-93. Epub 2002/04/11.

[116] Nakagawa, K; Yamashita, H; Shiraishi, K; Nakamura, N; Tago, M; Igaki, H; et al. Radiation therapy for portal venous invasion by hepatocellular carcinoma. *World journal of gastroenterology: WJG*, 2005, 11(46), 7237-41. Epub 2006/01/27.

[117] Ota, H; Nagano, H; Sakon, M; Eguchi, H; Kondo, M; Yamamoto, T; et al. Treatment of hepatocellular carcinoma with major portal vein thrombosis by combined therapy with subcutaneous interferon-alpha and intra-arterial 5-fluorouracil; role of type 1 interferon receptor expression. *British journal of cancer*, 2005, 93(5), 557-64. Epub 2005/08/18.

[118] Hata, M; Tokuuye, K; Sugahara, S; Kagei, K; Igaki, H; Hashimoto, T; et al. Proton beam therapy for hepatocellular carcinoma with portal vein tumor thrombus. *Cancer*, 2005, 104(4), 794-801. Epub 2005/06/28.

[119] Dawson, LA; Ten Haken, RK; Lawrence, TS. Partial irradiation of the liver. *Seminars in radiation oncology*, 2001, 11(3), 240-6. Epub 2001/07/12.

[120] Hashimoto, T; Tokuuye, K; Fukumitsu, N; Igaki, H; Hata, M; Kagei, K; et al. Repeated proton beam therapy for hepatocellular carcinoma. *International journal of radiation oncology, biology, physics*, 2006, 65(1), 196-202. Epub 2006/03/28.

[121] Potters, L; Kavanagh, B; Galvin, JM; Hevezi, JM; Janjan, NA; Larson, DA; et al. American Society for Therapeutic Radiology and Oncology (ASTRO) and American College of Radiology (ACR) practice guideline for the performance of stereotactic body radiation therapy. *International journal of radiation oncology, biology, physics*, 2010, 76(2), 326-32. Epub 2010/02/02.

[122] Siva, S; MacManus, M; Ball, D. Stereotactic Radiotherapy for Pulmonary Oligometastases A Systematic Review. *Journal of Thoracic Oncology*, 2010, 5(7), 1091-9.

[123] Tse, RV; Hawkins, M; Lockwood, G; Kim, JJ; Cummings, B; Knox, J; et al. Phase I study of individualized stereotactic body radiotherapy for hepatocellular carcinoma and intrahepatic cholangiocarcinoma. *Journal of Clinical Oncology*, 2008, 26(4), 657-64.

[124] Andolino, DL; Johnson, CS; Maluccio, M; Kwo, P; Tector, AJ; Zook, J; et al. Stereotactic body radiotherapy for primary hepatocellular carcinoma. *International*

journal of radiation oncology, biology, physics, 2011, 81(4), e447-53. Epub 2011/06/08.

[125] Sanuki, N; Takeda, A; Oku, Y; Mizuno, T; Aoki, Y; Eriguchi, T; et al. Stereotactic body radiotherapy for small hepatocellular carcinoma: A retrospective outcome analysis in 185 patients. *Acta Oncol*, 2013. Epub 2013/08/22.

[126] Choi, BO; Jang, HS; Kang, KM; Lee, SW; Kang, YN; Chai, GY; et al. Fractionated stereotactic radiotherapy in patients with primary hepatocellular carcinoma. *Japanese journal of clinical oncology*, 2006, 36(3), 154-8. Epub 2006/03/08.

[127] Bujold, A; Massey, CA; Kim, JJ; Brierley, J; Cho, C; Wong, RK; et al. Sequential phase I and II trials of stereotactic body radiotherapy for locally advanced hepatocellular carcinoma. *Journal of clinical oncology: official journal of the American Society of Clinical Oncology*, 2013, 31(13), 1631-9. Epub 2013/04/03.

[128] Goodman, KA; Wiegner, EA; Maturen, KE; Zhang, Z; Mo, Q; Yang, G; et al. Dose-escalation study of single-fraction stereotactic body radiotherapy for liver malignancies. *International journal of radiation oncology, biology, physics*, 2010, 78(2), 486-93. Epub 2010/03/31.

[129] Louis, C; Dewas, S; Mirabel, X; Lacornerie, T; Adenis, A; Bonodeau, F; et al. Stereotactic Radiotherapy of Hepatocellular Carcinoma: Preliminary Results. *Technol Cancer Res T*, 2010, 9(5), 479-87.

[130] Kwon, JH; Bae, SH; Kim, JY; Choi, BO; Jang, HS; Jang, JW; et al. Long-term effect of stereotactic body radiation therapy for primary hepatocellular carcinoma ineligible for local ablation therapy or surgical resection. Stereotactic radiotherapy for liver cancer. *BMC cancer*, 2010, 10, 475. Epub 2010/09/04.

[131] Seo, YS; Kim, MS; Yoo, SY; Cho, CK; Choi, CW; Kim, JH; et al. Preliminary Result of Stereotactic Body Radiotherapy as a Local Salvage Treatment for Inoperable Hepatocellular Carcinoma. *J Surg Oncol*, 2010, 102(3), 209-14.

[132] Choi, BO; Choi, IB; Jang, HS; Kang, YN; Jang, JS; Bae, SH; et al. Stereotactic body radiation therapy with or without transarterial chemoembolization for patients with primary hepatocellular carcinoma: preliminary analysis. *BMC cancer*, 2008, 8.

[133] Taguchi, H; Sakuhara, Y; Hige, S; Kitamura, K; Osaka, Y; Abo, D; et al. Intercepting radiotherapy using a real-time tumor-tracking radiotherapy system for highly selected patients with hepatocellular carcinoma unresectable with other modalities. *Int J Radiat Oncol*, 2007, 69(2), 376-80.

[134] Jung, J; Yoon, SM; Kim, SY; Cho, B; Park, JH; Kim, SS; et al. Radiation-induced liver disease after stereotactic body radiotherapy for small hepatocellular carcinoma: clinical and dose-volumetric parameters. *Radiat Oncol*. 2013, 8(1), 249. Epub 2013/10/29.

[135] Castro, JR. Results of heavy ion radiotherapy. *Radiation and environmental biophysics*, 1995, 34(1), 45-8. Epub 1995/03/01.

[136] Linstadt, DE; Castro, JR; Phillips, TL. Neon ion radiotherapy: results of the phase I/II clinical trial. *International journal of radiation oncology, biology, physics*, 1991, 20(4), 761-9. Epub 1991/04/01.

[137] Tsujii, H; Kamada, T. A Review of Update Clinical Results of Carbon Ion Radiotherapy. *Japanese journal of clinical oncology*, 2012, 42(8), 670-85.

[138] Nikoghosyan, A; Schulz-Ertner, D; Didinger, B; Jakel, O; Zuna, I; Hoss, A; et al. Evaluation of therapeutic potential of heavy ion therapy for patients with locally

advanced prostate cancer. *International journal of radiation oncology, biology, physics,* 2004, 58(1), 89-97. Epub 2003/12/31.

[139] Kanai, T; Furusawa, Y; Fukutsu, K; Itsukaichi, H; EguchiKasai, K; Ohara, H. Irradiation of mixed beam and design of spread-out Bragg peak for heavy-ion radiotherapy. *Radiation research,* 1997, 147(1), 78-85.

[140] Ishikawa, H; Tsuji, H; Kamada, T; Akakura, K; Suzuki, H; Shimazaki, J; et al. Carbon-ion radiation therapy for prostate cancer. *Int J Urol,* 2012, 19(4), 296-305.

[141] Hamada, N; Imaoka, T; Masunaga, S; Ogata, T; Okayasu, R; Takahashi, A; et al. Recent advances in the biology of heavy-ion cancer therapy. *Journal of radiation research,* 2010, 51(4), 365-83. Epub 2010/08/04.

[142] Fukumura, A; Tsujii, H; Kamada, T; Baba, M; Tsuji, H; Kato, H; et al. Carbon-ion radiotherapy: clinical aspects and related dosimetry. *Radiation protection dosimetry,* 2009, 137(1-2), 149-55. Epub 2009/10/09.

[143] Denekamp, J; Waites, T; Fowler, JF. Predicting realistic RBE values for clinically relevant radiotherapy schedules. *International journal of radiation biology,* 1997, 71(6), 681-94. Epub 1997/06/01.

[144] Kato, H; Tsujii, H; Miyamoto, T; Mizoe, JE; Kamada, T; Tsuji, H; et al. Results of the first prospective study of carbon ion radiotherapy for hepatocellular carcinoma with liver cirrhosis. *International journal of radiation oncology, biology, physics,* 2004, 59(5), 1468-76. Epub 2004/07/28.

[145] Kato, H; Yamada, S; Yasuda, S; Yamaguchi, K; Ohno, I; Ohto, M; et al. Four-fraction carbon ion radiotherapy for hepatocellular carcinoma: Results of a phase II clinical trial. *Journal of Clinical Oncology,* 2004, 22(14), 335s-s.

[146] Ohno, T; Kanai, T; Yamada, S; Yusa, K; Tashiro, M; Shimada, H; et al. Carbon Ion Radiotherapy at the Gunma University Heavy Ion Medical Center: New Facility Set-up. *Cancers,* 2011, 3(4), 4046-60. Epub 2011/01/01.

[147] Imada, H; Kato, H; Yasuda, S; Yamada, S; Yanagi, T; Kishimoto, R; et al. Comparison of efficacy and toxicity of short-course carbon ion radiotherapy for hepatocellular carcinoma depending on their proximity to the porta hepatis. *Radiotherapy and Oncology,* 2010, 96(2), 231-5.

[148] Combs, SE; Habermehl, D; Ganten, T; Schmidt, J; Edler, L; Burkholder, I; et al. Phase i study evaluating the treatment of patients with hepatocellular carcinoma (HCC) with carbon ion radiotherapy: the PROMETHEUS-01 trial. *BMC cancer,* 2011, 11, 67. Epub 2011/02/15.

[149] Habermehl, D; Debus, J; Ganten, T; Ganten, MK; Bauer, J; Brecht, IC; et al. Hypofractionated carbon ion therapy delivered with scanned ion beams for patients with hepatocellular carcinoma - feasibility and clinical response. *Radiat Oncol,* 2013, 8, 59. Epub 2013/03/19.

[150] Ikai, I; Arii, S; Okazaki, M; Okita, K; Omata, M; Kojiro, M; et al. Report of the 17th Nationwide Follow-up Survey of Primary Liver Cancer in Japan. *Hepatology research: the official journal of the Japan Society of Hepatology,* 2007, 37(9), 676-91. Epub 2007/07/10.

[151] Kuhlmann, JB; Blum, HE. Locoregional therapy for cholangiocarcinoma. *Curr Opin Gastroen,* 2013, 29(3), 324-8.

[152] Sulpice, L; Rayar, M; Boucher, E; Pracht, M; Meunier, B; Boudjema, K. Treatment of recurrent intrahepatic cholangiocarcinoma. *The British journal of surgery*, 2012, 99(12), 1711-7. Epub 2012/11/08.

[153] Wang, YZ; Li, J; Xia, Y; Gong, RY; Wang, K; Yan, ZL; et al. Prognostic Nomogram for Intrahepatic Cholangiocarcinoma After Partial Hepatectomy. *Journal of Clinical Oncology*, 2013, 31(9), 1188-95.

[154] Ebata, T; Kamiya, J; Nishio, H; Nagasaka, T; Nimura, Y; Nagino, M. The concept of perihilar cholangiocarcinoma is valid. *Brit J Surg*. 2009, 96(8), 926-34.

[155] Ohtsuka, M; Ito, H; Kimura, F; Shimizu, H; Togawa, A; Yoshidome, H; et al. Extended hepatic resection and outcomes in intrahepatic cholangiocarcinoma. *Journal of hepato-biliary-pancreatic surgery*, 2003, 10(4), 259-64. Epub 2003/11/05.

[156] Valle, J; Wasan, H; Palmer, DH; Cunningham, D; Anthoney, A; Maraveyas, A; et al. Cisplatin plus gemcitabine versus gemcitabine for biliary tract cancer. *The New England journal of medicine*, 2010, 362(14), 1273-81. Epub 2010/04/09.

[157] Andre, T; Reyes-Vidal, JM; Fartoux, L; Ross, P; Leslie, M; Rosmorduc, O; et al. Gemcitabine and oxaliplatin in advanced biliary tract carcinoma: a phase II study. *British journal of cancer*, 2008, 99(6), 862-7. Epub 2009/02/25.

[158] Riechelmann, RP; Townsley, CA; Chin, SN; Pond, GR; Knox, JJ. Expanded phase II trial of gemcitabine and capecitabine for advanced biliary cancer. *Cancer*, 2007, 110(6), 1307-12. Epub 2007/07/14.

[159] Ray, CE; Jr. Edwards, A; Smith, MT; Leong, S; Kondo, K; Gipson, M; et al. Metaanalysis of survival, complications, and imaging response following chemotherapy-based transarterial therapy in patients with unresectable intrahepatic cholangiocarcinoma. Journal of vascular and interventional radiology: *JVIR*, 2013, 24(8), 1218-26. Epub 2013/06/04.

[160] Fu, Y; Yang, W; Wu, W; Yan, K; Xing, BC; Chen, MH. Radiofrequency ablation for postoperative recurrences of intrahepatic cholangiocarcinoma. *Chinese journal of cancer research = Chung-kuo yen cheng yen chiu*, 2011, 23(4), 295-300. Epub 2013/01/30.

[161] Shinohara, ET; Mitra, N; Guo, M; Metz, JM. Radiation therapy is associated with improved survival in the adjuvant and definitive treatment of intrahepatic cholangiocarcinoma. *International journal of radiation oncology, biology, physics*, 2008, 72(5), 1495-501. Epub 2008/05/13.

[162] Chen, YX; Zeng, ZC; Tang, ZY; Fan, J; Zhou, J; Jiang, W; et al. Determining the role of external beam radiotherapy in unresectable intrahepatic cholangiocarcinoma: a retrospective analysis of 84 patients. *BMC cancer*, 2010, 10, 492. Epub 2010/09/16.

[163] Gohongi, T; Tokuuye, K; Iida, H; Nakai, R; Gunji, N; Akine, Y; et al. Concurrent proton beam radiotherapy and systemic chemotherapy for the metastatic liver tumor of gastric carcinoma: a case report. *Jpn J Clin Oncol*, 2005, 35(1), 40-4. Epub 2005/02/01.

[164] Kanemoto, A; Oshiro, Y; Sugahara, S; Kamagata, S; Hirobe, S; Toma, M; et al. Proton beam therapy for inoperable recurrence of bronchial high-grade mucoepidermoid carcinoma. *Japanese journal of clinical oncology*, 2012, 42(6), 552-5. Epub 2012/04/12.

Index

I

M

U

V

W

Y

X